# Partnerships in family care

D0512881

# Partnerships in family care

edited by
Mike Nolan, Ulla Lundh, Gordon Grant and
John Keady

**Open University Press**
Maidenhead · Philadelphia

Open University Press
McGraw-Hill Education
McGraw-Hill House
Shoppenhangers Road
Maidenhead
Berkshire
England
SL6 2QL

email: enquiries@openup.co.uk
world wide web: www.openup.co.uk

and
325 Chestnut Street
Philadelphia, PA 19106, USA

First published 2003

Copyright © Mike Nolan, Ulla Lundh, Gordon Grant and John Keady 2003

All rights reserved. Except for the quotation of short passages for the purposes of criticism and review, no part of this publication may be reproduced, stored in a retrieval system, or transmitted, in any form or by any means, electronic, mechanical, photocopying, recording or otherwise, without the prior permission of the publisher or a licence from the Copyright Licensing Agency Limited. Details of such licences (for reprographic reproduction) may be obtained from the Copyright Licensing Agency Ltd of 90 Tottenham Court Road, London, W1T 4LP.

A catalogue record of this book is available from the British Library

ISBN 0 335 21261 1 (pb)    0 335 21262 X (hb)

Library of Congress Cataloging-in-Publication Data
CIP data applied for

Typeset by RefineCatch Limited, Bungay, Suffolk
Printed in Great Britain by Bell and Bain Ltd, Glasgow

To Jacinta Evans for bringing vision, insight and integrity to the world of publishing

# Contents

# Acknowledgements

We would like to offer our sincere thanks to all the innumerable carers, cared-for persons and professionals who have given their time over the years. Their generosity has made this book possible.

Particular thanks are due to Helen Mason for the energy, professionalism and dedication she displayed throughout the production of this manuscript. It could not have seen the light of the day without her efforts.

# Notes on contributors

*Dr Christine Bigby* is a Senior Lecturer, and Director of Undergraduate Programs in the School of Social Work and Social Policy at Latrobe University, Melbourne Australia. She has particular interests in policy development for people with intellectual disability, ageing with a disability and case management. She is a member of the Victorian Disability Advisory Council and author of a book *Moving on Without Parents: Planning, Transition and Sources of Support for Older Adults with Intellectual Disability*, published by Maclennan & Petty.

*Louise Brereton* is a Lecturer in Nursing in the Department of Community, Ageing, Rehabilitation, Education and Research (CARER) in the School of Nursing and Midwifery, University of Sheffield. Louise's particular research interests, and her current PhD studies, are related to the needs of new family carers following a stroke.

*Denise Chaston* qualified as a State Enrolled Nurse (Mental Health) in 1981 and then as a Registered Mental Nurse in 1984. She is currently employed by Doncaster and South Humber NHS Trust as a Clinical Nurse Specialist, working with younger people with dementia and their carers/families. Denise is an active member of her local Alzheimer Society.

*Chris Clark* qualified as RMN in 1981 and successfully completed a diploma in Community Health Care Nursing (CPN) in 1992, and has spent most of her professional career working with, and on behalf of, people with dementia and their carers. She is currently employed as a Community Mental Health Nurse for Older People with Doncaster and South Humber NHS Trust. Her special area of interest has been to encourage early recognition of the signs of dementia and promote early referral to specialist services.

*Sue Davies* is a Senior Lecturer in Gerontological Nursing in the Department of Community, Ageing, Rehabilitation, Education and Research, University of Sheffield. Sue's research interests focus upon the needs of older people in care homes and the development of conceptual and theoretical frameworks to inform practice with older people in a range of care settings, and to guide education for service providers.

*Iréne Ericsson* has experience of nursing people with dementia, and of counselling and educating families and professional caregivers. Her present work is at the Institute of Gerontology in Jönköping, where they have recently developed a two-year dementia course on the Network University. Iréne is also involved in research and development works.

*Gordon Grant* holds a Research Chair in Cognitive Disability in the School of Nursing and Midwifery, University of Sheffield, and Doncaster and South Humber Healthcare NHS Trust. His main interests concern family caregiving of vulnerable groups and the support needs of people with severe and complex learning disabilities.

*Ingrid Hellström* has a background in gerontological nursing. She is now a postgraduate student at the Institute for the Study of Ageing and Later Life, Linköping University, Sweden. Ingrid's main research interest is older people with dementia and their spouses.

*Prue Ingram* is Manager of Support Services, Alzheimer's Association Australia. She is responsible for the management of a state-wide network of information, support and counselling services for people with dementia, their families and carers, as well as for the development of national resources for Alzheimer's Association Australia. She has strong interest in the development of services that are responsive to the self-identified needs of people with dementia their families and carers.

*John Keady* is Senior Lecturer in the School of Nursing and Midwifery at the University of Wales, Bangor. John's main interests are in the needs of people with dementia and their carers, and service responses to these needs.

*Gwynnyth Llewellyn* is an occupational therapist and family researcher, Sesquicentenary Professor of Occupation and Leisure Sciences and Director, Disability Studies Program at the University of Sydney, Australia. Her research interests include family and disability, caring and community care, parenting and social support, and disability policy.

*Ulla Lundh* is Docent and Senior Lecturer at the University of Linköping, Sweden. She has particular interests in the needs of older people and their carers and has been engaged in several studies that have sought to develop partnerships between family and formal caregiving systems.

*Professor Rhonda Nay* is currently Foundation Professor of Gerontic Nursing, Director of the Gerontic Nursing Clinical School and of the

Australian Centre for Evidence Based Aged Care at La Trobe University. She was elected President of the Australian Association of Gerontology in Victoria and has contributed widely to aged care through the International Congress of Nursing (ICN), research, teaching, publications, presentations and committees.

*Mike Nolan* is Professor of Gerontological Nursing at the University of Sheffield. He has long-standing interests in the needs of family carers and of vulnerable older people in a range of care environments, and has published extensively in these areas.

*Professor Alan Pearson* is the Professor of Nursing at La Trobe University, Australia and is the Editor of the *International Journal of Nursing Practice*. Professor Pearson is the Executive Director of the Joanna Briggs Institute, an International Research Collaboration for Evidence Based Health Care.

*Åsa Påulsson* is the Program Coordinator for the Nursing Program at the School of Health Sciences in Jönköping, Sweden, where she teaches on the care of older people. Her particular research interests are in the field of people with dementia and their family/carers.

*Jonas Sandberg*, PhD, RN, is a Senior Lecturer in Nursing at Mälardalen University, Eskilstuna/Västerås, Sweden. His research interests include family care, experiences of transitions to a nursing home, support to family carers when placing a relative in a nursing home, and collaboration between family carers and paid carers in the placement process.

*Professor Bev Taylor* is the Foundation Chair in Nursing at Southern Cross University, Lismore, NSW. She has been active in nursing practice, education and research for 34 years. She is the Editor of the *Australian Journal of Holistic Nursing* and the author of four books and multiple refereed publications relating to nursing.

*Roger Watson* is the Professor of Nursing at the University of Hull where he is responsible for leading research in nursing. His clinical experience was gained working with older people with dementia and he has a particular interest in the assessment of eating difficulty.

*Bridget Whittell* is a Performance and Planning Officer with Wigan Social Services. Prior to this point she was a Research Officer in the School of Nursing and Midwifery, University of Sheffield. She has been engaged in research concerning carers and people with learning disabilities and maintains a strong interest and involvement in these areas.

# Preface

> The title of this book reflects our belief that there is a need to 'break the mould' of the way that caregiving is conceptualized. In questioning some of the taken-for-granted assumptions about what constitutes family care, we are conscious that this process has only started. There is a need to follow new theoretical, methodological and empirical routes to a better, more holistic understanding.
>
> (Nolan *et al.* 1996a: 159–60)

So ended a book called *Understanding Family Care* (Nolan *et al.* 1996a) which attempted to bring together the existing literature on family care and integrate this with insights of our own which had emerged from research spanning several years. The aim was to present a more rounded view of 'this thing some call caregiving' (Gubrium 1995) which highlighted the dynamic interplay between the difficulties, satisfactions and coping strategies of family carers and suggested how these might change as caregiving unfolded. In doing so we hoped to promote a better understanding of the needs and circumstances of carers that would not only inform theoretical debates but also contribute to the development of better and more appropriate services. Central to such arguments was an indication of the temporal experience of care, which recognized that the need for support varied over time. We outlined a six-stage temporal model which had its early roots in work from the late 1980s but was more fully elaborated upon in the field of dementia (Keady and Nolan 1994a; Keady 1999).

Much has happened in the six years since *Understanding Family Care* was published and there have been significant developments in terms of policy and practice, particularly in the UK with the enactment of the Carers (Recognition and Services) Act (DoH 1995) and the Carers and Disabled Children Act (DoH 2000), together with the launch of the Carers National Strategy (DoH 1999). However, such developments have not been confined to the UK. Importantly there have also been concerted efforts to categorize support systems for family carers on a pan-European basis (see for example Philp 2001).

In addition to policy-related initiatives the research effort has continued apace and the 'explosion' of studies on family care that has occurred over the recent past (Fortinsky 2001) shows little sign of abating. Indeed, if anything, the published literature appears to be increasing. Why then, one might ask, do we consider that there is a need for 'yet another' book about family care?

We would suggest that while the 'mould' might not yet be broken, there are nevertheless visible and discernible signs that provide an early but growing indication of a 'paradigm' shift in the way in which services are conceptualized. This shift does not relate only to family care but is part of the wider movement evident throughout the 1990s towards a more participative and inclusive model based on empowering service users and carers (Bernard and Phillips 2000).

As a consequence some of the 'new theoretical, methodological and empirical routes' that we envisaged have been followed and the results are raising fundamental issues which question the 'perceived wisdom' about the 'when, who, what, how and why' of support for family carers (Nolan *et al.* 2002a).

This volume is intended to add further impetus to current changes so that the momentum is maintained. As such it should not be viewed as a 'second edition' of *Understanding Family Care*, although it does build on a number of concepts presented there, particularly the temporal model of caregiving. Indeed, the model lies at the heart of this book which incorporates studies that have either explored phases of caregiving in more detail or have focused their attention on issues more or less pertinent to a particular aspect of carers' lives at differing points in time.

It begins with a brief overview highlighting current tensions within the caregiving literature and locates these with reference to a number of the arguments presented in *Understanding Family Care*. This provides a context and rationale for the present book. Subsequently the book is divided into three broad sections which essentially address the early, middle and later phases of caring. These chapters draw on studies from a number of countries (the UK, Sweden, Australia) and consider varying conditions that herald the need for support (stroke, dementia, learning disabilities), within several differing relationships (spousal, child–parent, parent–child). Within these chapters we explore the nature of partnerships between family and professional carers in differing contexts. We recognize that this does not provide a comprehensive consideration of the full spectrum of caregiving circumstances, nor in applying the temporal model do we mean to suggest that the experience of caring can be placed into neat compartments that deny the variability and uniqueness of each situation. Indeed, as will hopefully become apparent, we would promote the opposite view and fully support the assertion that 'change is the quintessential element of caregiving' (Aneshensel *et al.* 1995: 92). However, despite such obvious variability we would agree with Montgomery and Kosloski (2000) that temporal approaches help to identify 'threads of continuity' that provide 'markers' as to when and in what way it is most appropriate to offer help and support to family carers.

The concluding chapter reflects upon the insights provided by both recent literature and the studies described in the preceding sections, and proposes a differing way of constructing partnership between people who need help, and those family and paid carers who provide support (Tresolini and Pew-Fetzer Task Force 1994).

# Introduction: why another book on family care?

## Mike Nolan, John Keady, Gordon Grant and Ulla Lundh

### Introduction

> With its strategic importance, and the unresolved issues surrounding it, we expect that the family will continue to be centre stage for many years to come.
>
> (Pearlin *et al.* 2001: 55)

> It takes no great philosopher, no expert practitioner and no outstanding researcher to work alongside people in a way that values them as people.
>
> (Clarke 1999a: 363)

> Paradigms are professionally established, deeply routinized in fixed litanies and potentially very far removed from the questions of urgency to those who are actually in need.
>
> (Post 2001: S18)

As Pearlin *et al.* (2001) rightly assert, there can now be no doubting the 'strategic importance' of family carers in making a reality of community care policies which aim to enable people, despite illness and disability, to remain in their own homes whenever possible. The resultant politicization of caring (Chappell 1996) has seen the needs of family carers move from the margins of social policy to a position where they now occupy 'centre stage' (Johnson 1998). Consequently services designed to support family carers have proliferated and their more widespread emergence in recent years has been described as one of the most 'striking developments' in the policy arena (Moriarty and Webb 2000). It therefore seems a safe bet that 'the family will continue to be centre stage for many years to come' (Pearlin *et al.* 2001).

Notwithstanding such developments there remain, as Pearlin *et al.* (2001) suggest, several 'unresolved issues'. Indeed, following a consideration of the recent literature it has been argued that several central issues relating to the support of family carers do indeed remain 'unresolved', including:

- *When* is the most appropriate time to offer support?
- *How* is support best delivered?
- *Who* is support primarily intended to benefit?
- *What* are the intended aims of support?
- *Why* support family carers?

(Nolan et al. 2002a)

It seems paradoxical that despite the 'explosion' of research into the field of family caregiving over the last two decades (Fortinsky 2001), the resulting 'voluminous literature' (Schulz and Williamson 1997) and the 'fervent hope' of most researchers that their findings will in some way 'make a difference' (Pearlin *et al.* 2001), we have very little evidence for the effectiveness of current methods of supporting carers (Zarit *et al.* 1999; Braithwaite 2000; Cooke *et al.* 2001; Zarit and Leitsch 2001).

A root of these difficulties is the fact that carers seem to find many existing services unacceptable. Respite care provides a prime example of this tension. Therefore, while some form of relief or break from the demands of caring is one of the most frequently requested forms of support (Briggs and Askham 1999), not all the available places are filled (Moriarity 1999; Zarit and Leitsch 2001). There are a number of potential explanations for this but the two most compelling are that carers either do not see services as relevant to their needs (Pickard 1999; Braithwaite 2000), or they do not consider that the service provides care of sufficient quality (Moriarty 1999; Pickard 1999; Qureshi *et al.* 2000).

In the case of respite care, while the need for a break is readily identified, services are often not sufficiently flexible or responsive (Moriarity 1999), and frequently fail to meet the quality standards that carers themselves set (Pickard 1999; Qureshi *et al.* 2000). As Qureshi *et al.* (2000) have recently pointed out, the primary motivation for most carers is to maximize the quality of life of the person they are caring for, and they expect services to do no less. While it may not take a 'great philosopher', an 'expert practitioner' or an 'outstanding researcher' to work alongside people in a way that values them as a person (Clarke 1999a), it often seems that services fail to appreciate, or at least to deliver upon, this simple maxim.

At an intuitive level why this should be the case seems perplexing, but in reality the reasons are often deep-seated and implicit, and therefore difficult both to identify and address. For although maximizing the quality of life of the cared-for person may be the most important attribute of services, carers also want their own expertise to be acknowledged and for services to be delivered in a way that values their contribution and treats them as partners (Qureshi *et al.* 2000). These underlying tensions are eloquently captured by Post (2001) above, when he notes the entrenched nature of the 'professional paradigm' and the consequent problems that can arise in identifying and responding to the questions seen as most urgent by those in need of support.

There can be no doubt that recently a far more holistic view of caregiving support has emerged, as seen, for example, in Askham's (1998) definition of support as any intervention which assists a carer to:

- take up (or not take up) the caring role;
- continue in the caring role;
- end the caring role.

Furthermore, possibly informed by such a definition, and driven by legislative changes in the UK, there is evidence that more innovative services are starting to emerge (Banks and Roberts 2001). But despite promising developments in certain areas, innovation continues to be limited by the conceptual ambiguity surrounding the purpose and intended outcomes of caregiver support, and the predominant focus on reducing carer burden, the upshot of which has been the development of services that carers have not always seen as helpful (Qureshi *et al.* 2000).

The main aim of this chapter is to explore some of the above contradictions and paradoxes in greater detail and to cast them within the context of the present volume. We intend to make explicit some of our assumptions and how we arrived at these. However, it would neither be appropriate nor possible to consider all the 'unresolved issues' here and, consistent with the goals of this book, we will focus primarily on how family and professional carers can work together most effectively in meeting carers' needs and those of the person they are supporting. The importance of creating working partnerships will be considered from a temporal perspective, highlighting how support must be responsive to circumstances as they change over time.

## Family care: beyond burden and stress

> Relatively little attention has been paid to the assessment of positive aspects of caregiving, the quality of care delivered by caregivers and the impact of caregiving transitions.
>
> (Schulz and Williamson 1997: 123)

At the beginning of the 1990s Kahana and Young (1990) suggested that the field of caregiving research had just started its 'search for commonalities which underline the caregiving process' (p. 26). They noted that the concept of burden had emerged as a 'unifying notion', which was shared by diverse groups of caregivers in diverse contexts. However, even at this relatively early stage they argued that there were conceptual limitations to, and only limited empirical support for, this relatively uni-dimensional view. They believed that 'it is becoming increasingly apparent that caregiving involves complex interactions with potentially positive and negative consequences for both care-recipients and caregivers' (p. 26). In suggesting a way forward they promoted the need to develop a conceptual framework that would allow for the consideration of differing dimensions of caregiving, and that also recognized its dynamic and changing nature and the varying interactions that occurred between caregivers and care receivers. Their main focus was on 'dyadic' interactions between caregiver and care receiver, but they also explored dyadic interactions between the family caregiver and professional caregivers, and between care receivers and professional caregivers, within the context of differing illnesses and their temporal dimensions. On this basis they argued that:

> Caregiving is part of a process of change in time, and dyadic inter-actions are likely to be affected by the course of the illness and the upward or downward trajectory of the patient, as well as the reactions and the changing life circumstances of the caregiver.
>
> (p. 91)

Consequently they contended that the needs of a couple dealing with Alzheimer's disease were likely to differ in important ways from the needs of a couple addressing the aftermath of a heart attack. Their arguments were eloquent and persuasive and, as will be apparent, exerted a considerable influence on many of the positions advanced in this book.

Notwithstanding the conceptual insights that Kahana and Young (1990) provided, a true measure of their grasp of current and future trends is best illustrated in their concluding section. Here they argued that the future research agenda in family care needed to consider more fully the 'triadic' interactions between family carers, care receivers and both professional carers as individuals, and the wider agencies of which they are part.

The prophetic nature of this suggestion only becomes fully apparent when it is realized that well over a decade later others are raising the same issues as if they were new.

For example, the considerable influence of a stress/coping paradigm on caregiver research is now fully evident (Schulz and Williamson 1997; Zarit *et al.* 1999; Fortinsky 2001) in terms not only of dominating the research agenda, but also of the impact it has had on the development of support services. As Zarit *et al.* (1999) note, the reduction of caregiver stress has become 'a major tenet of gerontological policy and practice', and while our interests in this book are not confined to the care of older people, such a conclusion would apply equally to all areas of caregiving research. As Qureshi *et al.* (2000) argue, this primary focus on burden has restricted innovation in the development of carer support services, resulting in several initiatives which carers themselves do not see as being particularly helpful.

Such an orientation has also limited the development of interventions designed to enrich caregiving relationships (Cartwright *et al.* 1994), or to view the creation of feelings of mastery and coping within carers as legitimate goals in their own right (Qureshi *et al.* 2000). Clearly then there is a need to move beyond 'the usual recitation of burdens experienced' (Ory 2000), towards more clearly focused and theoretically grounded interventions (Beck 2001; Dilworth-Anderson 2001; Fortinsky 2001). Future services need to be both theoretically sound (Bond 2000) *and* seen as meaningful by users and carers (Beck 2001; Schulz 2001) if they are to be optimal. To achieve this the theories upon which interventions are based must themselves be meaningful to carers, and reflect their views of the world. This raises important questions of knowledge and expertise, to which we will return later.

Whilst Kahana and Young (1990) raised very relevant questions about the constraining effects of adhering to a stress/burden model, their main contribution was to promote the belief that a better understanding of the needs of carers would only emerge if greater attention was paid to the way caregiving partnerships change over time.

## Partnerships: the 'new' rhetoric of caring relationships

As we have noted, Kahana and Young (1990) stressed the need for research to pay far greater attention to both relationships between caregiver and care receiver (dyadic interactions), and triadic relationships (between caregivers, care receiver and service provider/system). Recently several commentators have alighted upon the significance of both dyadic (Montgomery and Kosloski 2000; Zarit and Leitsch 2001) and triadic relationships (Brandon and Jack 1997; McKee 1999; Fortinsky 2001).

Our own thoughts on the nature of such relationships have been heavily influenced by the work of Rolland (1988, 1994), who proposed a model called the 'therapeutic quadrangle' which takes account of the perceptions of the cared-for person, carer and health care system/practitioner together with the influence of the illness/disease/disability that occasioned the need for care. Rolland contends that conditions vary along important dimensions, these being: onset (for example, sudden or insidious); course (for example, constant, remitting, relapsing); the degree of incapacity in several dimensions, and final outcome. So, for example, a stroke will differ widely on these dimensions from dementia and such differences have several implications for the caregiving situation and the need for support. Such a model is useful, not only as a conceptual device to promote a more holistic view of caring (see for example Nolan 1991), but also to set assessment into an appropriate context (see Nolan *et al.* 1994, 1998).

However, while a focus on partnerships and working together has now become an accepted part of the 'policy rhetoric', translating such ideals into practice is far more complex, and attempts to integrate partnerships into routine services have often been 'superficial in the extreme' (Adams and Clarke 1999). Difficulties have been identified in a number of areas.

As several authors have noted, the idea of the 'professional as expert' is deeply rooted (Brandon and Jack 1997; Qureshi *et al.* 2000; Paterson 2001) and consequently control and power are usually vested with those who hold the most 'prized' knowledge (Clarke 1999b). Essentially, as Thorne *et al.* (2000) argue, traditional models of professional working, at least in health care environments, are underpinned by three basic beliefs:

- The professional is the expert – this is a belief that professionals cling to and are reluctant to let go of.
- The professional is the gatekeeper to services – therefore expressing contrary views may well restrict access to services.
- The ideal patient is compliant – therefore those who raise questions are liable to be labelled as difficult.

To compound potential barriers to creating effective partnerships, others contend that even when debate does occur, it is confined largely to inter-professional and inter-agency concerns (Adams and Clarke 1999), and therefore, by implication, ignores the more fundamental tensions identified above.

Just how fundamental the potential differences between family and professional carers can be was highlighted by Clarke (1999c) in her exploration of professional/lay interactions in the field of dementia. Based on her work, Clarke (1999c) argued that family and professional carers bring to their meetings diametrically opposed viewpoints. Carers seek to 'normalize' their situation, a goal also noted by others (Pickard 1999), whereas professionals define the situation in largely pathological terms. The process of negotiating a shared set of expectations is termed 'inter-facing' by Clarke (1999c), and it is her contention that during this 'inter-facing' carers weigh up the potential 'costs' and 'benefits' of continued engagement with the formal service system. If the 'costs' are seen to outweigh the 'benefits' then services are rejected.

Clearly then dyadic and triadic relationships are complex, but good relationships are the key to better understanding, and have been variously described as a 'major factor' (Braithwaite 2000), the 'foundation' of caregiving (Pickard *et al.* 2000), and 'essential' to an understanding of the nature of family care (Montgomery and Williams 2001). But despite increasing recognition of the importance of such relationships in the academic literature, professional practice often overlooks, or fails to account for, the delicate reciprocities that characterize family care (Brandon and Jack 1997; Pickard *et al.* 2000).

In terms of the relationships between family and professional carers, these often turn, as noted above, on who is seen to hold the 'prized' knowledge, and where expertise is seen to lie. 'Expert' carers can be seen as threatening by professionals (Allen 2000a), yet this need not be the case, and the notion of 'carers as experts' does not *de facto* diminish the professional role but rather changes its orientation. The model of 'carers as experts' is underpinned by certain basic assumptions, which are:

- While an assessment of the difficulties of caring is important, a full understanding will not be achieved unless attention is also given to the nature of past and present relationships, the satisfactions or rewards of caring and the range of coping and other resources, such as income, housing and social support, that carers can draw upon.
- The stresses or difficulties of care can best be understood from a subjective rather than an objective perspective. This means that the circumstances of care are less important than a carer's perception of them.
- It is essential to consider both a carer's willingness and ability to care. Some family members may not really want to care but may feel obliged to do so. Conversely, while many family members may be willing to care they may lack the necessary skills and abilities.
- While recognizing the importance of services such as respite care, in-home support and so on, the primary purpose of the 'carers as experts' approach is to help carers to attain the necessary competencies, skills and resources to provide care of good quality without detriment to their own health. In this context helping a carer to give up care is a legitimate aim.
- 'Carers as experts' recognizes the changing demands of care and the way in which skills and expertise develop over time. A temporal dimension is therefore crucial, and this suggests varying degrees of 'partnership'. For carers new to their role professional carers are likely to be 'senior partners' in possession of important knowledge of a 'cosmopolitan nature' which is needed to help carers understand the demands they are likely to face. Conversely experienced carers, many of whom will have learned their skills by trial and error, often have a far better grasp of their situation than professionals, and acknowledgement of this is vital to a partnership approach. At a later stage the balance may shift again. So, for example, if it is necessary to choose a nursing home, carers may go back to a 'novice' stage, probably never having had to select a home before. They will therefore need additional help and support. Recognizing and achieving such a balance is the crux of the 'carers as experts' model.

(Nolan *et al.* 1996a, 1998)

Such an approach, as noted above, need not threaten the professional contribution as what is being proposed is that the carer be viewed as 'an' expert, not 'the' expert (Lundh and Nolan 2001). This highlights the need to see all knowledge as being equally important (Clarke 1999b), and to recognize that partnerships at all levels are essential to the development of better services (Qureshi *et al.* 2000). Fundamentally partnerships are based on relationships which are mutually trusting and respectful and 'in the presence of such a relationship caring can be an enriching experience, in its absence it becomes a custodial affair' (Zgola 1999: 2). However, relationships are not static, and explicit within the 'carers as experts' model is an acknowledgement of the temporal dimensions of caregiving.

## Caregiving: changing contexts over time

> The form, content and timing of interventions should depend to a considerable extent on where carers are in their careers, and involve an understanding of what has passed before, and what is likely to be ahead. That is, the problems encountered today should be viewed against the backdrop of yesterday, and with an eye towards tomorrow.
>
> (Aneshensel *et al.* 1995: 306)

Based on their extensive study of caregiving in dementia, Aneshensel *et al.* (1995) identified five principles for clinical interventions with carers as follows:

- Recognition that the multiple dimensions of caregiving interact in diverse and complex ways. Interventions should therefore be preceded by a multi-dimensional assessment that 'identifies the unique constellation of issues found within a particular family'.
- Subsequently goals should be based on 'the particular configuration of conditions that exist for each individual caregiver at a specific time in his or her caregiving career, . . . therefore goals for treatment should emerge from caregivers themselves'.
- On the basis of the above broad and comprehensive interventions are needed.
- Multiple evaluative criteria must be used which account for particular circumstances.
- It should be recognized that the interests of the carer and person with dementia may sometimes diverge.

In light of the above it seems particularly ironic that the proposed solutions to the failure of existing intervention studies to detect 'significant' differences are primarily methodological, consisting of calls for ever more robust 'measures' or larger, more powerful trials, with bigger samples (Thompson and Briggs 2000; Beck 2001; Cooke *et al.* 2001; Pusey and Richards 2001). And although some have now begun to question the appropriateness of the 'trial' paradigm (Zarit and Letisch 2001), the way forward is still nevertheless viewed mainly in terms of ever greater statistical sophistication. This seems contrary to the growing realization that caring can only be fully understood in its own unique context (McKee 1999; Pickard 1999; Downs 2000; Ory 2000; Dilworth-Anderson 2001; Montgomery and Williams 2001). Dilworth-Anderson (2001) assert that context is the 'pivotal connecting point' in family care and identify several 'types' of contexts that exert an influence on the way carers respond to their situation. These are:

- the socio-cultural context – including the values and beliefs that the caregiver and care receiver hold;
- the structural context – referring to the level and type of support/help that the carer needs to provide;

- the interpersonal context - relating to the quality of the relationship between carer and care receiver;
- the personal context – comprising the resources available to the carer;
- the temporal context – which concerns the timing of caring in terms of the life course of the carer/cared-for person, and the way caring unfolds over time.

All of these contexts are important and we have already alluded to the interpersonal context, that is the quality of relationships, in some detail. But in the 'context' of this volume it is the 'temporal' perspective that is particularly significant.

Rolland's (1988, 1994) model identifies one important temporal element of caring, that is the nature of the disease trajectory. As will become more obvious later, and throughout this book, this influences not only the way that caring is 'taken on' (Nolan *et al.* 1996a), but also how caring changes over time, and indeed how caring might end.

Similarly, Askham's (1998) definition of carer support as any intervention that helps a carer to: take up (or not take up) a caring role; to continue in a caring role; or to end a caring role, has implicit within it the idea of a temporal dimension. What is required, however, is a more detailed understanding of the way caring changes over time in order that services can provide the most appropriate type of support, at the most appropriate point.

The temporal experience of care has been the subject of interest for some time (see for example Wilson 1989a, b; Willoughby and Keating 1991; Kobayashi *et al.* 1993; Wuest *et al.* 1994). More recently several authors have suggested that there is a need to give greater attention to the nature of caregiving transitions (Aneshensel *et al.* 1995; Schulz and Williamson 1997; Montgomery and Kosloski 2000; Ory 2000; Qualls 2000; Whitlach *et al.* 2001). These authors do not contend that it is possible to 'predict' the course of caregiving, or that even for a given condition (for example, stroke or dementia) caring will follow a uniform path. Indeed, most are at pains to point out the diversity in caring circumstances. However, what they do argue is that, notwithstanding individual variation and context, it is possible to identify 'threads of continuity' (Aneshensel *et al.* 1995) or to 'discern consistency' (Montgomery and Kosloski 2000), which provide an indication of when might be the best time to offer support, and what type of help is most likely to be useful at a particular point in time (Montgomery and Kosloski 2000). Indeed, as the quote which began this section stresses, 'the form, content and timing of interventions should depend to a considerable extent on where carers are in their career' (Aneshensel *et al.* 1995).

The metaphor of a 'caring career' was used by Aneshensel *et al.* (1995) to conceptualize the transitions and role changes that carers experience over time. They identified three broad phases to such a 'career' which were:

- preparation for, and acquisition of, the caregiving role;
- enactment of caregiving;
- disengagement from caregiving.

More recently others have also likened caring to a career with a 'beginning, discernible temporal extension or direction, and an end' (Montgomery and Kosloski 2000). These latter authors contend that despite great diversity in caregiving circumstances, conceptualizing caring as a 'career' is helpful in better understanding the nature of relationships and how these change over time. In elaborating upon their arguments they suggest that the use of a temporal approach helps to identify 'markers' which highlight when carers may be more in need of, or more receptive to, support. They provide what they consider to be seven critical markers, which develop sequentially as follows:

- performing tasks previously undertaken by others;
- self-definition as carer;
- giving personal care;
- seeking assistance and formal service use;
- considering nursing home placement;
- nursing home placement;
- termination of caregiving either by the death of the cared-for person, the recovery of the cared-for person, or because the carer 'quits'.

While potentially useful, in our view such a conceptualization is rather too mechanistic and instrumental. For instance, it equates caring primarily with 'performing tasks' or 'giving personal care', thereby failing fully to acknowledge the less visible, but often more important 'types' of care (see Bowers 1987, 1988; Nolan *et al.* 1996a).

We would, however, agree that temporal models are useful, indeed they are the *raison d'être* for this book, which is largely structured around the temporal model first described in detail by Nolan *et al.* (1996a). This model had its roots in early studies (Nolan 1991; Nolan and Grant 1992a) but, building on the work of Wilson (1989a, b), was more fully developed and elaborated upon by Keady in the field of dementia (Keady and Nolan 1994a; Keady 1999). The model proposed that caring can be considered to comprise six 'stages' termed:

- building on the past;
- recognizing the need;
- taking it on;
- working through it;
- reaching the end;
- a new beginning.

Although not a stage of caring *per se*, 'building on the past' highlights the importance of prior relationships to an understanding of the caring situation. 'Recognizing the need' refers to the processes by which carers become aware of their changing relationship with their relative or friend. This may be a subtle process which evolves over several years and comprises differing types of care (Bowers 1987; Nolan *et al.* 1996a). 'Taking it on' describes the realization by the carer of a fundamental change in their relationship, with a cognitive shift towards greater recognition of a caring role. Once again, how carers 'take on' their role varies. In the event of a sudden health crisis, for instance a stroke, both 'recognizing the need' and 'taking it on' may happen very rapidly. Ideally before 'taking it on' carers should be helped to make important decisions about both their willingness and ability to care (Nolan *et al.* 1996a). However, this rarely occurs and carers frequently 'take on' their role with little understanding of its longer term implications (see for example Stewart *et al.* 1993; Opie 1994). In other situations, for example dementia, 'recognizing the need' and 'taking it on' unfold, often with little or no awareness, over a period of time.

'Working through it' is intended to capture the proactive way in which carers respond to their role, and the active strategies they develop in order to feel 'in control'. This is the period in which carers gain 'expertise', usually through a process of trial and error.

'Reaching the end' is in some respects a misnomer, as apart from the death (or recovery) of the cared-for person, most carers do not 'reach the end' *per se*. This phase is primarily concerned with the process by which alternative caring arrangements are established, usually by the placement of the cared-for person in a care home. Once again, carers often receive little help during this difficult and stressful period.

Finally, a 'new beginning' is intended to capture the importance of helping carers to 'move on' with their lives, either following the death of the cared-for person, or to reconstruct caring roles following placement of the cared-for person in a nursing home. It is the further elaboration of this temporal model that is the primary aim of this book.

## Why another book on family care?

An epistemology of humility insists that only the constituency will define the questions . . .
(Post 2001: S18)

Methodologies such as grounded theory offer perhaps the greatest hope of obtaining the true essence of users' views, since theoretical insight and interpretation follow, rather than precede, data collection.
(McKee 1999: 152)

The intention of this introductory chapter has been to provide the 'context' for the remainder of this book and in so doing hopefully to answer, at least by implication, the question 'why another book on family care?' We have attempted to highlight several of the 'unresolved' issues in family caregiving (Pearlin *et al.* 2001), particularly as they relate to the provision of support and the design of interventions intended to help family carers to 'take up, continue in, or end' a caregiving role (Askham 1998). We have focused in particular on the notion of partnerships, and stressed the importance of the nature and quality of 'dyadic' and 'triadic' relationships. It seems to us that central to such debates is the conundrum raised by Post (2001), that is, 'who asks the questions?' In other words, are agendas driven primarily by the concerns of researchers or service providers, and couched largely in their terms, or is it only the 'constituency', that is family carers and cared-for persons, that should be defining the questions? We would contend that in any genuine partnership the views of all three major 'constituencies' must be seen as equally relevant.

However, we also believe that despite the signs of on emerging 'paradigm' shift, it is still the voices of researchers and their search for ever more 'sophisticated' methodologies, or policy makers/practitioners who determine what counts as 'evidence', that still hold sway. That is why we need 'another book on family caring'.

The aim of this book is to consider caregiving as a temporal experience and in so doing, to draw upon studies which, as McKee (1999) suggests, are more likely to capture the 'true essence' of, in this case, carers' views. In so doing we are acutely aware that in most instances it is primarily the voice of the carer that is heard, with the perspective of the third member of the so called 'triad', the cared-for person, being rather muted. It is in no way our intention to marginalize such a perspective, indeed our commitment to the valuing of all perspectives in the 'therapeutic quadrangle' has been evident for some time, and reinforced on several occasions (Nolan 1991; Nolan *et al.* 1996a, 1998). We will reiterate this commitment, as well as providing a potential framework for promoting better triadic relationships, in the concluding chapter. In this way it is our hope that the emerging 'paradigm' shift will gain yet further momentum.

# SECTION ONE

## 'Recognizing the need' and 'taking it on'

Family caregivers deserve to be informed and assisted in their
adaptations to the new responsibilities and demands of care, and to
be informed how to provide care at home in an effective manner.
(Given *et al.* 1999: 83)

This section comprises three chapters each of which provides differing but
complementary insights into the early stages of caring that have been
called 'recognizing the need' and 'taking it on' (Nolan *et al.* 1996a).

The opening chapter by Keady and Nolan considers the subtle and often
hidden ways in which the early stages of dementia are experienced by
both carers and people with dementia. There are several reasons why it is
particularly appropriate that this chapter should be the first major contribution to this volume. First, as will become apparent, much of the early
and important work exploring the temporal dimension of caring emerged
from the dementia care literature. Second, the temporal model, which
provides the structure for this book, is built explicitly on the work of
Wilson (1989a, b), again in the field of dementia. This chapter provides a
vehicle which places the theoretical elaboration and subsequent empirical
testing of this model in context. Perhaps most importantly of all, however,
the chapter clearly highlights the pivotal contribution of Keady's work
in shaping the temporal model first described in detail in *Understanding
Family Care* (Nolan *et al.* 1996a).

This first chapter is in some respects unique as, unlike most other work
in the area of family care, it draws explicitly on data from both the carer
and the cared-for person and in so doing allows for a far more nuanced
understanding of the delicate interdependencies that characterized the
best caring relationships, termed by Keady and Nolan 'working together'.
It also explicitly reinforces the importance of prior relationships in largely
determining the context of caring (building on the past) and highlights
how in the absence of a solid foundation caring can be experienced as
'working alone' or 'working apart'.

The second chapter represents an interesting extension of the first, and
again concerns itself with the early experience of dementia. Drawing on
case study material it provides a counterpoint to the chapter by Keady

and Nolan as it focuses primarily on innovation service responses, something that was often tellingly absent in the experiences recounted in the initial chapter. Here, the main authors are practitioners who were closely involved in establishing the initiatives upon which this contribution is based. They were supported in this endeavour, and particularly the evaluation component, by an academic link to Gordon Grant at the University of Sheffield, whose post is co-funded by the Trust within which the work was conducted. Therefore, this chapter illustrates how creative partnerships between practice and academia can help to narrow the so-called 'theory–practice gap'. In this chapter Clark, Chaston and Grant focus on the development and evaluation of two forms of early intervention in dementia. One concerns a service designed to support carers and people with dementia who are over the age of 65, the second turns attention to a still reduced neglected area, support for those who develop dementia at an early stage in the life cycle.

In terms of Rolland's (1988) typology, and the way in which 'recognizing the need' and 'taking it on' manifest themselves, Chapter 3 provides a marked contrast to the initial two chapters. Its subject matter is the experience of 'new' carers of stroke survivors who, compared to caregivers in dementia, are suddenly confronted with a major health crisis and have to 'take it on', often with very little time to prepare. Methodologically the study adopted a 'grounded theory' approach, as did Keady and Nolan in Chapter 1. However, there are important and significant differences, for while Keady and Nolan's work was underpinned by a temporal model, their data were collected cross-sectionally. Although theoretical sampling was used and carers were strategically sampled across the various phases of their caregiving career, cross-sectional data inevitably requires an inferential leap in moving from 'taking it on', to 'working through it', to 'reaching the end' when these experiences have not been described by the same people. Such a limitation does not apply to the contribution by Brereton and Nolan, as data were collected longitudinally from the same carers every 2–3 months over a period of up to 18 months. Drawing on data from 78 interviews Brereton and Nolan are able to provide a rich and detailed description of several caring 'transitions'. They focus in this chapter on the period of hospitalization and the immediate post-discharge support (or often lack of it) that carers experience at home.

Interestingly, despite the very differing contexts of these three initial chapters, it is already possible to begin to discern 'threads of continuity' and to identify 'markers' as to when professional support might be most relevant, and the form that support might take. For example, during the 'taking it on' phase, Keady and Nolan describe how carers ask the question 'can I do this?', that is take on care, highlighting the uncertainty carers feel about their ability to care. Similarly, for carers in Brereton and Nolan's study, one of their primary concerns was whether or not they were 'up to the job' of caring. It is such 'threads of continuity' that surface throughout the book that we will draw together in the concluding chapter.

# 1

# The dynamics of dementia: working together, working separately, or working alone?

## John Keady and Mike Nolan

### Introduction

There has probably been more research into the needs of family members caring for a person with dementia than in any other field. As with the wider literature, a stress/burden model has been the predominant theoretical frame of reference but other, more positive and holistic orientations have had their roots in dementia care. So, for example, Hirschfield's (1983) important contribution was to develop the concept of mutuality, defined as: 'the caregiver's ability to find gratification and meaning from the caregiving situation' (p. 26), and to demonstrate that in situations of high mutuality, caregiving was less stressful and more likely to be sustained. This early work highlighted the importance of the quality of prior and current relationships in providing a context for caregiving. Later Motenko (1989) explored further the delicate interplay between the frustrations and gratifications of caring for someone with dementia and his work further belied the belief that caring was necessarily all 'bad news'.

Other important insights have also been gained from research in the field of dementia. For instance, Bowers's (1987, 1988) exposition of the differing types of care that daughters provide for their mothers with dementia moved the focus away from an 'instrumental' or hands-on caring role and suggested that other, often invisible types of care were seen by caregivers to be both more important and more stressful. Bowers (1987, 1988) argued that it was not so much what carers did that mattered but rather that the important consideration was the motivation or purpose underlying differing types of care. Building on this she identified several types of care that developed over time including: anticipatory care; preventative care; supervisory care; instrumental care and protective care (Bowers 1987). In a second study she began to explore the interplay between family and professional carers following placement of the person with dementia (PWD) in a care home. On the basis of this work she identified a further type of care, 'preservative care', by which the family tried to maintain the PWD's family connections, dignity, hope and sense of control. She argued that the family wanted to collaborate actively with staff in ensuring that the PWD's needs were met. However, staff were often not conscious of, or did not respond to the families' efforts to work together.

Hasselkus (1988) similarly suggested that family carers considered that they had expertise and knowledge that they wanted to share with professionals. Once again, however, such knowledge was often overlooked or ignored, which frequently resulted in families rejecting the support they were offered.

These differing but complementary insights provided a wider perspective on family care, and each in their own way has been influential in the evolution of our own approach to 'understanding family care' (Nolan *et al.* 1996a). However, in the present context it is the development of the six-stage temporal model of care (Keady and Nolan 1994a; Nolan *et al.* 1996a; Keady 1999) that is the primary focus of this chapter.

Several temporal models have emerged to help identify and better understand the changing experiences of families providing support to a PWD (see, for example, Kobayashi *et al.* 1993; Wuest *et al.* 1994; Aneshensel *et al.* 1995), but our own work was most influenced by the model developed by Wilson (1989a, b). The purpose of this chapter is to outline briefly the way in which Wilson's model was further elaborated upon by Keady (Keady and Nolan 1994a; Keady 1999), and then to focus on the early caring period, particularly the process of 'recognizing the need'. However, we will not concentrate solely on the views of carers but also incorporate those of the PWD, and in so doing map out the ways in which these two key figures interact and help to shape the nature of caregiving. This interaction largely determined whether carers and PWD 'work together', 'work separately', or 'work alone'. We will highlight in particular the often prolonged, subtle and sometimes divisive interactions that both carers and PWD engage in during the period before a formal diagnosis of dementia is provided. In order to portray an accurate sense of the temporal sequence in which Keady's (1999) work unfolded, this chapter will describe the carer's perspective first, then add that of the PWD before seeking to integrate the two.

In order fully to acknowledge the influence of Wilson's (1989a) work, and to provide a context against which to consider our adaptation of it, the chapter begins with a quite detailed summary of the published work that informed our own. For the purposes of this chapter the greatest emphasis is placed on the first of her two studies (Wilson 1989a).

## A temporal model of caregiving in dementia

Wilson (1989a, b) used a grounded theory method to explore the experience of living with a PWD and to interpret the processes and coping patterns of family carers. She adapted an analytical approach first described by Hutchinson (1986) to outline an eight-stage model of the course of Alzheimer's disease as experienced by family members.

Her temporal model begins with the initial stage of 'noticing', where family carers gradually become more aware of the bizarre, or aberrant, behaviour of the person they live with. This stage was reported as only being recognized in retrospect and no particular cognitive deficit or behaviour was cited by family caregivers in this study as alerting them to the fact that something was wrong. Noticing, therefore, was as a result of cumulative behaviour which was initially discounted and normalized. The processes of 'discounting and normalizing' formed stage two of the model, and at this point carers attributed changes mainly to old age until two conditions emerged:

- the unusual behaviour worsened;
- a particular event took place which was sufficiently serious to make discounting it very difficult.

Wilson (1989a) gives an example of one family noticing changes for three or four years until one behavioural cue made it impossible to discount. This led to stage three, 'suspecting'. Wilson (1989a) suggested that 'pervasive uncertainty' characterized this stage with family members speculating about what was going wrong. This suspicion fuelled a realization that something more serious was happening and prompted family carers to search for explanations. In stage four, 'searching for explanations', Wilson (1989a) suggests that the decision to seek confirmation of a diagnosis was undertaken 'reluctantly' as families were increasingly aware of the financial costs and stress involved. The discovery that the person had probable Alzheimer's disease led some families to avoid further medical investigations, fuelled by the belief that nothing could be done anyway.

Stage five, 'recasting', describes how, once the diagnosis had been tentatively confirmed, families engaged in a range of tactics which involved reappraising, retrospectively, various experiences with their demented relative; that is, they reflected back on their experiences to date within the context of the diagnosis. In stage six, 'taking it on', 'recasting' provides the basis for making informed decisions about whether to 'take on' care. Wilson (1989a) describes this as being a decision taken without full knowledge of the likely demands and implications of the role. Rather, the decision to take on family care was motivated by a sense of moral duty. Stage seven, 'going through it', describes how dementia presents the family caregiver with a 'seemingly unending list of problems' (Wilson 1989a: 43) which require resolution. These are tackled on a trial and error basis, with little or no practical help, support or respite. The experience is characterized as 'living on the brink' of the family carer's tolerance, with carers being continually confronted by negative choices in which decisions must be made, but without desirable alternatives. Wilson suggests that most family caregivers then come to terms with the erosion of their own physical and emotional well-being and start to consider institutionalization. This leads to stage eight, 'turning it over'. At this point family caregivers consciously and reluctantly let go of the direct care of their relative and entrust that care to an institution. Wilson (1989a) suggests that carers continue their role in a less visible capacity by under-taking daily visits, taking care of financial management and 'being there' during crises and transfers in and out of institutions. Wilson (1989a) acknowledged that this study offered 'a beginning knowledge basic to interpreting the meaning associated with their (family carers') experience' (p. 44). While she went on to elaborate upon the theory in another study (Wilson 1989b), it is the above account that most influenced our work, and the way in which Wilson's (1989a) study was further developed is described below.

## Taking the model further

Our interest in the dynamic nature of caregiving, the quality of relation-ships, and the interface between family and professional carers from a temporal perspective has been long-standing (see, for example, Nolan and Grant 1989; Nolan 1991; Nolan and Grant 1992a, b). However, it was Keady's efforts to extend Wilson's work further that underpinned the six-stage model upon which this book is based. As already noted, the six stages of this model are:

- building on the past;
- recognizing the need;
- taking it on;
- working through it;
- reaching the end;
- a new beginning.

                                                                    (Nolan *et al.* 1996a)

The influence of Wilson's work on this model is obvious. For example, we adopt Wilson's phrase 'taking it on' as an explicit part of our model. Moreover, 'working through it' is analogous to Wilson's 'going through it', but this stage was renamed and 'going' replaced by 'working' to capture the much more proactive stance adopted by carers, as suggested in Keady's study (Keady and Nolan 1994a; Keady 1999). However, it is the prior elem-ents of the model, particularly 'recognizing the need' that are explored in greatest detail here.

   In building on Wilson's (1989a, b) studies, Keady too adopted a grounded theory methodology (see Keady 1999 for a detailed account). The original aim of the study was to explore further the temporal experience of care using the prior literature, and especially Wilson's (1989a, b) work, not as an explicit theoretical framework, but as a heuristic device that would help to recognize 'leads' in the data but without 'leading' data collection (Morse 1994). To this end a series of interviews were conducted with family carers. During a small number of these the PWD also asked to contribute, and on this basis a tentative temporal model from their perspective was also developed (see Keady and Nolan 1994b). Subsequently further joint interviews (n = 11) were conducted that explicitly included and focused on the perspective of the PWD. This allowed for an integration of the two temporal models and a resultant grounded theory which suggested that the primary aim of both caregiver and the PWD was to try and maintain the involvement of the PWD as an active agent in the world (Keady 1999). This was best achieved by the carer and PWD 'working together' (ideally in concert with the formal services) but occasionally they would also 'work apart', or the carer was left to 'work alone' (Keady 1999). The nature of the 'working' relationship which predominated was heavily influenced by the type and quality of prior relationships (building on the past) and the interactions that occurred prior to the formal diagnosis of dementia. This is what we will focus on here.

In doing so we will draw explicitly on Keady's (1999) original grounded theory but will further elaborate and reconsider the subtle interplay that occurs during 'recognizing the need', and suggest that in addition to 'working together', 'working alone', or 'working apart', another process, 'working separately', also occurs, of which 'working apart' is a variant. As modifiability is one of the key characteristics of a good grounded theory (Glaser and Strauss 1967; Charmaz 2000) we believe that this subtle change provides a further elaboration upon the original processes identified by Keady (1999).

## Results

Just as with Wilson's (1989a, b) studies, early data collection suggested that it was often a seemingly insignificant but either unusual or repeated event that caught the carer's eye and first alerted them that something was perhaps not quite right. This 'noticing' took a variety of forms and often involved a daily event, for example, driving:

> The first thing I noticed? His [carer's husband] driving. My husband had always been such a careful driver and then he suddenly started to hit the kerb and drive too close to the car in front. He also didn't seem to understand traffic lights anymore. They would turn to green and I would be sitting there waiting to move off but he didn't go. He

would just sit there and I would have to tell him to go in the end. I just thought he was getting on and that he couldn't see as well as he used to. That's what I told myself anyway, but I thought it was a little strange.

Other examples included forgetting to pay bills when previously this had always been done punctually, or not being able to calculate a darts score when this had always been second nature. Wilson's study suggested that in the early stages these events would be discounted and normalized (stage two) until this was no longer possible, when carers moved onto stage three of her model – 'suspecting'.

However, close consideration of data from the interviews did not fully support such an interpretation. First, it became apparent that carers did not 'discount and normalize' but rather that they first normalized and only then discounted. These processes were therefore related but distinct and had a differing temporal sequencing than Wilson (1989a) had suggested. Initially carers would ask themselves 'what am I seeing?' and 'why is this happening?' 'Normalizing' the unusual behaviour usually involved finding a rational explanation, for instance stress at work, acute illness, or often 'just old age'. This would allow carers to come to the conclusion that 'this (the behaviour) is okay' and could be 'discounted'. However, as the behaviour was either repeated or became more obvious carers began to 'suspect' that something might be wrong and it became more difficult to 'discount' the behaviour. Carers then began a more active process than 'noticing' and specifically began to 'keep an eye' on their relative, in some respects a process akin to the preventative care described by Bowers (1987). This could often go on for a prolonged period of time:

> What did I first notice about Mum? Well, the first nine months I was down there [her mother's house situated a short walk away] virtually from the time I got up in the morning to the time I went to bed. I'd run home, get a quick snack, and I would have to spend more and more time down there because . . . I think it really started that we noticed . . . I mean I noticed there was things she was forgetting and I put it down to old age and she, I mean my sister, she came up once a year for a week. So the first year she came up she was fine, the second year she started to say that 'Mum is definitely forgetful, isn't she?', and the third year she came up I said, 'Yes she is.'

As will be highlighted later, the extended nature of this process of 'suspecting' was in part due to action on the part of the PWD (undiagnosed at this point) to 'cover their tracks'. However, carers eventually began to realize that 'this might be serious' and therefore 'increased vigilance' (Keady 1999), and began to observe their relative far more rigorously. However, despite the increasing severity of the symptoms several carers still hoped to find another explanation for their concerns:

In the early days I wanted my mum to be better. I knew it was not getting any better, but I wanted her to, if that makes any sense to you. She was so forgetful by then. Calling me the wrong name all the time, not doing the shopping and the like. It was so unlike her. And her temper! I knew then I had to do something, but early on I always hoped that she would come back and be my mum again.

The data also suggested that 'noticing' was not a stage in caregiving, but rather a process that was not confined to the first episodes of odd behaviour but occurred throughout the caring trajectory, that is, carers continued to 'notice' things even after the diagnosis. This strategy was used to alert them to yet further changes in the PWD:

... isn't it funny. Just this morning I '*noticed*' [emphasis added] that he [her husband] didn't dry his face with the towel. He just sat there with it in his hands and looked at me – he didn't seem to know what to do. I always help him in the bathroom, with his shaving and that, but he has always dried his face afterwards. Normally, I just hand him the towel and he gets on with it. So this morning when he didn't do that I thought it was a little strange.

Prior to diagnosis the time would come when carers could no longer sustain a belief that 'this is okay' and moved from the notion that 'this might be serious' to 'this probably is serious'. Prior to this, children in particular often tried to get external confirmation for their concerns from siblings, but eventually carers' concerns were such that they sought more concrete confirmation. This tended to happen in one of three main ways:

• they might raise their concerns directly with their relative – 'have you noticed anything?';
• some event would occur that was so bizarre or unacceptable that the carer's patience would 'snap' and they would directly confront the PWD – 'bringing things to a head';
• they would seek medical confirmation – 'asking the experts'.

As we will discuss later, 'working together' began much earlier and was more successful when: the PWD agreed that they too had 'noticed' something; both the carer and the PWD 'asked the experts' early, and the expert (usually the GP) was receptive and well informed and acted upon the concerns that had been raised. Unfortunately this was not the usual pattern of events.

In instances when the carer asked their relative 'have you noticed anything?' (originally termed 'open confirmation', Keady 1999), this was often denied, thereby effectively closing off further discussion:

I tried to tell my mother about what she was doing and ask her if she recognized it too, but she didn't want to know. I thought I had done all the right things, you know, planned what I was going to say and I waited until there was no one else in the house. She seemed happy enough at first but I couldn't get through to her. She just stopped me stone dead and said there was nothing wrong with her . . . [pause], but I knew there was.

In such instances the 'issue' might not be raised again until an event occurred that 'brought things to a head' (originally termed 'confrontation confirmation'):

*Carer*:      I remember coming home from the shops to find my husband on his knees trying to put soiled toilet paper into a plant pot. At the time I felt sick and disgusted, I was just so tired of having to chase after him all the time. I remember shouting at him, 'Why don't you flush it down the toilet like everyone else!' I then said something like 'You're a grown man' and 'You're not normal'.

*Researcher*: What happened after you said those things?

*Carer*:      Nothing much, he just sort of looked at me strangely and started to walk away.

*Researcher*: Did you chase after him?

*Carer*:      Yes. I went running after him. I remember I was still shouting at him, things like 'You've ruined my life', that sort of thing. I feel terrible telling you all about this now because he [carer's husband] really isn't well. But it is what happened. When he didn't answer me I told him I was 'going to do something about it', so I remember leaving him by himself and I went straight to the doctors. I couldn't cope any more. I felt so angry and I knew something had to be done.

When something like this happened carers usually felt very guilty afterwards, but at least this unexpected event highlighted the need to 'ask the experts'.

Of course, not all carers had their first contact with their doctor following such a dramatic event. Nevertheless, in many instances, initial medical contact was made without the knowledge of their relative, either because they had not responded to the carer's question, 'Have you noticed anything?', or because the carer wanted to talk things through before raising it with their relative. As already noted, 'working together' began earlier and was more effective when both the carer and the relative went to the 'expert' together and he/she responded appropriately. All too often, however, and irrespective of the events prior to the consultation, the medical response was inadequate:

I went to the doctor because my wife was doing things that I just did not understand. I knew she was ill but nobody would believe me – she couldn't go with me you see and they had to go on what I said. All the doctor said to me was, 'Come back again in six months if things have not improved.' Some help that was.

*Carer*:      All I knew was that he would do funny things and fiddle with things in the house. It was when he started to put the gas on and forget to light it, that I knew something had to be done. We discussed it as a family and we all agreed.

*Researcher*: When you say you discussed it as a family, did the discussion include your husband?

*Carer*:      No.

*Researcher*: So it was when your husband began to be unsafe in the house you felt you had to do something?

*Carer*:      Yes, that's it. I went to the doctor then and he gave me a booklet – one with a black cover. He asked me to read it and come back again if I was having trouble managing. He also gave me a booklet telling me who to contact and, you know, that's just about it until I went back again to see him.

*Researcher*: So how long did you live with this knowledge, and your husband, before you returned again to your doctor to ask for more help?

*Carer*:      About two years.

Ironically many of the encounters with GPs resulted in the family doctor adopting the same tactics as the carer had earlier, and both 'normalizing' and 'discounting' the carer's concerns, usually by attributing the behaviour to old age and telling the carer that it was 'okay'. By this stage, of course, the carers were usually quite sure that it was not okay but their belief that 'this might be serious' was discounted by the 'expert', thereby adding to their stress and the emerging feeling that they were 'working alone'.

Eventually, however, a diagnosis was provided and the carer's 'needs' were recognized by the 'experts', leading to a situation where the carer had to decide if they wanted to 'take it on'.

The decision-making processes involved in choosing to become or not to become a 'carer' at the time of the diagnosis constituted the next stage of care, one Wilson (1989a) had previously named 'taking it on'. While the time dimension for this stage of care is brief, it is, nonetheless, a crucial phase of the caregiving experience. The data suggested that this stage was not particularly well understood by carers, and it was a period in which professional intervention played a major role in the life of both the person with dementia and also the carer. Formal (medical) explanation of the cause of the person's behaviour/actions marked a critical juncture, leading the carer out of 'recognizing the need' and into a stage that propels the family member towards the more formally recognized role of 'carer'. The data would suggest that this period of further decision making confronts the carer with a number of questions, such as:

- Is this for me?
- Can I do it?

- What will it mean?
- Should I 'go through with it'?

The decision to take on the caring role is a result of a number of complex dynamics, which are related directly to the context of previous relationships and to the opportunities provided by professional care agencies. How carers weigh up the options at this time is crucial, and yet there was not one carer in the sample that had been made aware of potential alternatives to them 'taking on' the caring role. From the perspective of helping agencies, it was expected that caregiving would continue and that, when offered, professional support would simply assist in this process; it was through this narrow and circumscribed view of the world that carers took on their role. From the data it appeared that Wilson (1989a) had accurately represented and named this stage as 'taking it on', and it seemed inappropriate to change the title simply for cosmetic purposes.

To a significant extent 'taking it on' was shaped by 'building on the past' and the length of time it had taken to work through the stage of 'recognizing the need'. For some carers, reaching the point of a diagnosis was a relief as it validated their concerns about the relative and put their future into some form of context. Conversely, other carers approached 'taking it on' with misgivings, uncertain about the future and their relationship with the person with dementia.

## Adding another perspective

As we noted at the start of this chapter, in four of the later interviews with the family carers the PWD had also asked to be present and gave their account of their experiences to date. Based on these, and a consideration of the literature, a tentative temporal model from the perspective of the PWD was published (Keady and Nolan 1994b) comprising nine stages:

- slipping;
- suspecting;
- covering up;
- revealing;
- confirming;
- surviving;
- disorganization;
- decline;
- death.

It is the first five stages that are particularly relevant here, and these are described more fully below.

*Slipping*

The process of dementia was seen to begin with a stage of slipping where the person gradually became aware of minor and seemingly trivial 'slips and lapses' in his/her memory and/or behaviour. These 'slips and lapses' were initially ignored, but as they became more frequent could no longer be so easily dismissed. At this time emotion-focused coping behaviours such as 'discounting' and the 'normalizing of events' were used to deny the significance of the symptoms. The stage was then seen to shade into:

*Suspecting*

Here the incidences occurred with greater frequency/severity so that they could no longer be rationalized or ignored. The 'discounting' and 'normalizing of events' became less successful coping strategies and the individual began to suspect that something could be quite seriously amiss.

*Covering up*

This strategy was employed when the person made a conscious and deliberate effort to compensate for his/her difficulties and actively to hide them from family members, friends and colleagues. As the condition progressed and covering up became more problematic, the person began to restrict activities in certain areas where his/her competence was difficult to sustain. If they had not noticed before, it was often at this point that the individual's partner/family may have begun to notice changes in the behaviour of their relative.

*Revealing*

A stage of revealing is then reached where the individual's difficulties are revealed to those closest to him/her. This may be as a result of a conscious decision, or as a result of being confronted with patterns of loss. At this point shared knowledge might still be kept within the immediate family and a formal confirmation of suspicions may be delayed.

*Confirming*

Next is a stage of 'confirming' where open acknowledgement of the problem is made and the process of diagnostic conformation begins. This is usually the first point of contact with formal services.

It was the desire to explore these stages in greater detail that resulted in interviews being undertaken with ten people with dementia (PWD) and their carers. This provided a number of methodological and ethical challenges (see Keady 1999 for more detail) but also produced a rich source of data that allowed for a far more detailed understanding of the caring dynamic to emerge.

## Hearing the voice of the person with dementia

Analysis of data from these interviews indicated that while the initial stages of slipping, suspecting and covering up were broadly descriptive of the early experience of dementia, they failed fully to capture the subtle and proactive actions taken. It emerged that during the stage of 'slipping' the PWD 'noticed' something unusual in their normal behaviour and, as with the carers, initially normalized and discounted such events. Only when the behaviours or events reoccurred, increased in severity, or new lapses occurred did the PWD begin to suspect that something quite serious might be happening. However, at this stage people generally kept their fears hidden:

> At the beginning it was so dark. I couldn't believe I was doing these things. I felt so stupid and didn't want to share it with anyone else. I had trouble getting the right word out and forgetting people's names. It was awful.

Therefore none of these early experiences were shared; rather the PWD began to engage in a 'secret' process of 'testing' themselves out to see if their performance would return to normal. During these early stages they therefore actively 'worked alone' to try and maintain a veneer of normality. However, this could not be sustained indefinitely and, as the PWD feared that they would be 'discovered' they began a process of 'closing down' (Keady 1999) in order to 'keep it (their suspicions and failing memory) hidden'. 'Closing down' was a prolonged process that could go on for several months and allowed for two main things to occur. It gave the PWD:

- time to adjust to their situation;
- space to reflect and try to make sense of what was happening.

'Closing down' can therefore be seen as a protective mechanism aimed at maintaining the person's integrity and sense of 'who they are'. It was also an intensely private experience, often accompanied by a lowered mood and feelings of depression. 'Closing down' comprised a number of tactics, all of which were designed essentially to limit exposure to 'threatening' situations where the PWD might no longer be able to cope. Two broad categories of activity could be identified, termed here:

- playing it safe;
- making excuses.

'Playing it safe' involved sticking to a limited number of behaviours and activities that the PWD felt that they could complete effectively. Hiding their failing abilities, or 'making excuses', is descriptive of the PWD's need to justify why they were not undertaking activities that they would previously have completed with no difficulty. It was often at this point that carers began to notice the increasingly limited social world of the PWD, as it also began to impact on them. The following interchange illustrates this well:

*Person*:   Well, it was the simple things really. I couldn't remember where the shopping went in the cupboards so I said something to [my wife] and would let her do it [playing it safe]. She used to get angry with me about that. I also got scared driving as I couldn't work out the way to the shops, so I told her my eyesight wasn't good and I stopped [making excuses].

*Carer*:   [to researcher] That's true. I used to think he was doing it on purpose. I never stopped at the beginning to think that something was wrong with him. I just thought he was trying to annoy me all the time, and that he had lost his confidence.

Eventually as the PWD felt certain that things were not going to return to 'normal', they began a brief process of 'regrouping', which again was an active process of seeking to maintain their involvement for as long as possible. Several tactics were adopted, for example:

- taking things one day at a time;
- keeping any further memory loss to myself for as long as possible;
- engaging in mentally challenging activities such as puzzles and crossword;
- using lists and other memory aids;
- constantly repeating things to myself to help me remember;
- keeping my real fears and feelings secret;
- trying to keep calm and relaxed at all times;
- making up stories to fill in the gaps;
- fighting the memory loss and trying not to let it get the better of me.

At this point the PWD used a variety of adaptive and creative coping tactics, such as writing down significant matters of concern such as: important birthdays, ages of (your) children, date of (your) anniversary, directions to the local shop, where important keys are kept and what they are for, a pictorial representation of the value of money and so on. These lists were usually secreted in places of as near absolute safety as possible where their chances of discovery were minimal; although, even in this scenario, there was an associated fear that their discovery could reveal the depths of an individual's loss and perceived sense of failing. Interestingly, in carrying out this adaptive coping strategy, there were gender differences in places of concealment. For men a common hiding place for the lists was usually outside the house in places such as the garden shed or inside the car, while for women inside a handbag or inside clothes hanging in a wardrobe were frequently cited as 'secret places'. Wherever it was hidden the purpose of the list was to maintain the veneer of normality and to preserve feelings of self-worth, identity and control.

The active nature of such activities was termed 'covering your tracks', and this could go on for months or even years, and eventually, in some cases, was even accepted as 'normal' by the carer:

> After a while I began to think what he [her husband] was doing wasn't a problem. He wasn't doing any harm, you know. I got frustrated at first not being able to go out as often as I would have liked, to get the shopping mainly, but I just thought he had gone off the idea of driving. That's what he told me anyway, and there are worse things in this life than not going out in the car, don't you think? I picked up some old interests of mine and life just went on.

How long 'covering your tracks' could be sustained depended on whether it was questioned by carers. In some cases carers unwittingly began to collude with the stories and behaviours of their partner, thus twisting their meaning and making a seemingly abnormal situation 'normal' again.

Eventually, however, 'covering your tracks' became an increasingly fraught and difficult process to manage. In time the PWD started to react to events rather than shape them, and others then began to 'notice' the 'slips and lapses' and note their frequency. For the individual with dementia, long-held coping mechanisms aimed at concealment also began to break down and their cognitive skills were not sufficient to reshape them successfully.

Eventually the PWD needed to 'open up' to the fact that something was wrong and, as noted earlier, carers often initiated this process themselves, or alternatively the PWD raised their concerns with the carer. Paradoxically, reversing the situation described in the carer interviews, in two cases when this occurred the carer initially denied that there was anything wrong, and when the PWD asked, 'Have you noticed anything?', they said no.

However, from the interviews conducted with PWD, in three out of ten cases the carers made the initial contact with the GP, and in seven out of ten cases it was a joint approach. The data from the larger set of carer interviews would suggest that this pattern was not typical and that fewer couples make an initial joint approach. The greater numbers approaching the GP together from the second set of interviews may well have been an artefact of the sample, as by definition these couples were willing to discuss their situation openly. Clearly there is a need for more research in this area.

However, in the situations where there was mutual acceptance of the situation, the PWD entered a new and less stressful phase termed 'sharing the load' (Keady 1999). This meant that the PWD and their carer could begin to 'work together' in making sense of, and responding to the future:

I know I have Alzheimer's disease, but what can anyone do about it? I do silly things now but we just try and laugh about it. We have a saying, 'Pick up the pieces and start again.' It's the only way we manage.

However, even now the PWD would still keep their deteriorating abilities 'secret' for as long as possible, but the motivation was usually one of wishing to protect the carer for as long as possible from knowledge of their worsening condition. Interestingly this seemed to be a reverse of the 'protective' caring described by Bowers (1987).

## Mapping experiences: when do trajectories cross?

A comparison of the early experience of the signs and symptoms of dementia from a carer's perspective, and that of the PWD, clearly indicates that this is a time of great uncertainty for both parties. Moreover, this uncertainty can be prolonged and is often not helped by the ways in which behaviours are kept hidden, particularly in the early stages. Furthermore, even when professional support is sought the reaction is often not particularly helpful thereby further prolonging an already difficult period.

As the focus of this book is on how partnerships can be created both within dyadic (carer/cared-for person) and triadic (carer/cared-for person/professional) relationships, the ways in which these early experiences unfold is very important. Within the context of the situations described above we have adopted the term 'working' to capture the largely proactive, but frequently covert, strategies adopted by both PWD and their family carers. While 'working through it' is an explicit stage in our temporal model it is apparent that several types of 'work' also occur during the 'recognizing the need' stage. We would suggest that, depending on the extent to which carers and PWD experience a shared early trajectory, then four main types of 'working' can emerge. These are:

- 'Working together' – describes the 'best' case scenario when there is shared and early recognition of the symptoms and help is sought jointly. Fears and concerns are recognized by the GP, and appropriate specialist advice is taken.
- 'Working alone' – occurs even when there is a shared and early recognition of the difficulties that the PWD has, as he/she is likely to have kept his/her initial concerns secret for some time and will have been 'working alone' to hide them. Furthermore, both carers and PWD are often left to feel that they 'work alone' when their efforts to seek professional help do not get the appropriate response.
- 'Working separately' – describes the instances where the PWD is working alone to 'keep things hidden', and the carer is also actively 'increasing vigilance' so that a situation occurs where both parties are investing considerable effort but are 'working separately', each trying to

make sense of and respond to their circumstances. When the PWD is very adept at 'keeping it hidden' and carers accept this behaviour as normal, then this period of 'working separately' can be prolonged.

- 'Working apart' – usually occurs when prior relationships between the carer and the PWD have not been good, or when difficulties in the 'working separately' period lead to strained interactions. Consequently the carer and the PWD can 'work apart' so that their relationship deteriorates and the carer feels increasingly trapped in his/her role:

> We've been married over 60 years. I took her on for life and we made vows to each other. That meant everything to me and no one is going to take her away from me. I would have to be dead first. I'll put up with all this because I love her and she's my wife. I take everything day by day and I thank God for every day we are alive. As long as I get someone to help me with a bath for her, I don't need anything else. Ever.

This obviously represents a particularly fraught set of circumstances and provides testimony to the importance of prior relationships, 'building on the past', in framing the early caregiving context. Clearly the goal should be to try and ensure that all parties 'work together' as soon as possible, and we would suggest that certain conditions are likely to determine this. These are:

- a good prior relationship;
- a willingness by the person with (undiagnosed) dementia openly to disclose their fears, concerns and coping behaviours with a trusted person;
- a willingness by the trusted person (carer) to hear these concerns, validate and act upon them;
- a mutual decision to do something about it, where both parties recognize and agree that 'this is (might be) serious';
- a reasonably quick decision to seek a medical opinion;
- primary health care teams taking the reported signs and symptoms seriously, and having the necessary knowledge and skills to facilitate an early diagnosis of dementia. Alternatively, the primary health care team response may be to refer the person/couple to more specialized support services, such as a memory clinic, for a more detailed assessment;
- an early diagnosis being made and the person with dementia and the carer being informed of the diagnosis and prognosis;
- An understanding by the person and carer of the implications of the diagnosis;
- an explicit willingness by the person/carer/family to work through the processes involved in living with the experience of dementia in a supportive manner;
- specialist services being available on a continual basis to help support 'the partnership' – and the family – through this transition;

- ability of the carer to 'maintain involvement' even when the person with dementia reaches the time when he/she can no longer play an active role but the carer is still able to gain satisfaction and meaning from the act of caring itself (mutuality).

## Discussion

The purpose of this chapter has been to explore the early stage of caring ('recognizing the need' in particular) from the perspectives of both family carers and the PWD. Using a grounded theory method, 'working' has been identified as one of the key processes, with the PWD and the carer often being proactive in terms of both trying to hide and to make sense of their early experiences. As a result much emotional and cognitive energy is invested, particularly by the PWD in 'keeping things hidden'. Consequently, they are often working alone in the first instance. Later, as carers begin to suspect that all may not be well, they too engage in an initially rather passive, but eventually more active process of noticing and becoming increasingly vigilant. At this point both parties are working hard, but 'working separately'.

The point at which PWD and their carers begin to work together, or even if they do successfully work together, depends in no small measure on the way in which they 'open' up the discussion and both acknowledge the difficulties they are facing. As we have indicated, in the best cases people begin to work together at an early stage, but all too often working separately is prolonged, and in the worst situations this can lead to a process whereby the caring dyad 'work apart'.

Much of the above would seem to turn on the extent to which there is open discussion and a willingness to share concerns and fears. In many instances our data and results resonate with those of Hutchinson *et al.* (1997) who carried out a similar study involving both carers and PWD, but who used Glaser and Strauss's (1968) concept of 'awareness contexts' as a heuristic to explore and interpret their data.

'Awareness contexts' were initially developed as a model to help understand awareness of death in hospitals, with Glaser and Strauss (1968) identifying four differing awareness contexts:

- open;
- mutual pretence;
- suspected;
- closed.

In an open awareness context all parties are aware of the situation and discuss it openly. In a mutual pretence context all parties are similarly aware but 'pretend' that things are different. A suspected awareness context refers to circumstances where parties only suspect that something is wrong. A closed awareness context does not relate simply to whether all parties have knowledge of the situation, but also requires that they are all willing to discuss the matter openly. Hutchinson *et al.* (1997) argues that the idea of awareness contexts relates equally, but in differing ways, to Alzheimer's disease, and our data would support such a conclusion.

As we have described above, during the early stages the most common and most lengthy form of awareness context was a 'suspected' one. This reflects the diffuse and difficult nature of early symptoms. Similar to our own conclusions, Hutchinson *et al.* (1997) argue that if a suspected context is prolonged then it can result in a competitive situation whereby the PWD is working hard to 'keep it hidden' and the carer becomes 'hyper vigilant' (Hutchinson *et al.* 1997) in trying to find out what is wrong. As Hutchinson *et al.* (1997) contend, this is not conducive to 'interpersonal closeness' which, as we have noted, can result in carers 'working apart'.

We were also able to discern 'mutual pretence' contexts when, for example, spouses will pretend that everything is normal for their children. However, more often than not closed contexts exist either because the diagnosis is kept from the PWD or one or other party (PWD/carer/professional) 'discounts' the knowledge/concerns of the other, thereby maintaining a closed dialogue.

Clearly then the extent to which carers, PWD and professionals can 'work together' in the best relationships mandates an open awareness context and establishing this should be one of the priorities in the 'recognizing the need' stage, if during 'working through it' the PWD is to maintain involvement as an active agent for as long as possible.

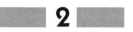

# 2

# Early interventions in dementia: carer-led evaluations

## Chris Clark, Denise Chaston and Gordon Grant

### Introduction

This chapter sets out to highlight and discuss some of the difficulties people with suspected cognitive impairment and their carers have in accessing timely and appropriate support and to consider the nature of the difficulties. Early assessment and diagnosis are complex issues that remain the subject of debate. However, to be successful early intervention depends on the ability to detect early cognitive changes, a willingness and awareness of the individual to seek medical intervention and a general practitioner who is willing to consider that early signs of memory impairment may indicate the need for further investigation and treatment. In response to concerns about timely and appropriate access to specialist support for people with suspected dementia, two studies aimed at raising awareness of the early signs of cognitive impairment and promoting early referral to specialist services were developed in Doncaster, South Yorkshire, UK. In this chapter we review why early intervention was considered important, how the two early interventions in dementia were operationalized, and what lessons have been learned to date from associated monitoring and research.

### What do we mean by early interventions and early stage support?

Early recognition of symptoms affords options for treatments to arrest the illness, alleviate symptoms, reduce morbidity and ultimately improve quality of life (DoH 2001a). The philosophy of health promotion is well researched and documented with an emphasis on empowering people to take care of themselves and enabling them to do so by giving them information, advice and support on which to make informed choices about their health and their future. Pender (1996) suggests the importance of primary preventative health promotion in mental health, especially counselling individuals and families to help them to recognize, avoid or deal constructively with problems or situations that may pose a threat to mental health. In the case of a person with dementia this may well include the mental health of family carers. Secondary preventative efforts may include assisting family members to deal with the stress of mental illness and tertiary measures may include continued health supervision and actions to maintain stability in cognitive and social functioning. These descriptions were further reinforced recently in *Making It Happen: A Guide to Delivering Mental Health Promotion* (DoH 2001a), which went on to highlight the importance of early intervention and reinforce the link between stress and the physical health of carers.

By comparison with early intervention work in other fields such as cancer care (Emmanuel and Cass 1993; *Cancer Bulletin* 2002), early interventions in the care of the person with dementia are relatively new. Until recently the most significant issue facing family physicians when presented with a person with possible dementia was the exclusion of potentially treatable aetiologies (Santacruz and Swagerty 2001). Although the introduction of treatments for dementia has seen an encouraging trend towards 'earlier' referral of people with suspected dementia for assessment, current practice often results in support being offered at a relatively late stage of the person's illness, and too late to consider some preventative or education-orientated interventions. However, the recognition of early signs of dementia is difficult. Early signs are often so insidious that they may go unnoticed for some considerable time with the result that often the early signs of the disease are well established before help is sought. Even at this stage, given the nature of the illness, the person with dementia may be unaware of the problem or reluctant to admit to difficulties, both of which may result in further delays or failure to access early advice and support.

A study by Ruston and colleagues (1998) commented on people receiving help for cardiac problems and suggested that delays were often attributed to patients being uncertain about the meanings of their symptoms, and to the GP. General practitioners have long been criticized for their part in delayed access to specialist services. Carers of people with dementia frequently criticize GPs for delays in confirming diagnosis and providing support services (Alzheimer's Disease Society 1995).

The Audit Commission (2000) in their *Forget Me Not* report specifically mentioned that many GPs see no point in early diagnosis of what they view essentially as an untreatable condition. GPs' failure to recognize dementia and determine a diagnosis has been attributed to many factors including a reluctance to diagnose difficulties (although it has been argued that most GPs have good diagnostic skills (Iliffe 1994)), problems in differentiating dementia from other psychiatric disorders (O'Connor *et al.* 1988), as well as the clinician's own emotional response to the diagnosis of dementia (De Lepeleire *et al.* 1994). The Alzheimer's Society report *Right from the Start* (1995) looked at the experience of GPs and carers of people with dementia and suggested that there was increasing evidence in medical journals highlighting that it is more likely to be GP attitudes and practices rather than medical knowledge that caused most concern. The report commented that GPs felt they had little to offer people with dementia, that early referral was unhelpful and that the difficulties experienced by people with dementia and their carers were mainly social.

In regard to early interventions for dementia GPs appear to hold a very important key and unfortunately come in for a great degree of criticism. They are criticized for slow and inaccurate diagnosis (O'Connor 1988), delays in access to specialist services (Glosser *et al.* 1985) and 'choosing' not to refer for help until carers and relatives insist that something is done (O'Connor 1988).

The National Service Framework (NSF) for Older People (DoH 2001b) appears to defend under-detection of mental illness in older people, including dementia, by suggesting that as physical and mental health problems frequently occur together in older people these make diagnosis more difficult. The report then goes on to say 'mental health problems may be perceived by older people and their families, as well as by professionals, as an inevitable consequence of ageing, and not as health problems that will respond to treatment' (p. 90).

Early signs of cognitive impairment in younger people with dementia can present major difficulties in diagnosis with the initial signs of poor memory linked often to poor work performance (DoH 2001b). Sperlinger and Furst (1994) found that 73 per cent of people in their study had to retire early as dementia affected their ability to continue in employment. GPs frequently fail to consider early onset progressive memory problems, preferring to attribute the symptoms to depression (Fossey and Baker 1995; O'Donovan 1999) or work-related stress with the result that diagnosis can frequently take several months to be established (Chaston and Shpylka 1999; O'Donovan 1999).

When considering early symptoms of cognitive decline in older adults, too frequently mild memory lapses are attributed to normal ageing and the potential benefits of early screening and diagnosis are lost (Drickamer and Lachs 1992; Iliffe 1994). As experienced Community Mental Health Nurses (CMHNs) (Christine Clark and Denise Chaston) we recognize the numbers of people referred who have demonstrated progressive signs of memory impairment often for two years prior to being seen. Many of these people or their family carers have seen their GP about their memory problem but have not been referred on for specialist support. In contrast Wolfe *et al.* (1995) cited research suggesting that even when a diagnosis was known it was rarely recorded in the practice records. Both of these actions clearly deny people access to appropriate support.

The potential benefits of early intervention are not dependent on a formal diagnosis of dementia. However, those people who do recognize the very subtle early signs of progressive cognitive impairment have the opportunity to seek out a formal diagnosis and with it the option for treatment and long-term support. Dementia is at present incurable but treatable. Treatments need to be considered and offered as soon as possible to gain maximum benefits. Treatment with acetyl cholinesterase inhibitors offers choices not previously available and for those for whom treatment is advised it offers the prospect of slowing down the inevitable progression of the disease (Clafferty 1999; Cameron *et al.* 2000; Cummings *et al.* 2000).

Early intervention and early stage support also provide potential opportunities to provide individuals and their families with a greater understanding of the disease, to consider the likely prognosis but most importantly review options for future planning and decision making (Clafferty 1999).

Family carers too have a responsibility with early intervention as they frequently have a tendency to protect and compensate for their loved one and as a result only seek help when faced with the unexpected consequences of the disease. Research confirms that in most cases it is family members who bring the client to the GP consultation in light of their suspicions about the possibility of dementia (Drickamer and Lachs 1992; O'Connor *et al.* 1993).

Caring for a person with dementia often begins long before the person is recognized as requiring or being a recipient of care. At this stage the symptoms suggesting the onset of dementia are insidious and difficult to identify, and carers can be left bewildered and doubtful that the changes they think are happening are actually real (Wilson 1989a and b; Wuest *et al.* 1994). This may lead to subtle changes, which may be picked up by the GP, being frequently dismissed and denied (De Lepeliere 1994). When carers do seek to confirm the changes and the reality of the confirmation and likely prognosis dawns, they often find themselves bombarded with a whole range of feelings and emotions and many unanswered questions as they seek to gain understanding and attribute meanings to behaviours (Keady and Nolan 1995; Keady *et al.* 1995).

Many of the early interventions begin before the patient receives a formal diagnosis. Referrals for people with suspected cognitive impairment are quite frequently seen by the CMHN. At this point there is a more formal acknowledgement of the difficulties and in a sense the journey then begins. The initial contact with the CMHN may be the first time that family carers have been able to express their concerns fully and disclose their fears to another person. This experience, dependent very much on the interpersonal skills of the CMHN, will prompt a relationship, based on mutual respect, trust and caring (Benner 1984), that will encourage an honest exchange of information to take place. The initial contact with the CMHN may also be an essential point in the process of acceptance and mark the beginning of a lay–professional partnership.

Timely and accurate information, communicated in an acceptable way, can have a beneficial effect on how carers and the person with dementia understand and work with the disease over the remainder of the life course. Advice, signposting and working through problems and finding solutions, empower and enable successful caring. CMHNs for Older People frequently are the providers of such support. Two studies attempted to identify the interventions used by the CMHN when working with people with dementia and their family carers, highlighting the diversity of needs among family carers and the range of skills employed by professional 'carers' to help and support them (Gunstone 1999; Ho 2000). For example, both studies focus on the nature of the intervention providing emotional support and advice, liaison and networking, but Ho in particular attempts to identify the personal qualities and skills of the CMHN as identified by family carers, highlighting listening skills, confidence, maturity, caring and sensitivity.

Information and support about the nature of the disease and its course are essential (Murphy *et al.* 1995; DoH 2001b) and should be offered to both the person with dementia and their family carers, while advice and help may be necessary with problem solving and in accessing other sources of help. Younger people with dementia and their carers may need additional information and advice, for example about working with dementia, mortgages, specific relationship difficulties or young siblings as carers (Alzheimer's Disease Society 1996; O'Donovan 1999). Support, especially from professionals, also appears to work best when it carries an affective content and encourages an understanding of dementia and the development of effective coping strategies (McHaffie 1992; Gunstone 1999; Ho 2000).

Support may also include arrangements for practical help with caring and help with financial management. All information, advice and support should be offered based on the belief that carers, if informed about what to expect as time goes by, and given the tools to face the challenges that will inevitably arise, will be more able to achieve a satisfactory outcome for their relative and for themselves (Nolan *et al.* 1996a). Ultimately the aim is to encourage a realistic awareness of a deteriorating illness. Satisfactory is not to imply judgement of good or bad caring but merely that the way of caring is successful, acceptable and rewarding to both the person delivering the care and to the person receiving it. Successful caring tends to happen when a carer adapts positively to the changing demands of the person they care for (Willoughby and Keating 1991). Conversely, without information carers are more likely to suffer from stress and consequently be less able to continue to care (DoH 2001b: 28). In general, advice, information and support have the potential to 'buffer' the negative effects of stressful events by influencing interpretation of events and the emotional responses to them, thereby decreasing illness-producing potential (Pender 1996).

Written and verbal information seems to be highly valued by all carers as well as people with early symptoms of dementia, as has been found in other studies of family carers (for example, Nolan *et al.* 1990; Keady and Nolan 1995; Murphy *et al.* 1995). Most carers asked about dementia, its effects, the prognosis and who can help. Many have a thirst for knowledge. Others, on the other hand, only wanted information about the 'here and now' and did not want to look too far ahead. This underlines the importance of understanding people's own conceptions of time horizons in family care. That is, people usually want to know what the future holds for them in order that they can plan, anticipate, stop worrying unnecessarily, deal with things with greater certitude, knowing that their efforts are recognized and supported by others. For some this is short-term while for others the time horizon is much longer. Professionals need to recognize this and not assume that temporality is fixed. This finding is consistent with other research on ways of working with older people with mental health problems or those with dementia and their carers, which stresses the importance of temporality or caregiving stages that are commonly experienced (see Kobayashi *et al.* 1993; Ferguson and Keady 2001).

Information needs to be delivered to carers in a meaningful way, in an appropriate language, that is understandable and personal. In both of the studies to be discussed next, the CMHNs delivered information personally, using their experience and expertise, and/or acted as an information gateway to other sources. Information may need to be broken down into 'manageable chunks' and repeated or reinforced using different mediums. For example Mr D requested written information about aspects of Alzheimer's disease, which was then used to facilitate individualized questions and discussion with the CMHN. The information was retained for reference at a later time. Whereas Mrs F.'s understanding of Alzheimer's disease was enhanced by one-to-one, topic-specific discussions with the CMHN who used visual diagrams and pictures. The nurses' unique professional relationship with the family allows them to gauge how much, when, and by what method information should be shared. Having information enables carers to make appropriate decisions. When a solution cannot be found, carers may then use strategies to reframe meanings or perceptions.

So far the chapter has considered some of the difficulties and barriers to early interventions in dementia and discussed the positive view of providing early stage support. Recognition of, and response to, such difficulties and a wish to promote a more proactive response led to the development of two studies undertaken by CMHNs for Older People in Doncaster, South Yorkshire, UK.

## The Early Intervention in Dementia (EID) and Younger Person with Dementia (YPD) studies

We now outline the two projects, developed and implemented in Doncaster, in order to understand how they influenced a change in referral practice and afforded a unique opportunity to work with people with dementia and their carers at the beginning of their journey at a time when they were coming to terms with a diagnosis of dementia.

The Early Intervention in Dementia (EID) study developed from reflection and awareness that CMHNs for Older People were frequently accepting referrals for people with dementia at times of crisis or extremes of carer stress. It was felt that many of the difficulties could have been avoided or significantly reduced had interventions begun earlier. The study aimed to encourage GPs to be more proactive in their management of people with symptoms of progressive poor memory by referring earlier for specialist assessment and nursing support. For the purpose of the study 'early' was interpreted to mean from the initial presentation to the GP requesting help and advice for cognitive difficulties.

People with suspected cognitive impairment who were referred to the study received a full initial assessment (carried out by the CMHN and GP) that led to the exclusion of any concurrent or treatable causes for memory problems and ultimately a diagnosis of probable dementia (people with atypical presentations were referred immediately for assessment by a consultant psychiatrist). At this point they and their carers were offered ongoing interventions by the CMHN. Interventions included both the person with dementia and their carers although most were carer-led and addressed issues of diagnosis, legal and financial planning and learning to live with dementia.

The study was planned on the understanding that preparing families as early as possible to respond to the changing needs and requirements of their relative or friend would lead to more effective coping strategies by them. Three main types of support were offered:

- emotional support and advice;
- liaison and networking;
- training and information.

Carer stress in these circumstances is quite common (for example Zarit *et al.* 1980; Gilleard *et al.* 1984; Nolan *et al.* 1990; Pearlin *et al.* 1990). At intervals throughout the EID study, the overall level and nature of carer stress was formally assessed and carers were asked to complete the General Health Questionnaire 28 item (GHQ28) (Goldberg and Hillier 1979). In addition to assessing psychological distress among carers, and the effects of efforts to provide families with support, it was also considered important to identify the strategies used by carers to help them to cope and highlight how useful these had been. The Carer's Assessment of

Managing Index (CAMI) (Nolan *et al.* 1995) was used effectively for this purpose.

The EID study was undertaken by a Community Mental Health Nurse (CMHN) for Older People who, in addition to working with people with early signs of dementia and their carers, worked closely with GPs and members of the primary healthcare team in supporting them to recognize the signs and symptoms of early dementia, encouraging more proactive referral and raising awareness of the services available. Pre-study information was sent to all GP practices along with an invitation to discuss the study in more detail. Not all GPs accepted the offer and overall the number of referrals to the study was lower than expected. As a result GPs were asked about their appreciation of the scope of early intervention work with people with dementia and in doing so gave a valuable insight into their awareness of and attitude to dementia. A questionnaire and semi-structured interview were designed for this purpose, though the results are not discussed in detail here.

The Younger Person with Dementia (YPD) study began in response to a number of professionals identifying common themes running through their work with younger people. These suggested that the needs of younger people with dementia (aged less than 65 years) were different to those identified for older people and that this made them a distinct client group. Tindall and Manthorpe (1997) have made similar observations and examined the case for specialist service provision and the social impacts of early onset dementia.

With the YPD study, an audit was carried out to identify the prevalence of dementia among younger people in the study area (Doncaster). The main themes to emerge were:

- lack of awareness of dementia in younger people, information and education;
- no central point for referrals and no defined pathway of care;
- lack of cohesive working between agencies;
- isolation and exclusion faced by both younger people with dementia and their families.

The audit and subsequent study were carried out once again by a CMHN, this time with a special interest in younger people with dementia and a specific remit to develop services for younger people and their families. A multi-agency steering group was convened, which included members from the professional and voluntary sectors, and later carer and user involvement. The aim of this group was to support and encourage development of the study. Building on the outcome of the audit, this study explored family carers' perceptions of existing service provision. Semi-structured interviews were used to explore carers' experiences and although people with dementia themselves were not formally interviewed, in some cases they were present and they were encouraged to contribute their views and experiences. Stories told by carers of younger people with dementia highlight the struggle and frustrations to access appropriate diagnosis and then appropriate support. This is one story as written by a carer, reproduced with his permission. Names have been changed to protect anonymity.

## Joan and Richard's story

My wife was diagnosed in 1991 at the age of 54 with Alzheimer's disease. These are some of the obstacles I have encountered since her diagnosis, a few of many, as there are too many to mention in this small space.

After the initial diagnosis my family received no help or advice, be it medical or financial. We were left alone to deal with this to our best ability. During the early years, looking after my wife was like looking after a naughty child; you needed eyes in the back of your head and a good pair of running shoes to catch her as she tried to make her escape. At times this meant her heading across town to where she was born, not able to communicate with anyone, as at this point she was not able to tell you her name or where she lived.

It was at least three years after diagnosis that I received help from any care professional. My first contact was with the CMHN who organized day and respite care at the local hospital. As her condition deteriorated day care staff were unable to cope with her behaviour and this resulted in them refusing her permission to attend. This was only resolved when a promise to find alternative care was brokered by the CMHN. This was duly found. The problem arose because they did not have a facility that could deal with a younger person with dementia.

During this period my wife received Disabled Living Allowance and I receive Carer's Allowance. The government rules for entitlement to the care allowance benefit are that you have to care for a person for 35 hours a week. This meant we had to calculate exact timings for her admission/discharge for respite to stop my benefit being withheld or reassessed. At this point my wife was in respite care for two weeks and at home for eight weeks.

As the years since the initial diagnosis have passed my wife's condition has worsened and more support and care are needed. Again this has been a battle with the local authority although it must be said that Doncaster do provide more than other authorities. You just have to fight for it.

After nine years of struggle I have finally got the care package and support my wife deserves. The only obstacles I now face are the ones of filling out forms to keep up to date with the allowances. My care allowance has stopped on my 65th birthday. As I am in receipt of my state pension I am no longer entitled to both though my wife still needs looking after.

Because Alzheimer's is not a 'fashionable disease' like AIDS or cancer you face a lack of understanding and in some instances pure ignorance of what this condition is. If I had a £1 coin for every time I have had to explain to a faceless bureaucrat that my wife cannot fill out the mountains of paperwork needed to claim her allowance I would be a wealthy man. Things need to change or care in the community will continue to be a fallacy.

This story does not explain all the difficulties that Richard and his wife encountered in obtaining a diagnosis. It also highlights frustrations often experienced by carers. Right at the beginning of their journey there is a sense of abandonment: 'We were left alone to deal with this.' There was recognition that early medical and financial advice was not offered, suggesting retrospectively that it would have been beneficial. What is equally clear are the effects on individuals of uncoordinated health, social care and social security provision.

In an attempt to highlight such difficulties and assess how best to bring care services together, two conferences were subsequently organized to raise awareness and understanding of the specific needs of younger people with dementia and their families. The second of these saw a turning point for the development team with the involvement of a key representative from Social Services who made a commitment to look at the current service provision, for example home care services and residential care, and consider how they may need to change and adapt to meet the needs of younger people. This multi-agency involvement has been crucial.

Both studies worked and developed closely together and in both cases several common themes emerged. At the point of seeking professional help carers often found reluctance among GPs to recognize and accept that problems existed. Once a memory problem had been identified there was a lengthy delay in referral to appropriate specialist services and support networks. In part this was due to being unclear about what services were available for people with dementia as well as the nature of the access route to those services.

## What are the difficulties in accessing early stage support?

Too often valuable opportunities are lost by a failure to seek advice at an early stage of the dementia. There appear to be a number of reasons for this. As alluded to earlier, the early signs of dementia are often very subtle and insidious with minor lapses in memory attributed to 'normal' ageing. From the authors' experience it is not uncommon to find people, who have been with a partner for many years, unknowingly compensating for the deficits of their partner. It is only when that person acts wholly out of character that they begin to question, reflect on, and acknowledge the changes that have taken place. Fear of the unknown is a great disincentive when considering seeking help and often comes after long periods of uncertainty and speculation. Wilson (1989a, b) suggests that carers work through many experiences before searching for explanations. The first stage she describes is *noticing*, which leads to *discounting and normalizing*, where relatives eventually reflect on isolated incidents and 'having noticed the changes . . . tend to initially discount and normalize them' (p. 42). An example of this would be making excuses for a lapse in memory or accepting personal responsibility for the result. 'No wonder he forgot, I probably should have reminded him.' Wilson goes on to describe *suspecting*. Suspecting that something more serious was wrong and being unable to offer explanations for change can lead carers to search for explanations as the following case example illustrates from the EID study.

## Mary and John's story

The first signs that John was beginning to have problems with his memory were so subtle that Mary was not sure herself if she was imagining the changes. She recalls their story. John had been quite fastidious about paying bills to the extent that they were almost always paid the day they were received. When a red letter arrived about an unpaid bill it was the first of several minor 'hiccups' that she was to become more aware of over the next few weeks. John was always the last to bed and would follow a 'night time' security check. However, he went to bed leaving the TV on, and regularly forgot to turn off the lights and lock the door. Mary began by asking John if he had remembered to lock the door and so on, which almost always resulted in John becoming defensive and angry. To prevent such confrontation, Mary then began checking when John went to the bathroom before bed and maintained this habit until well after it became clear that John was not able to perform this task at all. She recalls other lapses in memory, which appeared almost transient, an example being John forgetting the name of his grandchild, only to recall it quite spontaneously and 'normally' on a subsequent visit. These incidents on their own did not mean much but when Mary thought about them and recalled them all she felt certain something was happening to John.

Mary kept these fears to herself for some time and attempted to check them out with close friends. However, John always seemed to be his usual self around company and suggestions that his memory was failing were refuted by close friends. Mary was left more confused than ever and dealt with her fears initially by continuing to compensate for John's minor failings. She checked things after him, started to take more interest in the household finances and protected them both from the subtle effects of change.

This kind of compensatory behaviour is quite common in relationships where one partner has a growing dependence on the other. Bowers

(1987) adopted the term *supervisory caregiving* when talking about adult caregivers and their ageing parents but this term could equally apply to older carers as it describes a conscious process of active and direct involvement of the carer. This involves activities such as 'making sure', 'checking' and 'setting up', all of which may be done without the care recipient's knowledge.

When the progressive signs of the disease can no longer be dealt with by compensatory practice alone this usually prompts the carer actively to seek help and advice. Quite often though they are unsure where to go to seek help and again, in the authors' experience, family carers in particular do not always associate this kind of help with their GP. People with early signs of cognitive impairment are often aware of a progressively failing memory and this in turn adversely affects their self-esteem and self-confidence (Fearnley *et al.* 1997). They too are frequently unsure about whom to contact for advice and, in the authors' experience, they often have a fear of 'opening the floodgates' by exposing the problem.

## Outcomes and lessons

*The EID study*

The EID study asked carers of people with dementia to complete the GHQ 28 item (Goldberg and Hillier 1979) as a measure of the level of psychological distress among carers. Using GHQ scoring, where 0–5 is determined to be within 'normal' limits, over 75 per cent of the carers in the sample group had scores in excess of 10, suggesting their psychological health was poor. Following as few as six interventions by the CMHN and concentrating on provision of information, advice and support, all carers' GHQ scores had improved with only 40 per cent scoring above threshold at this point.

The nature of the distress similarly changed with carers following intervention reporting a lessening of somatic symptoms and anxiety although reports of social dysfunction remained high. Even at this early stage, carers commented that following diagnosis they felt less able to leave the person with dementia to pursue their own social needs. The diagnosis, for some, had the effect of changing the relationships as one partner adopted a parental role over the other:

> I can't go out alone now. I wouldn't know what I was coming home to. What if someone comes when I'm out, he wouldn't be able to deal with it.

Many carers needed help to consider how much help and supervision was actually needed to balance this against the realistic consequences of their actions. Anecdotal evidence from the EID study suggested that carers wanted to tell their story, to be understood and to have their needs and fears acknowledged. They frequently sought reassurance: 'Is the diagnosis correct?', 'Will I be able to care?', 'Why is this happening to us?' Confirmation that 'someone' was taking notice and trying to help provided a sense of relief for some:

> I knew something was happening but wasn't sure why he was behaving like this. I thought I was imagining the problems with his memory and mood. I thought I was to blame in some way.
>
> (Mrs W.)

Again, anecdotal evidence from the EID study suggests that providing information to carers greatly reduces levels of anxiety, as does confirmation of the problem. Confirmation of the problem and diagnosis (when confirmed) appeared to have the most beneficial effect initially:

> We've struggled on for 18 months not really being sure if he had a memory problem or not. Now we know what's wrong I'm sure we can deal with it. At least now we know where to start.
>
> (Mrs B.)

Using CAMI, the EID study found that most carers valued the benefit of having someone trusted to talk over problems with, having professional help and getting as much information as possible about the disease.

These preliminary results of measuring the outcomes suggest that early intervention work can have a beneficial effect on both the psychological well-being of carers and their ability to cope with caring for a person with the early symptoms of dementia.

In response to lower than expected numbers of referrals, the EID study consulted with local GPs (n = 92) and asked them, using a multiple-choice questionnaire, to identify the reasons why they would not refer a person over 65 with suspected cognitive impairment for early intervention work. 'Forgetfulness is seen as a part of normal ageing' was the most frequent response for 43 per cent of those questioned. Forty per cent suggested that it was because patients and carers refuse interventions and 36 per cent felt early signs of dementia were difficult to recognize. These figures point to the difficulties of isolating early signs and symptoms of dementia from 'normal' ageing, as discussed earlier. Worryingly, they also suggest that people may not be getting referred because of the perceived likelihood of their refusing a service. Semi-structured interviews with a sample of GPs was equally revealing but will not be discussed in detail in this chapter. However, the comment that 'nothing can be done' was repeated often and the feeling among GPs that they had little to offer people with dementia is not new. Wolfe *et al.* (1995) recall similar expressions from GPs surveyed about their attitudes to referral for people with suspected dementia.

The CMHN has since been working closely with GPs and members of the Primary Health Care Team to promote early referral for people with suspected cognitive impairment by increasing awareness and understanding of the early symptoms of dementia and developing clearer pathways of care. As a result GPs are generally more proactive in their management of suspected dementia, more likely to ask for advice, with a noticeable increase in referrals for people with early symptoms and subsequently increased access for treatment.

*The YPD study*

The YPD study similarly found that younger people with dementia were less likely to be referred for assessment of cognitive impairment because of lack of knowledge among GPs and a failure to attribute the presenting symptoms to early onset dementia. The YPD audit carried out in Doncaster consulted GPs about their understanding of early onset dementia. Only one GP responded that he was aware of early onset dementia and that he felt sufficiently confident to refer on to appropriate services. Other responses suggested that GPs did not always consider progressive memory problems in younger people, had difficulty recognizing signs and symptoms and when these were suspected were unsure where and to whom to refer for diagnosis and advice.

The difficulties do not stop here. Younger people with dementia and their carers face increased difficulties as dementia is still largely viewed as a problem of older adults. If cognitive difficulties are acknowledged they are frequently attributed to depression or work-related stress. The experience of the YPD project suggests that patients may find themselves being treated by their GP or, in some cases, psychiatrists for working-age adults, for up to 18 months before consideration that the cognitive impairment may be linked to early onset dementia. The consequences of delays in providing support to their carers are self-evident.

The YPD project, as part of awareness raising, produced a simple but effective leaflet highlighting the possibilities on early onset dementias and suggested how and where help and advice could be accessed. The leaflet was left at GP surgeries to be taken by the public and was subsequently picked up by a young couple who had been visiting their GP for some time about the husband's poor memory, increasing lack of concentration and loss of confidence. They presented the leaflet to the GP with the result that he was referred for appropriate assessment and received a diagnosis of early onset dementia.

Prior to the study referrals for younger people were directed to numerous services including neurology and psychiatry. Post study, referrals are being directed more appropriately to the YPD service and anecdotal evidence suggests a reduction in the time taken to confirm a diagnosis.

The YPD study was unique in that following on from gathering information about experiences, it asked younger people with dementia and their carers to consider and identify what services or alternative services they would prefer. Twenty carers and younger people were consulted. The following are their 16 preferences, listed in priority order.

- a named key worker with 'expert' knowledge;
- a defined pathway of care;
- an information leaflet;
- carers' social group;
- flexible day/evening activities;
- flexible respite services;
- a home-based personal/terminal care service;
- night sitting service/overnight facilities;
- special home support team for challenging behaviour;
- befriending service;
- work-based schemes;
- one-stop shop for diagnosis and support;
- specialist benefit advice;
- specialist legal advice;
- specialized unit/adapted house or bungalow for challenging behaviour;
- intensive physiotherapy/speech therapy.

There was a clearly identified need for a shift from hospital-based services towards community provision and for a clear referral pathway. The overwhelming expression by carers of feelings of isolation and the need to talk to others in similar situations led to the development of a 'Coffee Shop' which provided an informal setting in which family carers could meet on a regular basis and, with the help of a facilitator, provide each other with support and friendship. This has been extremely successful and the PROP (People Relying On People) group has since formally established its unique identity and formed its own committee. The development of a resource centre for younger people and their carers is an ongoing project and the centre hopes to establish a clear identity and will, among other things, be able to provide flexible respite in line with carers' requests.

The project funding for the second study came in part from the Alzheimer's Society and is currently being evaluated by the Society and Dementia North.

## Conclusion

In both of the studies several common themes emerged. At the point of seeking professional help carers often found reluctance among GPs to recognize and accept that problems existed. Once a memory problem had been identified there was a lengthy delay in referral to appropriate specialist services and support networks. In part this was due to lack of clarity about what services were available for people with dementia and the access route to those services.

Results from both studies also suggest that very few GPs initially considered referral for early stage support, preferring to wait until the symptoms of dementia were more established or a time when advice was needed to deal with the consequences of the disease, which could not be managed effectively in primary care. Diagnosis and risk assessment by GPs is obviously challenging. Interestingly, McIntosh *et al.* (1999) concluded that many GPs also find dementia management 'a difficult, stress-provoking experience' (p. 42), suggesting by implication that it might be an experience some would prefer to avoid, though with disastrous consequences for patients and family carers.

Evidence gathered for inclusion in the earlier part of this chapter highlighted the difficulties people with dementia and their carers experience in accessing support and the difficulties of the GP experience. Anecdotal evidence from both the EID and YPD studies clearly supports the need for training to improve GPs' response to dementia and to promote more positive management of dementia in primary care. Dementia presents a challenge to primary care both in terms of early detection and improving primary dementia care services (Eccles *et al.* 1998; Downs 2002; Iliffe *et al.* 2002).

O'Connor *et al.* (1993) reinforce the need for improved screening tools, emphasizing the importance of their proper and controlled use, and insisting that they are used to complement a thorough assessment of informant history. Promoting early intervention and screening for dementia in primary care has reinforced the need to refine quick screening tools and has led to the development of the 6-CIT (Cognitive Impairment Test) (Brooke and Bullock 1999) and the GPCOG (General Practitioner Assessment of Cognition) (Brodaty *et al.* 2002), both of which are well validated.

The recent Access to Health Care report (Gulliford *et al.* 2001) suggests that there is 'evidence of a significant mismatch between professional expectations, patients' needs and patterns of uptake of services' (p. 7) and this was certainly the case with the services for younger people with dementia. Their choice of services to meet their needs was very different to the services currently being provided.

The *National Service Framework for Older People* (DoH) 2001b sets out guidelines for developing a comprehensive mental health service for older people and reinforces the need for early diagnosis and access to drug treatments. People with dementia and their family carers need to be a part of this development to ensure that the services are what are actually wanted. GP training is again highlighted but raises the question of who will provide the training and how much of it will involve people with dementia and their carers as facilitators. As O'Connor and colleagues state, 'dementia cannot be managed, however, if doctors fail to detect it' (O'Connor *et al.* 1993).

The literature, carers' narratives, case studies and our own clinical experience in seeking to fashion and evaluate early interventions suggest that best practice will only emerge when practitioners across all health and social care services strike partnerships with people with dementia and their families. This means involving them as partners and experts in planning, providing and reviewing early intervention work. More robust and larger scale evaluations are called for to validate and consolidate elements of good practice identified in this chapter.

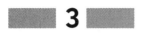

# 3

# Seeking partnerships between family and professional carers: stroke as a case in point

## Louise Brereton and Mike Nolan

### Introduction

Over a decade ago Nolan and Grant (1992b) suggested that one of the most significant, but often ignored, challenges for practitioners working in acute health care environments was to help prepare 'new' family carers for their role, particularly those who become carers suddenly and unexpectedly. This situation is typified in the event of a stroke which, as has been suggested, represents a 'paradigm' case, highlighting the tensions that arise when lives are interrupted by entirely unanticipated health care crises (Brereton 1997). This chapter focuses on the experiences of family carers in the aftermath of a stroke and describes the significance of events that occur during and shortly after hospitalization. In line with the aims of this book, emphasis is placed on carers' needs and the extent to which these were addressed during their interactions with professional carers. The chapter draws on data collected as part of a longitudinal, grounded theory study, which charts the caregiving trajectory over a period of 18 months (see later under methods). The chapter begins with a brief consideration of the literature available at the time data collection commenced in 1997 so as to provide a context for the study.

### The current situation

Stroke is the third leading cause of death in the UK (Wolfe 1996) and a major cause of morbidity. While early mortality is relatively high, subsequently individuals may live for many years, and over a third of those who survive are not functionally independent after a year (Wolfe 1996). Despite this there have been relatively few longer term studies which have charted the experience of living and caring after a stroke. The psychological consequences of stroke are significant, with a number of authors highlighting the 'long-term misery' that stroke can cause (Young and Gladman 1995; Parker *et al.* 1997). As stroke is 'unanticipated and devastating' (Farzan 1991) and as there is so little time to prepare, coming to terms with the effects poses particular difficulties (Lewinter and Mikkelsen 1995a). For example, Tyson (1995) suggests that while the prospects of physical recovery might be moderately optimistic, psychological recovery is often more limited and the social outlook is 'bleak'. Rehabilitation following stroke therefore presents a number of challenges, and is recognized as an important public health issue (Wolfe 1996).

Given the sudden and often devastating nature of stroke and the long-term physical, psychological and social consequences, there has been relatively little qualitative and longitudinal work describing the experiences of those most affected, that is stroke survivors and their families. Doolittle (1988) has argued that our knowledge of how stroke survivors adapt over time is sparse and although she and others (Doolittle 1991, 1992, 1994; Häggström *et al.* 1994; Lewinter and Mikkelsen 1995a) have attempted to redress the balance, these accounts are not as fully developed, nor as sophisticated, as our understanding of other chronic conditions such as multiple sclerosis or spinal injury (Nolan *et al.* 1997).

However, what emerges most clearly from the available studies is the importance of focusing on the values, goals, aspirations and meanings of stroke survivors and their families (Doolittle 1991, 1992, 1994; Lewinter and Mikkelsen 1995a; Pound *et al.* 1995). As Doolittle (1991) has noted, more emphasis needs to be placed on the impact of stroke on the person's life rather than simply focusing on the neurological damage. Moreover, the crucial role played by the family (Farzan 1991; Evans *et al.* 1992a, b, 1994; Brummel-Smith 1994) must be acknowledged, with stroke typically being depicted as a 'family illness'.

It is argued that family carers should not be viewed simply as resources (Evans *et al.* 1992a, b, 1994), and Wolfe (1996) contends that they are the most important members of the multidisciplinary team. Several authors suggest that interventions targeted at carers should address a range of issues such as education, skills training, emotional support and counselling (Anderson 1992; Evans *et al.* 1992a, b, 1994; Williams 1994; King *et al.* 1995), with skilled assessment of family dynamics being essential to help prepare carers for role changes and increased responsibilities (Jongbloed *et al.* 1993; Enterlante and Kern 1995). Consequently preparing carers for their role is actively promoted (Kernich and Robb 1988; Best 1994), particularly around the time of hospital discharge (Redfern 1990; Rosenthal *et al.* 1993, Moore 1994; Wellwood *et al.* 1995).

However, despite considerable rhetoric about helping family carers following stroke, there is rather less in the way of concerted support, and despite the fine sentiments noted above, practice lags some way behind these ideals. Studies suggest that carers are rarely actively involved in patient care in hospital, even when they wish to be (Anderson 1992; Rosenthal *et al.* 1993; Nydevik and Eller 1995). Moreover, carers' needs for both information (McLean *et al.* 1991; Anderson 1992; Wellwood *et al.* 1995; Bunn 1996a) and emotional support (Farzan 1991; Wellwood *et al.* 1995) are not addressed adequately and they often lack the preparation and skills to provide care (McLean *et al.* 1991; Bunn 1996b).

There is little improvement, for either stroke survivor or family carer, upon discharge from hospital. Despite the emphasis placed on careful discharge planning, arrangements are often haphazard and ad hoc, engendering feelings of abandonment (Doolittle 1992; Lewinter and Mikkelsen 1995b). Follow-up arrangements and long-term aftercare are similarly fragmented (Anderson 1992; Corr and Bayer 1992; Young and Gladman 1995; Wilkinson 1996). Even efforts to effect better liaison, such as home visits prior to discharge, are often poorly organized with too much duplication of effort (Clarke and Gladman 1995). Continuity is generally found wanting and the ideal of seamless care, often promulgated, seems utopian in comparison to the reality of existing arrangements. The desire to understand better the experiences of 'new' carers of stroke survivors was the motivation for the study upon which this chapter is based. Due to the dearth of previous research a qualitative approach using a grounded theory method was adopted.

## Method

In order to inform the main study data were initially collected from seven experienced carers of stroke survivors, all members of a stroke and carers' club, who had been caring for between two and four years. These seven spousal carers volunteered to be interviewed and the sample consisted of two male and five female carers between 65 and 84 years of age. Tape-recorded, semi-structured interviews took place in the carers' homes. Following each interview, tapes were fully transcribed and a detailed content analysis undertaken in order to identify key themes. A constant comparative approach was adopted in which data were systematically compared both within and between informants.

Following these initial interviews, prospective data were collected from 18 'new' family carers recruited from two hospitals in the north of England – one city hospital and one district general hospital serving a more rural area. New carers, over 18 years of age and who spoke English were eligible for inclusion in the study provided that the stroke survivor consented to their involvement. Informants were purposively sampled from three areas: general acute medical admission wards (eight carers); a specialist stroke unit (eight carers); and the community when stroke survivors did not enter hospital at all (TIA clinic) (two carers). The sample included eight males (six husbands and two sons) and ten females (four wives and six daughters) whose ages ranged from 32 to 93 years of age. Two carers were themselves nurses and another two carers had previously suffered a stroke themselves.

Apart from two people who suffered a Transient Ischaemic Attack (TIA), stroke survivors had all been hospitalized. Two died in hospital, ten returned home and four were admitted to a nursing home, although one subsequently returned home and another subsequently died.

Data were collected using prospective serial in-depth, semi-structured interviews with the same informants every two to three months over a period of up to 18 months. This chapter draws on data from 78 interviews. Informants were invited to describe their needs relating to becoming a carer in their own words and the interview was primarily under their control. An initial analysis of the interviews was undertaken immediately afterwards in order to inform theoretical sampling for subsequent interviews. Data were transcribed for analysis which evolved through a process of constant comparison (Corbin and Strauss 1988; Charmaz 2000). Having read the transcripts, the initial open codes were identified before being grouped into categories. Line-by-line analysis was then undertaken to identify the properties and dimensions of each category. To aid analysis and constant comparison, tables of relevant data were developed for each category. Data from subsequent interviews were analysed in the same way and relevant data added to the tables. Through an ongoing process, memos and diagrams were used to assist the development of axial codes, which link categories and sub-categories together. The results of the ongoing analysis were discussed with interviewees who provided further information to illuminate and challenge the emerging themes. This ensured that the themes reflected their needs as family carers, and that the emerging theory was precise and conceptually dense. Furthermore, this process enabled identification of carers' changing needs throughout the transition to caring to be reflected in the results.

## Results

From the initial set of interviews four main themes emerged which between them captured the complex factors that influence family carers' experience following a stroke (see Brereton and Nolan 2000). These were termed:

- What's it all about?
- Up to the job?
- Going it alone
- What about me?

'What's it all about?' captures the uncertainty and confusion that most carers felt following the stroke, and depicts their efforts to gain insights into what had happened by collecting information that would help them to make sense of their rapidly changing situation:

> You need to know what a stroke is and what it does to a person and . . .
> all the things you'll have to do . . . what to expect . . . and I think you
> need to know from Day 1.
>
> (Husband)

However, despite carers' best efforts to obtain information and help from
professional carers, they often received inadequate or inappropriate
advice, which left them feeling that they were 'going it alone'. Consequently, carers directed their attention to other sources of knowledge
such as books, family and friends, more than one describing their efforts as
a 'Do it Yourself' job:

> You get such a lot of bad communication I'd say there's a lot of a lack
> of communication because nobody tells you anything at all. It's a DIY
> job and I've said this all along and I'll still say it that it's Do It Yourself
> because if you don't fight nobody's bothered.
>
> (Wife)

The initial interviews suggested that as discharge approached, carers
wanted to gain the skills they might need in order to support their relative
at home, as they particularly wanted to feel that they were 'up to the job'
of caring and could provide the most appropriate care:

> . . . what worried me was . . . I was making him do all these things
> with his hands, was I doing right? I didn't know and that really
> frightened me and all I wanted to know was that what I was doing for
> him was right.
>
> (Wife)

Once again, however, there were few systematic efforts to assist carers to
obtain the skills they needed, and most learnt these by a process of 'trial
and error'.

The final theme to emerge from the initial interviews, 'What about me?',
comprised two elements. The first concerned the lack of attention to
the carers' own need for help and support, and the second described
the failure by professionals to recognize carers' intimate knowledge of the
stroke survivor. Carers considered this to be an essential element of a
comprehensive rehabilitative package:

> I think the nurses need to know what type of person they're dealing
> with, which no one asked me . . . He's a very quiet gentleman. If you
> know the type you're dealing with, you know how to deal with them.
>
> (Wife)

These initial interviews provided some important insights into the
experience of family carers following a stroke, that were further elaborated
upon in the subsequent longitudinal interviews. These generated extensive data which allowed for a much more sophisticated understanding of
the above four themes. This analysis identified 'seeking' as the key activity

undertaken by carers during the early post-stroke period (Brereton and Nolan 2002). Reinforcing the preliminary data the second set of interviews highlighted the sense of bewilderment that carers experienced and their search to understand 'what's it all about?'. In order to begin to make sense of the apparent chaos they were experiencing they actively sought partnerships and help/support from both their family and professional carers. However, these 'seeking' behaviours were often not recognized or responded to by staff, reinforcing carers' sense that they were 'going it alone'. Their response was to seek information from other sources such as books and the internet, and also to observe, listen and absorb any information they could collect while visiting their relatives in hospital:

> Some [nurses] are quite helpful and do come and tell me about my dad and how he has been, others don't talk to me at all . . . They know I have read the [medical] notes, but I don't think I would have been told anything if I hadn't. I find out most things by reading the notes about his condition. It would be nice if the nurse could find a couple of minutes just to speak to me . . . instead of me having to find the information out for myself.
>
> (Daughter)

> Nobody will tell you anything . . . I need to know now . . . you listen and you can hear everything that's going off . . . we read everything [if they leave her notes by the bed].
>
> (Husband)

This feeling of 'going it alone' was exacerbated by the relative lack of attention given to family carers' own needs ('What about me?') and the failure of staff to draw actively upon carers' knowledge and expertise. This was seen to compromise the primary goal of carers, which was to ensure that both professional carers and they were 'up to the job' of providing the best possible care for the stroke survivor.

Their desire to 'seek best care' was multifaceted and involved several types of 'seeking' behaviour, which varied in emphasis over time. In respect of the care provided by professionals, carers sought both: 'influence' by providing staff with information that they thought would improve the care that their relative received; and 'continuity' – in other words, carers wanted consistently high standards of care to be delivered, preferably by a limited number of staff who had got to 'know' their relative.

However, carers' attempts to seek to influence care often went unrecognized:

> My mum has never ever eaten potatoes, greens, eggs. She never sits down to a hot meal. Now she is on a diet that's got to be pureed and when we tell them that mum has never eaten that type of food they say, 'Well there is nothing else she can have, she's got to have it.' Now if my mother was a vegetarian or a diabetic, they'd have to find

something for her ... but for me, I'm putting food in my mother's mouth that I know she doesn't like ... a lot of dignity goes.

(Daughter)

When staff failed to act upon carers' knowledge they began to observe and monitor the care that was provided in order to try and ensure an element of continuity:

I just needed to know that people were going to look after him when I wasn't there. I was so afraid to leave him for a little while because [cries] the way he was presented when I went back onto the ward – mismatching pyjamas and nothing on that was his, lolling out of the chair.

(Daughter)

Particular anxiety was aroused when carers felt that some staff provided good care but others did not:

That was the most wonderful thing one day when he had the dental hygienist and she cleaned his mouth out and it was fantastic. She left instructions that his mouth was to be cleaned with distilled water and cotton swabs ... then the next time I went all the things she had left had gone and there were some foam sticks and some Corsodyl and they said, 'Well, we're using this now.' So it worried me that she had said definitely use this, showed me what to do and here was something different that they [nurses] had decided should be used. I didn't want to say anything to them because I didn't want to criticize them but these things kept falling on the floor and I thought they are using these in his mouth and they have been on the floor.

(Wife)

## Discharge – bringing things to a head

As carers became more familiar with the hospital environment, and as they perceived that discharge was approaching, some sought more active involvement in caregiving. This served two related but distinct purposes. One was to try and ensure that their relative received 'best care', and the second was to begin to learn the skills that they felt they needed to provide care at home (seeking skills). Once again, however, their efforts were often thwarted:

I wanted to be involved more [in my wife's care in hospital] but they kept saying 'No'. If they had shown me how to do it without hurting her, I would have done it. Like last night she wanted to go to the loo and there was nobody to move her. I would have done it. You're waiting because there's not enough staff to take her and I could do it . . . I need to start doing that now [because] it's me that's got to be ready when [wife] comes home.

(Husband)

As discharge approached carers naturally wanted to be prepared to give care at home. Thus 'seeking skills' became an important activity for informants but they usually had to take the initiative, describing how they had to overcome apparent resistance on the part of staff:

I think they [staff] thought I was intruding, I felt as though I was intruding as well because when we went down to physio . . . I felt a bit of tension there too with me wanting to go in there all the time.

(Husband)

I want to get just some idea of what I'm going to need at home . . . I asked them yesterday . . . today they [nurses] said, they'll [physio and occupational therapist] let you know when they are ready. But I want to be ready.

(Husband)

This desire to be 'ready' for discharge again led carers to ask, 'What about me?', as their efforts to be involved in care and to learn the skills they felt they needed often went unheeded, or were sometimes actively thwarted:

I feel cross . . . that I am being shut out of his treatment by them [physiotherapist and occupational therapist]. They had meetings at the hospital where they sat together and talked about all the patients. You would think that they would say this is where we have got to and this is where you have to go.

(Wife)

In addition to learning the practical skills of caring, family members were also acutely aware that discharging their relative home would inevitably mean adjustments to the home environment. Once again several informants indicated how their efforts to prepare for this in advance were either played down or ignored by staff:

I want to start [getting ready for his wife's discharge home]. I've asked them yesterday, I need to know what I'm going to need at home. I want to get it going now, just some idea, even if I don't end up with it, just some idea of what I'm going to need . . . because I still don't know about taking her home and things like that. How am I going to get her upstairs and things like that. So actually I need to talk to somebody about things like that. So I asked yesterday and they said, 'Yes we'll sort something out', and I've come today and they come straight up to me and they said, 'Oh no, you don't need to know anything like that', and I do.

(Husband)

As discharge loomed, carers became increasingly concerned that they had not prepared the home environment, nor could they obtain advice as to what might be needed. Even relatively simple information such as the practicalities of using a wheelchair caused carers concern:

> Now I'm thinking that he is going to come home I want to get cracking on things to make it all right for him when he does come home. Yet nobody will say – they wait until he's about ready, don't they, until they talk to you about it. By then it's too late. I need central heating putting in and a downstairs lavatory putting in, and, I mean, that's going to take time . . . I've got to do major stuff at home to make it right for him yet nobody will come down to it and say, 'This is what you need.' I don't even know until I ask one of the physios, but I'm having to ask, 'How wide is a wheelchair?'
>
> (Wife)

In addition to advice about home adaptations, carers also wanted an indication of the benefits and allowances they might be entitled to:

> I had started the ball rolling by asking, 'Well, what happens with Attendance Allowance, and what happens about the disabled badge?', and I was sort of told 'Whoa', basically that isn't important for the stage that we are at. But to me I needed to know that it could be addressed, but nobody has mentioned it at all.
>
> (Daughter)

For some the frustration eventually became too much and they initiated action themselves, either by contacting local service agencies or occasionally pressing ahead and arranging for their own home adaptations:

> It seems as though you have to challenge [staff about the level of services offered on discharge] to get anywhere near acceptable service – so . . . once I had got through to the right place I rang and he [Social Services' planning officer] didn't ring back but I wasn't thwarted. I rang again and I got through to the man and I said, 'Look, I am not being pushy but I have got to have time off work to meet you . . .'. You don't want to have to agitate and you play this game with yourself about how long shall I wait before I ask somebody else? How long should I wait before I ask again? Should I leave it a week or two weeks? But then we are two weeks further down and, you know, what is a reasonable amount of time to make a phone call and get a response? It is like a DIY discharge – you just feel, Oh blow it, I might as well get on and do it myself, or find out what I can do for myself. It is very frustrating . . . why isn't anybody helping me, sort of thing. I shouldn't have to spend my time trying to track this man down.
>
> (Daughter)

> He [social worker] forced us into making a decision and paying for it ourselves really [putting in a new bathroom], because we were told that it would be a two-year waiting list and we would have to fund it ourselves, and so you are forced into doing something because that is not acceptable for somebody to wait that long for a bath.
>
> (Daughter)

In some cases adaptations proved to be costly mistakes as they were impractical and of little benefit. In such instances families felt understandably let down by the system, which had not provided the advice and information they sought:

> It would be nice for him just to be able to have a shower too. We have just given up on the idea really, it doesn't bother us because it doesn't come into the equation any more. I just use the shower thing for filling the washbowl really. The only thing that is annoying is that we spent all that money, and just a toilet and a large washbasin would have been fine. We were in their hands and they are supposed to be the experts but they haven't really helped us at all.
>
> (Wife)

Not surprisingly, many of the carers interviewed felt ill-prepared for discharge and were unsure about what to expect at home, and the type of help and support that was available. Even when help had been organized carers often received minimal information and had very little idea of what had been arranged:

> Like they've [ward staff] said to me there's people who come out to do some physio [community rehabilitation team]. I don't know who they are, where they come from, whether they're based here, whether it's a team that just work this area, or how many times they're going to come in. I'd like to know that now.
>
> (Husband)

Unfortunately, on some occasions, the amount of help seemed overwhelming, and carers' limited understanding of who was coming and why meant that services were sometimes seen as intrusive and consequently cancelled:

> She [wife] was coming home on the Wednesday and I found out who they [community rehabilitation team] were on the Monday afternoon. I didn't meet them; I was just told their names, what they did and how often they came in. And then they'd got this 24-hour nursing – well, I've done away with the 24-hour nursing, they just come in at the weekends. It was just unbelievably intrusive . . . we've actually finished with the night nurses, we've had the last night nurse last night because . . . when they were here, they were just sat here and I was still taking her to the toilet, doing everything . . . It was just too much for us to come out of hospital and have six people

in here sometimes, the nurse, physio, district nurse was coming sometimes for the insulin in case I wasn't here with working. I'd got six or
seven people in here one morning, all come to see what was going off
in them first two or three days and with me and [wife], well it was just
making it worse for us. We didn't need them and when they walked
in, there was mud all over as it had been raining and I had to go round
with the hoover and that was upsetting. It was just too much.

(Husband)

Despite the difficulties some carers experienced, one key task during
the early discharge period was to seek partnerships with a new group of
professionals. This meant considering if they were 'up to the job'.

## Seeking partnerships – are they 'up to the job?'

As in hospital, the primary goal for carers was to ensure that the stroke
survivor received the best possible care (seeking best care), and most of
them recognized that this was best achieved in partnership with professional carers. However, while carers again actively sought such partnerships they also wanted reassurance that the professionals were 'up to the
job'. This judgement hinged on two key factors: first, whether or not carers
had confidence in professional carers, and secondly, if they trusted them
or not. Confidence and trust were distinct but related attributes and there
was a delicate interplay between them. Confidence was based primarily on
whether informants felt that professionals had the necessary knowledge
and skills to deliver safe and competent care. Confidence was a prerequisite of trust, but trust was only 'earned' when carers believed that
professionals had the best interests of the cared-for person at heart, and
also responded in a positive way to carers' own expertise and knowledge.
Therefore, while it was not possible to trust professional carers without
being confident in their abilities, it was possible to feel confident without
necessarily trusting them. In essence, confidence was a judgement about
professional skill and ability, whereas trust relied on the interpersonal
dynamic within the triadic caregiving relationship.

If carers had confidence in professional carers then they respected their
judgement and could learn from them:

I think I'm learning from these staff because I'm confident about
them. I think that if I wasn't confident about them, I might do it a
different way. But I really am happy with them.

(Husband)

Trust required that professional carers acknowledged carers' understanding of the situation, and, where appropriate, took action. For
example, the quote below relates to a carer's perception that a recently
fitted foot support was not suitable:

Well, we said to her, 'It's not uncomfortable but it doesn't feel right for [wife]'. She said, 'All right, I'll sort you something out', and she brought this one and that's spot on.

(Husband)

Such mutual respect laid the foundation for a trusting relationship and the development of fruitful partnerships. Such partnerships flourished if professionals gave family carers positive feedback on their efforts (thereby reinforcing for carers that they themselves were 'up to the job'), and made the time to clarify expectations:

And she actually said to me [physiotherapist], 'Your dad has done so well because you have been here and been able to do the things we have asked, and you have encouraged him', and that has made me feel better because obviously I wasn't running around like a twit – I actually had a role in all this. At one time we actually wanted to talk to her about outcomes and she made time, she came back after her other patients and talked to us and she said, 'In my opinion this is what your dad will probably achieve', or, 'This is what we will aim for', and she has been very sensible and open and honest and I have said to her – we have worked together.

(Daughter)

The final prerequisite for a well-functioning partnership was a belief that professionals actually 'cared' about what they did and conveyed this in the way they interacted with the stroke survivor and family carer:

I can't praise them enough . . . they [community rehabilitation team] want to be here . . ., they want to be part of [wife's] life, and that comes across, every one of them that comes in wants to be here . . . Because of the way they communicate and the way they treat [wife] and how they talk to her, how they talk to me – they have even got time for the dog. It's simple things like that that come across and the more you get to talk to them, the more you realize that they love it, what they are doing.

(Husband)

It could reasonably be argued that confidence and trust are no more than should be expected of any good service but all too often one or the other proved elusive. Confidence was destroyed and services rejected when it was apparent to family carers that paid carers not only lacked the skills and competencies to give 'best care' but they could not even provide adequate care:

The physios have come in and shown [sister-in-law] how to move her better than the nurses were doing because the nurses were doing it three or four times before they realized how to because they've never been trained . . . when the physio came to show [sister-in-law], that nurse said, 'That's the first time I've ever been shown how to move someone properly.' The carer that this team provide, she said, 'That's the first time we've ever been shown how to do it [moving and handling a patient] properly.' And that made me think God . . . God, what's happening when I'm not here? So we did away with the day [nurses] – afternoon and morning and we just had the night shift . . .

(Husband)

Moreover, both confidence and trust were eroded when carers felt that they had been misinformed about the status of paid carers, as the following quote succinctly captures:

They [nurses] weren't caring for her properly and then they weren't even nurses. That was a terrible thing when I found out that they weren't even nurses. I felt tricked. We were told that they were nursing staff and they came in a uniform and that wasn't true. So when you're told that at the beginning and you find out that they are not nurses, then you are on your guard all the time then. You are on your guard because I didn't feel that she was treated right. Even now I won't let her out of my sight because I felt that things weren't right from the beginning.

(Husband)

A lack of continuity, with a frequent change of paid carers, was another major impediment to both ensuring confidence and establishing trust:

Like I say, you bond, you get to know those first three nurses who walk through that door and then when they don't come the day after, you've already expressed yourself to them and told them how you feel because they've asked. You've talked to them when [wife] has gone to sleep, I've sat here and I've talked to them before I've gone to bed, I've talked to them and the next time it's somebody else and you don't want to do it again.

(Husband)

The first weekend of rapid response they tried to farm Dad out to an agency – it was hopeless, they didn't brief them properly on the amount of time that they needed and so they came expecting a 20 minute call, and of course it is like an hour and 20 minutes in the morning and so they spent the whole call huffing and puffing, and so of course Dad was on edge because he knew – he could tell what was going on and then they finally got it all together and off they went and they told Dad what time they would be back – well I had been shopping and called in on my way back and they didn't turn up when they said they would and they weren't there an hour later and when it got to 2 o'clock I sorted out the meal for him.

(Daughter)

A lack of continuity made it difficult to 'bond' with paid carers (an important element of trust), and prompted carers to pass on their own knowledge to staff so that they would know what was required:

> I want to protect him. I make a point of saying to them, look this is how we move him and handle him like this because I don't want anything to damage him or halt his progress really. So whenever there is a change [in staff caring for her father], I go in there [to see staff at her father's home] . . . until I can tell from Dad that he has trust and confidence in them, I know that Dad will get anxious and worried about it and because he has said that is what happens – he has said that he hates it when he has somebody new and he has to tell them how to do things and what is best to do – but he doesn't always remember all the finer points of it and if they don't know what to do then it is a bit hit and miss really.
>
> (Daughter)

In the above instance the carer's desire to ensure continuity was realized because one of the professional staff was sensitive to the issues involved, and worked actively with the carer to try and ensure that there was continuity of care:

> I must say the physios have been very good this time – they know about all this aggro we have had with all the different providers and they have said, 'Look, tell me when it happens because we want to meet with them and show them how to handle your dad because we are not having any of this belt lifting business again.' So I have felt that they were there and I don't feel that I have to go over the top with these new people – I feel that they [physiotherapists] are going to be there and I felt supported then. I think if I tell them when these new people are going in then they will make a point of being there and meeting these new people and showing them what they can do to help . . .
>
> (Daughter)

Here the presence of a professional carer who was alert to the carers' concerns helped to alleviate the situation. However, this did not always happen and many carers felt that professionals did not value or acknowledge either their concerns or their expertise:

> They think I'm just a carer, not a professional. There is a big barrier between carers and professionals because they just think that you are in the way. They [professionals] don't think that you [carers] know what you are doing – they just see you as a job. They see you as threatening their territory if you say anything.
>
> (Husband)

In the best relationships both confidence and trust were established and sustained, and creative partnerships forged between family and professional carers. All too frequently, however, these two essential components were compromised, sometimes due to the attitudes of professionals, but more often as a result of a system which seemed insensitive to the real needs of stroke survivors and their carers, and immune to their efforts to seek partnerships. Frequently the only option for carers was to 'go it alone' and bypass the structures putatively in place to provide help and support:

> Is there a system at all really? We have learned tolerance and we have learned that really it is up to yourselves to get on with it. Although people come at first, all they are doing really is . . . [pause] . . . fulfilling their liabilities.
>
> (Wife)

A graphic illustration of the difficulties that arose and the negative consequences that can occur is provided below in three excerpts taken from the third, fifth and seventh interviews with a husband who had been trying unsuccessfully to get services for his wife:

> I'm frustrated but I've got used to that now, I've had so many months of getting nothing that I'm used to it now. It [installing a handrail on the stairs] should have been done. I know money comes into it too, but that should have been done. They [community rehabilitation team] haven't just found out that it takes six weeks [to get a handrail delivered to the carer's house], they must have known. How long has the team been going? I would imagine that somewhere along the line one of them knows how long it takes to get a handrail.
>
> (Husband, third interview)

> You are definitely vulnerable. You feel let down because they won't let you do what you need to do. Going back to the woman from the adaptations, who's been today – she's left a rail. So I said, 'Right, I'll get that put up tonight.' So she said, 'Oh no, you can't fit it; you'll have to wait for me to send somebody from the Works Department to fix it, and that could be up to three weeks.' Well it won't be because I'll fit it tonight . . . Well it's the system, the system won't let you do things. You could do a lot more if they let you.
>
> (Husband, fifth interview)

> I've also learned not to trust anybody and do as much as you can for yourself. At first I left everything to see what would work and I trusted the system because I thought it would work and something would turn up to help out – but it doesn't. So you have to get out there yourself and sort things out for yourself more than I did – even though I did more than I think I should have done. I think you need to go out there and fight from day one for what you want. But people don't know that because they tell you Social Services will come out to you in a few days – but it takes them two weeks to get round to seeing

you. Then it takes another two weeks before anything happens – so that's a month gone. In that month you could have sorted more out.

(Husband, seventh interview)

The above carer did not have a uniformly bad experience of services but, as was apparent during the seventh and final interview, any remaining vestige of trust was gone. This was exacerbated by the abrupt way in which his relationship with the community rehabilitation team had ended. The impact of this is graphically portrayed below:

. . . we've come close to them all [the community rehabilitation team], more than I expected, a lot more than I expected. For them to be how they have been with us, I can't explain it to anybody. I've not even told them, I've not told anybody [looks upset] . . . I've even sat down and written things about them, that I've never done in my life before . . . For me to write things about people that I've only known for a few months, I haven't done that for people I've known all my life. They have been so . . . so much a part of my life over the past few weeks. It's hard to explain really . . . I've written a poem about them you know . . . I've not even told [wife] yet. It was for me but . . . I feel when they go I want to write it on a Christmas card for them. I don't know why, I've never done anything like it in my life before, but I feel that they have given me [wife] back and that's a big thing . . . [cries].

(Husband, eighth interview)

Other carers were also unprepared for the end of important and meaning-ful relationships, endings which often seemed to be dictated by arbitrary rules about the legitimate length of support:

Maybe they [professionals] should spell it out to you really [that rehabilitation is time limited]. Nobody has spelt it out to you and they just stop coming. Maybe at the outset – well, not at the outset because they don't know what will happen then – but half way through maybe they should say, 'Well, look, this treatment is for a limited period' and tell you how long they are likely to be coming for because they must have a standard and I know it will vary according to how people do but when we get to a certain point we will need to leave you – but they don't do that. . . and time flies by. We should have realized I suppose.

(Wife)

The community rehabilitation team has come to an end. They said, 'Your three months is up and now you move on to the centre and we will have all our equipment back' [laughs]. It was like the rugs were being pulled out from under us – it got to this date and it was just like that. There was none of this – if you feel that you are not getting on there come back to us – it was definitely you have had your twelve weeks.

(Daughter)

Even in the best of relationships it seemed that the 'system', as it was referred to, conspired to ensure that ultimately most carers were left with the feeling that they were 'going it alone':

> I think we feel really abandoned now ... I think maybe there is nothing more they can do for him [husband] at the moment ... But you still need the support... [cries].
>
> (Wife)

## Discussion

It is important to point out that at the time the data cited in this chapter were collected family carers in the UK who were 'providing (or intending to provide) regular and substantial care' had a statutory right to an assessment of their needs (DoH/SSI 1996). All of the carers in the study would have met the eligibility criteria for such an assessment; manifestly none had received one. As the study demonstrated, despite carers' best efforts to 'seek partnerships', most were ultimately left with the feeling that they were 'going it alone'. This is not to say that there were no examples of carers receiving sensitive and appropriate help; clearly this was not the case. However, almost invariably carers had to take the initiative and it often seemed that professionals were immune to their approaches, or that the 'system' was designed to thwart their efforts. Moreover, in those instances where creative partnerships had been forged, the time-limited nature of support and the often abrupt way in which help was withdrawn left carers feeling vulnerable, isolated and abandoned. In such circumstances both confidence and trust in the 'system' evaporated.

A decade ago Thorne (1993) explored the interactions between people with chronic illness and the formal healthcare system. She described a situation in which the real power lay with the professions and consequently chronically ill people often felt invalidated, with their own expertise being ignored. Frequently the initial 'naïve trust' people had, that the system would work in their best interests and that professionals understood their problems, was shattered, often by a single event, leaving many with a feeling of 'disenchantment'. Subsequently various types of relationship emerged, but the most successful partnerships were forged when both professionals and chronically ill people negotiated and shared responsibility, had mutual trust in each other's competence, acknowledged their own weaknesses and accepted the limitations imposed by the formal 'system'. In many respects such considerations are equally relevant to the carers in this study.

More recently, and specifically in relation to stroke rehabilitation, it has been suggested that up to a quarter of all the problems that stroke survivors and their carers experience are the direct result of 'system induced setbacks' (Hart 2001) caused by the inability of formal structures to acknowledge and account for the strategic actions taken by lay people. Clearly this figure might be an underestimate for our sample of 18 carers, although such 'system induced failures' may be affected by a number of factors such as locality, and there is a need for further work to elaborate upon the nature and type of such 'setbacks'.

This is essential as most stroke survivors are supported by kin (Low *et al.* 1999), and it is estimated that family carers of stroke survivors save the state approximately £672 million annually (Bosaquet and Franks 1998). Therefore on purely economic grounds there are pressing reasons to ensure they receive the support they need to enable them to care effectively and to meet their aim of providing the best possible care. More importantly, carers contribute significantly to the subsequent quality of life of the stroke survivor.

As Pryor (2000) notes, rehabilitation is primarily about reconstructing lives in the wake of injury or illness. This is a long-term project (Cardol *et al.* 2002) involving the reintegration of lives and relationships (Secrest 2000). Its success depends in no small measure on creating the right environment or 'milieu' (O'Connor 2000; Pryor 2000) which emphasizes not only *what* is done but also *how* it is done (O'Connor 2000), particularly in respect of managing relationships between individuals, families and practitioners.

Within the hospital environment the 'window of opportunity' is limited (Secrest 2000), particularly the time available to work with family carers. The situation is compounded by the fact that nurses focus almost exclusively on the patient, and often fail to see the family as a legitimate focus of care, and consequently they only provide information when asked for it (Smagt-Duijnstree *et al.* 2000). As the present study illustrates, family carers actively seek partnerships in order both to understand 'what's it all about?' and to gain the skills they need to be 'up to the job'. All too often their efforts go unrewarded.

Little improves upon discharge home and even in the best of cases the arbitrarily finite nature of rehabilitation ignores carers' need for longer term support. As Hochstenbach (2000) argues, functional recovery provides the most 'eye-catching' indication of success in rehabilitation, and professionals see rehabilitation as being realized when functional recovery is maximized. Others suggest that evidence-based care in stroke rehabilitation conveniently ignores 'difficult to establish evidence' and dresses up complex ethical debates in 'quasi-scientific' discourse (Wyller 2000). As a consequence the goals of care are frequently determined by the providers of services rather than those in receipt of them (Rodgers 2000). Small wonder then that psychological recovery from stroke is limited and the social outlook is 'bleak' (Tyson 1995). Clearly there is a need to look beyond disability and to gauge the success of stroke rehabilitation in terms of social participation (Cardol *et al.* 2002). 'System induced setbacks' (Hart 2001) are likely to remain prevalent until this happens.

However, changing the goals of the system must also be accompanied by a fundamental rethink about the way in which partnerships are construed. There may well now be a 'new language' of social policy (Bernard and Phillips 2000) but as Paterson (2001) notes, it is not enough simply to alter the language we use; there also needs to be a 'profound' change in complex power relations. The culture of 'practitioner as expert' may well be deep-rooted (Paterson 2001) but if one of the essential aims of a quality rehabilitation service is to ensure continuity of care in response to the long-term needs of patients and their families (Eldar 2000), then the way the 'system' operates and those who work within it will need to change. Both family and professional carers may believe that they are providing 'best care', but until confidence and trust can be established and maintained, 'best care' is likely to continue to be a case of 'going it alone'.

# SECTION TWO

# 'Working through it'

> Sensitive assessment where the carer is given the opportunity to think more broadly about their situation can open up whole new opportunities for carers.
>
> (Qureshi *et al.* 200: 4–35)

Rolland (1988, 1994) describes the experience of chronic illness as a 'long haul' and in many respects this aptly captures the indeterminate nature of family caregiving. This section of the book concentrates on the stage of caring that we have termed 'working through it'. This title reflects the proactive way in which families address the challenges they face. 'Work' in this context is not intended to suggest that family carers see their role in terms of a 'job', although in some cases this is true. Rather it denotes the active way in which carers develop expert knowledge of their situation. As the first chapter of the initial section suggested, ideally carers, the cared-for person and professionals should actively 'work together' in ensuring the best possible care. Unfortunately this is not always the case.

This section draws on studies from Sweden, Australia and the UK and highlights enduring challenges across such contexts. Sweden in particular provides interesting case material in that until recently state provision was such that there was little or no expectation that the family would provide care. This has changed significantly over the last decade, with several recent developments ensuring that family carers have become a policy priority (see in particular the chapter by Lundh and Nolan). As well as considering carers' needs and service responses in different countries, the contributions to this section also address quite differing caring contexts and, in illuminating the carers' experience in dementia and learning disability, provide some important insights.

At the heart of this section, however, lies the interface between family and more formal caregiving systems, and the extent to which the latter explicitly supports and builds on the expertise of the former. This is reflected in varying ways by each of the contributions here.

This section begins with a chapter by Lundh *et al.* which compares and contrasts family and professional carers' views of what constitutes good care for a person with dementia. While there is considerable agreement among informants, there are also subtle differences, particularly in the tactics that family and professional carers employ. In addition to these differences the study also suggests that in many ways the ability of professionals to deliver the quality of care they would wish is limited by a lack of resources and a system which is not as yet fully geared to the needs of carers. This is resonant of the 'system induced setbacks' highlighted in the case of stroke carers (Brereton and Nolan, Chapter 3).

The next chapter shifts attention to the area of learning disabilities and, drawing on extensive case study material, Grant and Whittell consider the influence of several key 'turning points' in the caring trajectory. Conceptually they make links between the wider 'life course' literature, the policy rhetoric and the experience of carers, and highlight how these differing 'calendars' are often out of 'synch'. The key messages would seem to be that services often provide 'too little, too late'. In particular the powerful case study material suggests how early interventions between families and professionals can exert a profound and lasting effect on future relationships and that if initial trust is lost, it is often difficult, if not impossible, to re-establish.

The next contribution takes a rather differing stance and focuses on the impact of professionals using a standard assessment format on their perceptions of family carers. In a novel approach Lundh employed experienced professionals (nurses, care managers etc.) as data collectors and used them to interview 245 carers using the three assessment instruments designed by Nolan *et al.* (1998). These consider the difficulties, satisfactions and coping strategies used by families. The results not only provide important insights into the type and range of services that need to be developed in Sweden, but also highlight the way in which a detailed and holistic assessment can provide a wider perspective on family carers. Therefore, while all of the 'professionals' interviewed felt that they understood the circumstances of family carers, these were challenged and modified considerably as a result of their involvement in the project. In particular professionals (mainly but not exclusively nurses) now felt that they had a fuller appreciation of the range of caring experiences and that as a result this would change their current ways of working and thinking.

The need to create a dialogue between families and other support systems is also stressed in the chapter by Nolan *et al.* This draws on data from Australia to explore the ways in which carers of people with dementia develop their coping strategies and considers whether services help or hinder this process. The results once again highlight the wide range of coping strategies that carers employ but also identifies gaps in current service provision. Consistent with research from other countries the need for better respite provision emerged as the single most requested service in a survey of carers of people with dementia drawn from members of the Alzheimer's Society. However, the results reinforce other studies which suggest that, in order to be acceptable, respite needs to be flexible, of high quality and delivered by consistent personnel.

The final chapter in this section most aptly covers the dilemma of older parents (60+) of people with learning disabilities when they consider the future for their children. Parent-carers, as Llewellyn notes, very rarely plan for the future despite the fact that their children will almost inevitably outlive them. She seeks to explain this paradox in terms of their caring biography and in so doing draws on experiences which span a lifetime of caring. Throughout this biography, often spanning 40 or more years, she notes both the tensions parent-carers experience in their interactions with formal carers and the often contradictory way in which public policy has evolved. This chapter vividly portrays how parent-carers are denied access to the 'inner circle of experts': the professionals, and as a consequence many do not use the support services available to them.

Several 'threads of continuity' emerge in this section and these concern the coping strategies that carers employ, their own perceived sense of expertise and the general failure of the formal 'systems' to respond appropriately to either of these. As Gilmour (2002) has recently argued, family and professional carers need to 'integrate' their efforts if optimal care is to be provided. This section provides some telling insights into the 'work' that remains to be done before such an integration can occur.

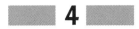

# 4

# Quality care for people with dementia: the views of family and professional carers

## Ulla Lundh, Mike Nolan, Ingrid Hellström and Iréne Ericsson

Person-centred care for people with dementia is an aspiration for both family and professional carers but what constitutes person-centred care and how it can be achieved are far from clear. Indeed, the views of family and professional carers on this matter can often be quite different, and both parties need to understand and value the perspective of the other if creative partnerships are to be forged. This chapter describes a Swedish study which explores the views of both family and professional carers of people with dementia as to what they considered constitutes quality care. Important areas of similarity and difference were identified and the results suggest that both groups of carers need to work closely together if person-centred care is to become a reality.

## Background

For many years research into dementia was dominated by a medical and disease-orientated approach (for example Marcusson *et al.* 1995), with symptomatology being understood in terms of pathological processes and therapeutic efforts directed at compensating for cognitive decline. However, building on the pioneering work of Tom Kitwood and colleagues (Kitwood and Bredin 1992; Kitwood 1997), the last decade or so has seen the emergence of an altogether more positive and person-centred view of dementia in which many of the problems people with dementia (PWD) face are attributable to the social environment they experience, which fails to acknowledge their personhood. The notion of person-centred care has become the watchword for a new culture of care in dementia which focuses on the residual strengths and abilities of the PWD rather than their deficits (Norman 1999; Morton 2000). There can be no doubting the impact that person-centred care has had in energizing and motivating staff working in residential care settings but such considerations apply equally to the community, where family and professional carers each have a key role to play.

Despite the stresses involved in caring for a PWD (Sällström 1994; Ory *et al.* 1999) significant numbers of people, even those with advanced dementia, remain at home with the support of close family members (Audit Commission 2000). Such family carers often view themselves as 'experts' in the care of their relative (Nolan *et al.* 1996a), emphasizing their ability to provide high-quality individualized care based on an understanding of the needs of the PWD not readily available to professional carers. This may in part explain the limited uptake of services, such as respite care, with carers expressing concerns about the quality of the support provided and its failure to recognize and sustain the 'personhood' of the PWD (Moriarty 1999; Pickard 1999).

Therefore while both family and professional carers place great store on the 'personhood' of the individual, professional support often fails to live up to the expectations of family members in this regard (Briggs and Askham 1999; Pickard 1999). This raises interesting questions as to whether families have unrealistic expectations, or if in fact family and professional carers have differing perceptions of what constitutes 'good care'. It was the desire to understand better the attributes of 'good care' as defined by family and professional carers that was the primary aim of the study upon which this chapter is based.

## Method

The study was conducted in two phases involving both qualitative interviews and a postal survey to a larger sample. For the qualitative study family carers were recruited from existing service users whose relative was receiving support from the local authority, that is day care or respite care. Interviews were completed with 20 family carers (nine wives, six husbands, three daughters, one brother and one sister), exploring their perceptions of what constituted good care. The interviews lasted about 45 minutes and were tape-recorded for later transcription and analysis. Interviews were also completed with 17 professionals who regularly worked with family carers; these included six nurses, six care workers, two heads of homes, two people working for the local authority and one occupational therapist. Following the interviews all the data were transcribed and subjected to a detailed content analysis to identify the main themes (Morse and Field 1994). The themes were then developed into statements for incorporation into a questionnaire comprising 33 items, which was sent to a purposive sample of 200 professionals working in the local community with dementia patients, and 200 relatives of PWD.

The response rate for relatives was 80 per cent and 60 per cent of residents were 65 years or older, with 16 per cent being 80 years or older. Sixty-one per cent were spouses and the remainder mainly children (34 per cent) or a sister, brother or friend to the cared-for person (5 per cent). The cared-for persons were mostly female (67 per cent), and the vast majority were 75 years or older (77 per cent) and had been ill for between three and five years (53 per cent). Most carers (64 per cent) lived with the cared-for person and had done so for a long time, 53 per cent for more than 40 years. Non-residential carers lived close to the PWD, usually within four miles. Sixty-nine per cent of respondents received some form of help with care, available from the voluntary sector (35 per cent) or organized home help (21 per cent) and respite care (11 per cent). The district nurse made regular visits to some of the PWD (22 per cent) and some participated in day care activities organized by the municipality (21 per cent). Eighty-two per cent of those who received help said they were satisfied with the support they received.

The response rate for professionals was 86 per cent, of whom only 2 per cent were male. Thirty-four per cent had a university degree (nurses, district nurses, occupational therapists), 46 per cent were staff nurses and 18 per cent had a less formal education and worked as home helpers. Most respondents worked in the home help sector or in primary care (47 per cent), with others working in care homes (36 per cent) or other kinds of support activities, such as day care. Respondents were generally very experienced: 37 per cent had worked 20 years or more in the care sector, and 60 per cent had more than four years of experience working with PWD. Forty-nine per cent worked solely in this area.

Having briefly described the methodology for the study, attention is now turned to the results, which highlight the main themes from the qualitative data and also identify a number of differing perceptions emerging from the quantitative survey.

## Results

The results of data collection are presented in three sections, beginning with a consideration of carers' perceptions of good care in dementia as identified from the in-depth interviews. Subsequently the perceptions of the professionals are presented before the quantitative data for both groups of respondents are highlighted. While in many respects there is considerable overlap between these data sets, indicating shared views as to the important dimensions of quality care, subtle and important differences also emerge which suggest the potential for tensions and conflict if issues are not addressed in an open and frank manner. Therefore although both family and professional carers lay great emphasis on maintaining the dignity, individuality and quality of life of the PWD, how this is to be achieved varies. Furthermore, the data also suggest that a lack of congruence between the views of family and professional carers may inhibit carers from accessing support. This is apparent when the perceptions of the family carers are considered.

## Quality of care – the views of family carers

The overwhelming motivation for family carers was to help the PWD remain within their own homes, and in close contact with family and friends. Being in a familiar environment, surrounded by shared memories, was seen to provide an element of security and belonging which was viewed as essential to a good quality of life. This notion of security within a familiar environment surfaced repeatedly in the data:

> It's security, I believe. Being able to be at home as long as possible makes him feel secure, when all's said and done. Sort of having his things and books and everything.
>
> (Wife)

> Well, I suppose, it's the feeling of security she gets from being here, that's the best quality of life for her. And that's because she and my older sister always spent their summers here at grandma and granddads when they were little. And that was sort of the best time of their life when they were little. And that's why she feels so positive about it, because she's back here again.
>
> (Sister)

As the quotation above suggests, familiar environments created a feeling of continuity, and helping the PWD to maintain links with their past were seen to be very important:

> It's important for them to have an environment they feel comfortable in and to have things they recognize from their earlier life perhaps. To just have something of their own that they feel belongs to bygone days perhaps.
>
> (Sister)

Intergenerational family ties were also highlighted as contributing to a feeling of belonging and continuity:

> Well, for him to be at home and be with us and . . . then the children and grandchildren and the little great-grandchildren come to see us and he enjoys that so much. And sometimes we go and see them and he goes with us, you know.
>
> (Wife)

Not surprisingly, temporary removal from a familiar environment often exacerbated difficulties and was one of the main reasons why services such as respite care were not embraced as enthusiastically as they might have been:

> I believe it's the security of recognizing things, as it seems like when she goes to other places, like when she's at the hospital at certain times and so on, she's a lot worse. So I think the security of the home environment is important, I really do.
>
> (Daughter)

As important as it was, a familiar environment was not of itself seen as sufficient to ensure a good quality of life. Rather this also required the sort of intimate knowledge that could only be obtained from a lifetime of shared experiences. For carers, and particularly spouses, such intimate knowledge was the foundation of their caring efforts, and the basis upon which they sustained their connectedness to the PWD. It also allowed them to make subtle judgements about the needs and preferences of the PWD, even if the PWD was unable to articulate them verbally:

> The person you've lived together with and loved. There's no one that can replace that person. You know each other, don't you? And well, you know how she's feeling and what you can do to help her and so on. That's important, in my opinion.
>
> (Husband)

> . . . but . . . everything seems so *natural* when you know each other so well. After all, we've been living together for over 40 years, almost a whole lifetime . . . we've grown together, know everything about each other . . .
>
> (Wife)

> Yes, I'm sure of that, I know his feelings and needs without him having to say anything. And I think that it is tremendously important to him to be able to be here at home. He's lived here all his life. I think I can see that he seems to feel best at home. He's been at respite care and he didn't like it there.
>
> (Wife)

This form of almost psychic connectedness was coupled with an in-depth appreciation of personal habits and preferences that was seen as being essential to maintaining quality of life:

> He knows me, I suppose, and I know him. By watching his face and body I can see what he's thinking. He makes it clear when he doesn't like something . . . but he likes sweet things, so if I put something really good and sweet on the table he looks really happy.
>
> (Wife)

> It's a matter of habit, her hair is so short now, but she had to have it put in curlers, 'cos that's the way she's always had it . . . Yes, I think it's important to her that I make her feel looked after.
>
> (Daughter)

So long as she gets her coffee . . . she can put it on herself but you can't leave her alone, you've got to keep an eye on her . . . she can go back to sleep and she sleeps until morning.

(Husband)

Clearly some of this information, such as a love of sweet things, or a liking for coffee, could be conveyed to others and in theory therefore could be replicated. However, it was the context within which such apparently mundane activities were enacted that was critical, as was the maintenance of lifelong routines and shared pleasures:

Well, it has an effect on the quality of life, I'm sure. We have an awful lot in common, singing and so on. I can't sing but still I sing with him [laughs], and he gets his mouth organ out and plays so I sing along. And he gets satisfaction out of singing and playing music, and we also play records and tapes and so on. That's real quality of life. And going out together and looking at all sorts of things. He's a great nature lover.

(Wife)

. . . we have our old habits and routines that we follow like we've always done, and of course I know what kind of life we've had and what we've done. And so it's obvious that it works best if we follow our normal routines. If I leave him just for a little while he wonders where I am. I'm the one that makes the food and so on and he likes what I give him [laughs].

(Brother)

However well-meaning professional carers might be, several family carers felt that it was simply not possible for them to provide the quality of care and level of commitment that the PWD experienced at home. This led some to resist offers of help, even when pressure was exerted by their families:

No, for heaven's sake, not as long as I can cope, no, I don't want that. I don't want anybody here among my belongings. I had home help for a while when I'd had an operation, but that was only for a few hours, but I still didn't like it.

(Wife)

We've never had any outside help and . . . we've not been ill very often, never been in hospital and so on. That can also have an effect on a person. They keep on at me to accept it, to ask for help . . . and it's so difficult for me. I sort of want . . . well, perhaps I want to protect my, or our, integrity. So I don't want to reveal private things about us, so to speak.

(Wife)

Other carers were more inclined to take a pragmatic view and to recognize that there were circumstances in which professional help was required, and indeed might even supersede family care. There was due recognition that aspects of role reversal could make it difficult for a family carer to question behaviour, while this might not be a problem for a professional:

> It can be difficult to do and say certain things in matters of care when it's a relative you're dealing with. It's an advantage knowing each other from the start but that's the disadvantage too. It's extremely difficult for me to tell her to do things, to wash herself etc., and that's when tension builds up. I mean when it's your mother, or your parents, it's quite different . . . well, it's this thing about the roles being reversed, and that's very hard to accept. Somebody from outside can more easily come in and say, 'You've got to have a shower now, you've got to do this and that . . .'.
>
> (Daughter)

> So that's why I think that nursing staff are better in certain circumstances, that's to say when the patient has reached a certain stage. It's easier for them to tackle this sort of thing.
>
> (Daughter)

However, while some carers recognized the need for outside help, and indeed valued it, they still stressed the value of negotiating care in order to ensure the best possible quality:

> . . . well, I'd perhaps like to have a meeting with that home help service, those people who are going to be in Mum's home . . . like about what's in her home, how she likes things done . . . I'd like to discuss these things with them.
>
> (Daughter)

## Negotiating care: the essence of partnership

Eventually most carers, despite their misgivings, realized that some form of professional help and support was needed and that they could no longer manage alone. When this occurred the extent to which carers willingly shared some of their responsibility depended in no small measure on the extent to which professionals actively sought their knowledge and experience:

> They really ask my opinion. It's like friends ringing up and saying, 'What do you think about your wife? Are things working out well, do you think?'
>
> (Husband)

> But they're very good at this day centre at making good use of us relatives as well, and they even ring us up the moment something happens. And I think that's really good and I call them if I think there's something that . . . if there's like something he wants . . .
>
> (Wife)

As well as a willingness to engage in genuine dialogue with carers it was important that staff demonstrated their commitment to ensuring the quality of life of the PWD, by attending to the 'little' things that extended beyond physical care. This was particularly important when the PWD had entered a care home:

> That there's staff there who've got time for them and that there are things to occupy them. That they don't just let them in and leave them to sit and watch TV. But that they try to do things together – partly such everyday things as making food and baking and so on, and partly things like excursions, experiencing things and so forth.
>
> (Daughter)

> Yes, in my mum's situation it's important that they tend to her hygiene properly in the mornings, in my opinion. And oh ... the right clothes for the right time of year. It's important what she looks like before she goes to her group ... to the day centre, I mean. So they don't just send her off looking, you know.
>
> (Daughter)

When such attention to detail was perceived as lacking quality of care and quality of life was inevitably compromised, services were either rejected or resisted until the last possible moment:

> Well, you see, it's small details that make the difference, that little extra bit, you can say. Looking after one or two patients' feet and legs, rubbing in some cream and fussing over them a bit, things I did automatically. And I noticed that things haven't been done quite the same way as I did them. I saw she had a callus and so on that bothered her. But she's shy and a bit quiet sometimes. She doesn't tell them. And, oh, it can never be the same as home no matter how hard they try. It just can't be and you know beforehand that that's how it is. And therefore you put off making the decision and so on ... [his voice breaks].
>
> (Husband)

One of the critical issues therefore becomes to what extent professional carers are aware of the values and aspirations of family carers and whether they are able to forge positive partnerships so that families feel that they can willingly share care. The data from the professionals provide some important insights.

## The views of professional carers

As with the carers, the interviews with professionals yielded rich and varied data which touched upon remarkably similar themes. Consistent with the views of family carers, professionals placed great store on maintaining the quality of life of the PWD. In order to do so they too recognized that it was essential to sustain their individuality and uniqueness, and that this required varied and diverse sources of knowledge:

> Well, just seeing the person behind the patient, that's a better way of putting it, seeing the person behind the illness, the individual. Not all cast in the same mould, so to speak. Not just doing things as you've done, but getting to the point where you can see each individual and care and nurse him according to his needs.
>
> (Assistant Nurse)

> Getting the whole picture of the person you meet, and that means not only the person himself but also the resources that are available around him, relatives, what sort of social network he has, as everything has to be taken into account, also what sort of life he has had earlier on and what sort of person he was before.
>
> (Occupational Therapist)

Knowing the 'person behind the patient', and applying such knowledge in a sensitive and informed manner was seen to enhance the quality of care, even when applied to such apparently 'basic' needs as 'personal hygiene':

> We've got an old gentleman here who's terrified of the shower, it's awful to see. But he's obviously had an accident some time in the past, so we know we have to be very careful with him – we start at the bottom with his feet and work our way up. That's the sort of thing that's very important to know about. If you don't know about it you just go straight in and turn on the shower.
>
> (Home Help)

A failure to recognize the importance of such aspects was seen by some as the antithesis of good care:

> When you don't see all these things I think you've forgotten the concept of good care. When all that matters is the work environment and rules and norms, then you've forgotten the individual human being, and definitely the relatives too, I think. You don't see good care and this leads to conflicts about aims of the different teams.
>
> (Home Care Assesser)

Many of those interviewed were well aware that knowing the 'person behind the patient' mandated that they actively drew upon the knowledge and experience of family carers, and indeed the PWD themselves:

> So certain times we've got relatives to give us the patient's life history to help us to try to find out from them what life was like before . . . so that we should perhaps listen to certain things and so on.
>
> (Home Care Manager)

It's very, very important to have contact with the relatives. They are the ones who know, they have the knowledge.

(Assistant Nurse)

You shouldn't forget that it's the relatives that are the professionals and the elderly person with dementia, they are the ones who've got all the knowledge and they've had to learn to cajole and sort of go roundabout ways to be able to meet his needs and make the day as good as possible for him.

(Home Care Assesser)

Generally there was recognition that gaining the trust of carers took an investment of time and energy, and the creation of an open, honest relationship:

The important thing is that they feel secure, both the relatives and the sick person. Secure within the framework of the help they can get and that they are well informed about what possibilities there are.

(District Nurse)

Moreover, there was a realization that such relationships could not be established unless there was an element of consistency in the professionals with whom carers had contact:

What it's all about is trying to build up their confidence in a few persons, preferably one, or there should be two contact persons at least and that they should meet as often as possible so they can have a secure relationship. And that's what we're trying to work on, to support the assistant nurses in this – it's a long-term goal in many cases, especially if there's a lot of suspicion about.

(Nurse from Support Team, with special education in dementia)

Unfortunately it seemed that the service systems often conspired to thwart the best intentions of the professional workers:

One husband was visited by as many as 29 people just over a period of a few days, I think 29 in eight days. He had to keep telling them how his wife was to be looked after so he gave up and declined the home help he was so badly in need of.

(Social Welfare Officer with special education in dementia)

Despite this many of those interviewed demonstrated an acute awareness of the need to work proactively with families in order to provide the best care. Furthermore, there was a recognition that their professional training and knowledge had to be accompanied by a genuine desire to work in the area of dementia care:

You can have the training, that's fundamental. I have to know what a dementia illness is, but then I have to learn how to understand the people who have the illness itself and how to understand the symptoms – that is very important.

(Community Nurse)

> The most important thing is that you want to work, the will to work must be the basis. I'm convinced of that. If I want to work but don't have the knowledge . . . well then, I'll be receptive to knowledge if the will is there, but I don't think the opposite is true. If you have the knowledge but not the will it will show. Especially when caring for dementia patients – I think this is important.
>
> (Community Nurse)

For some there was realization that they had to transcend their particular 'world view' and try to appreciate the broader picture:

> I think you've got to have a genuine interest – if you've got that then you acquire knowledge. And I think you have to have some sort of . . . well, you know, we talk a bit carelessly about our outlook on mankind . . . a sort of broad-mindedness about how we look upon an elderly person, see him as an important and valuable human being who has his rights . . . and realize that you can't apply your own set of values to another person, so to speak.
>
> (Dementia Nurse)

The above quote reflects many of the sentiments voiced by the family carers, and it attests to the fact that ultimately both professional and family carers are aiming for the same thing: 'a better quality of life for people with dementia'.

In comparing the data obtained from family and professional carers it is clear that both have the needs of the PWD as their prime concern and both are agreed that, whenever possible, the home environment is the one of choice. Moreover, both sets of respondents recognized that detailed knowledge of the PWD provides the building blocks of good care. However, family carers believed that such knowledge could only be fully obtained from a lifetime of experience, and that without this many subtle clues as to the needs and desires of the PWD are likely to be missed.

In marked contrast, professionals felt that, providing that they had access to a detailed historical account of the person's life before dementia, and that they were also able to build a good relationship with the person, they could provide better care than the family, combining, as they did, biographical knowledge with their own professional understanding and experience of the wider phenomenon of dementia.

These, and other differences in emphasis, were further highlighted in the quantitative data.

## The survey results

The survey provided an opportunity to explore further the views of family and professional carers using a larger sample. In this section responses to several of the questionnaire items derived from the interview data are presented in four tables, which respectively consider: the preferred location of care (Table 4.1); respondents' perceptions of involvement in care (Table 4.2); the management strategies adopted to provide good care (Table 4.3) and the type of knowledge needed to provide good care (Table 4.4).

With regard to the preferred location of care, Table 4.1 reinforces the qualitative data and the rather differing views of family and professional

**Table 4.1** The location of care

| Agreement with statements | RELATIVES | | | PROFESSIONALS | | | P |
|---|---|---|---|---|---|---|---|
| | Disagree | Partly agree | Mostly or totally agree | Disagree | Partly agree | Mostly or totally agree | |
| | % | % | % | % | % | % | |
| Good care is best provided in a familiar environment | 1 | 8 | 91 | 0 | 9 | 90 | NS |
| Good care is best provided in private homes | 2 | 32 | 66 | 11 | 72 | 16 | .000 |
| Best care is given in care homes for older people | 6 | 45 | 49 | 5 | 30 | 64 | .005 |

*Note:* P = probability, NS = Not significant.
Percentages do not sum to 100 due to rounding up decimal points.

**Table 4.2** Involvement in care

| Agreement with statements | RELATIVES | | | PROFESSIONALS | | | P |
|---|---|---|---|---|---|---|---|
| | Disagree | Partly agree | Mostly or totally agree | Disagree | Partly agree | Mostly or totally agree | |
| | % | % | % | % | % | % | |
| Good care is characterized by cooperation between professionals and family carers | 1 | 5 | 94 | 0 | 2 | 98 | NS |
| PWD should be able to influence their own care | 2 | 59 | 39 | 5 | 59 | 36 | NS |
| Support for relatives is an important part of the care | 1 | 8 | 92 | 0 | 2 | 98 | .000 |

**Table 4.3** Management strategies for good care

| Agreement with statements | RELATIVES | | | PROFESSIONALS | | | P |
|---|---|---|---|---|---|---|---|
| | Disagree | Partly agree | Mostly or totally agree | Disagree | Partly agree | Mostly or totally agree | |
| | % | % | % | % | % | % | % |
| **Establishing routines** | | | | | | | |
| Good care is best planned | 0 | 21 | 79 | 4 | 35 | 62 | .001 |
| Daily care is better when it is based on routines and regularity | 2 | 11 | 87 | 4 | 23 | 73 | .05 |
| A set time for activities is important | 4 | 42 | 54 | 21 | 44 | 34 | .000 |
| Good care is based on flexibility | 2 | 16 | 82 | 0 | 8 | 92 | .000 |
| It is good to improve and try new ideas | 3 | 44 | 53 | 1 | 26 | 72 | .000 |
| **Establishing boundaries** | | | | | | | |
| PWD go back to 'childhood' and need rules | 11 | 49 | 40 | 31 | 46 | 23 | .000 |
| It is important to correct PWD when they do things wrong | 10 | 47 | 43 | 35 | 43 | 22 | .000 |
| **Limiting stimuli** | | | | | | | |
| PWD are best cared for in a secure environment | 10 | 36 | 55 | 9 | 40 | 51 | NS |
| PWD understand less and need less information | 39 | 48 | 13 | 68 | 25 | 7 | .000 |
| Social interaction is tiring and should be limited | 21 | 62 | 17 | 23 | 65 | 12 | NS |

**Table 4.4** Knowledge for care

| Agreement with statements | RELATIVES | | | PROFESSIONALS | | | P |
|---|---|---|---|---|---|---|---|
| | Disagree | Partly agree | Mostly or totally agree | Disagree | Partly agree | Mostly or totally agree | |
| | % | % | % | % | % | % | |
| Good care is based on PWD's life history | 3 | 24 | 73 | 1 | 13 | 85 | .001 |
| Emotional ties facilitate understanding of the needs of PWD | 2 | 25 | 73 | 19 | 41 | 40 | .000 |
| Professionals have better and more important knowledge than relatives | 5 | 50 | 45 | 10 | 56 | 34 | .01 |
| Good care is best given by educated staff | 3 | 42 | 55 | 4 | 34 | 62 | NS |
| Professionals have best knowledge of the PWD's needs | 9 | 49 | 42 | 13 | 40 | 46 | NS |
| Knowledge is best gained through education and supervision | 1 | 24 | 74 | 4 | 41 | 54 | .000 |
| Education and supervision are needed for good care | 1 | 34 | 65 | 0 | 21 | 78 | .002 |
| Knowledge is best gained through experience | 2 | 24 | 74 | 4 | 30 | 66 | .002 |

carers. Both groups therefore endorse the view that care is best provided in a familiar environment. However, family carers are strongly of the opinion that this should be the home of the PWD, while professionals see advantages to care home placement. Such differences in perception may help to explain the limited 'preparation' for care home placement that carers receive from professionals, particularly with respect to the emotional consequences of the move (see Sandberg *et al.*, Chapter 11, this volume).

Turning to involvement in care, both sets of respondents strongly endorse the principle that good care is more likely to be achieved if families and professionals cooperate and that ideally the PWD should also play an active role in shaping their own care. Interestingly, professionals are more likely to see support for carers as an important part of care. However, it is not possible to determine whether this is because carers accord this less value, or if their responses reflect the fact that they actually feel they do not receive the support they would like. However, while this difference is statistically significant, the vast majority of both groups of respondents endorse the notion that supporting family carers is something to be desired.

The above results are encouraging insofar as cooperation is promoted, but to cooperate fully requires a shared set of goals and values. It has already been noted that improving the quality of life of the PWD is the main priority for both family and professional carers and this would seem to provide an encouraging start. On the other hand, differences as to the preferred location of care suggests a divergence of opinion as to how quality of life can be promoted and several other differences emerge when attention is turned to the preferred strategies for managing aspects of care.

The data in Table 4.3 indicates that there are often large and significant differences between the tactics that families and professionals view as being the best to promote high-quality care. Carers, for instance, assert the value of planning care carefully and sticking to routines and set patterns of activity, while professionals are more likely to promote flexibility and improvisation. Similar differences are apparent with regard to setting the boundaries of care, with family carers again preferring a clearer set of 'ground rules'.

The origins of such differences and their motives are difficult to interpret. For example, it could be argued that families tend to be overly protective and in so doing restrict the opportunities for self-expression by the PWD. However, the qualitative data would not support such an interpretation, indicating as they do that carers work hard to promote quality interactions and stimuli for the PWD that are consistent with their preferred and long-standing interests. Furthermore, management strategies are likely to be determined by a combination of both experience and circumstances, and as most family carers provide support to the PWD alone for the greater part of the day, then an element of order and consistency might not only help to ensure that essential care is provided, but is also likely to create the 'security' that carers feel is essential to the well-being of the PWD. Indeed, from their experience, when the PWD goes to an unfamiliar environment his/her perceived level of anxiety and agitation often increases significantly. It may therefore be the case that what professionals view as flexibility and improvisation is experienced as chaotic by the PWD.

Interestingly, both sets of respondents feel that the PWD is best supported in a secure environment and that he/she should not be exposed to too many interactions. However, carers, as opposed to professionals, are more likely to promote the value of limiting the flow of information to the PWD. Once again this could be interpreted as carers imposing unwanted restrictions on the PWD, or, conversely, as drawing on their greater personal knowledge and experience of creating a secure, calm, but high-quality environment.

Some of the most surprising, and at times paradoxical, data relate to the perceived sources of knowledge for providing good care. The qualitative data indicated that family and professional carers both promoted the value of 'knowing' the PWD, but that professionals thought that this knowledge could be gained by a thorough life history. Conversely families believed that intimate experience of the PWD, often gained over a lifetime, was also needed. To some extent these differences are reinforced in Table 4.4.

While both sets of respondents note the importance of knowledge of the life history of the PWD, this is accorded greater value by professionals. Conversely, family carers are far more likely to recognize the significance of emotional ties. Rather surprisingly, both groups believe that good care is best given by professionals and staff with an education, and families more than professionals feel that the knowledge held by professionals is better and more important than their own. Moreover, while both groups see the benefits of experience, education and supervision are also seen as being essential.

It appears from the data that while families intuitively feel that the knowledge and experience they have are the building blocks of good care, they still promote professional knowledge above their own. In large part this may be due to the way in which knowledge is constructed and understood by society. Knowledge is therefore likely to be seen in terms of 'facts and theories', as opposed to experience and emotion, which in the present context are the product of a shared life. The roots of these and other differences in our data are important to understand, as many of the difficulties and tensions that challenge the notion of genuine partnerships between family and professional carers can be attributed to subtle but important differences in values and goals.

## Discussion

As Fawdry (2001) notes, the current policy and practice rhetoric promotes the notion of family and professional carers working as equal partners, fully acknowledging and sharing their knowledge, skill and commitment. Such a vision emerged during the 1990s and yet early in that decade Davies (1992) cautioned that while partnerships were desirable, there was considerable potential for dysfunctional and competitive relationships to develop between family and paid carers. More recently Ward-Griffin and McKeever (2000) concluded that relationships between families and professionals remain essentially exploitative rather than being based on a true partnership, and are driven by economic rather than humanitarian concerns. Others have reached similar conclusions, arguing that a medically orientated discourse still dominates care, and that collaboration is equated with compliance, with partnerships being evaluated largely by the extent to which family carers work in support of professionally derived goals and outcomes (Tamm 1999).

Ward-Griffin (2001) contends that professional carers, while being more aware of the needs of carers, still tend to denigrate, and thereby fail to value the emotional and intellectual knowledge that carers hold. She further asserts that professionals often lack the skills needed to engage in the complex negotiations that are required to reconcile potentially differing expectations, values and goals. However, the hegemony of professional knowledge is further reinforced by the fact that both professionals and family carers see professional expertise as being superior (Ward-Griffin 2001).

To some extent our data reinforce such conclusions, for while both family and professional carers aspire to the same goal – improving and maintaining the quality of life of the PWD – differences are apparent in their means to achieving this end. Others have identified such disparities and have argued that carers view professional support as being either 'connected' or 'disconnected' from their own efforts (Wuest and Stern 2001), or 'integrated' or 'disintegrated' with their care (Gilmour 2002). Care is seen as 'connected' when there is congruence of goals between carers and professionals (Wuest and Stern 2001). We would endorse this but add that, although goals do need to be congruent, there also needs to be agreement as to how such goals can be achieved. In order for care to be integrated, as opposed to disintegrated, Gilmour (2002) suggests that professionals should recognize the expertise of family carers and seek to mirror the patterns of care they provide. She asserts that recognition of 'the family caregiver as the authority on the personal and intimate care of the person with dementia, rather than the nurse, is fundamental to the development of a meaningful nurse–family relationship' (2002: 522).

Fundamentally it has to be recognized that differences in emphasis between family and professional carers are to be expected, as both groups come to the caregiving situation with different histories and expectations. A number of authors have argued that professional and family carers need to work together so that each can build on the strengths of the other. For example, Harvath *et al.* (1994) talk of 'cosmopolitan' and 'local' knowledge, the former being the type of generalized understanding of conditions such as dementia that arises from formal education and experience of many individuals with dementia. Conversely, 'local' knowledge is confined to a limited but in-depth understanding of a single or small number of cases as a result of having experienced a condition yourself, or having cared for an individual with a certain condition over an extended period of time. In a similar vein Liaschenko (1997) describes 'case' and 'person' knowledge. Case knowledge is a disembodied, biomedical understanding of a condition as a series of signs and symptoms; it is decontextualized and impersonal. Person knowledge, on the other hand, is an intimate understanding of the impact of a condition at an existential and experiential level – what it means to live a particular kind of life. For Liaschenko (1997), person knowledge comprises at least three domains: agency – the capacity to initiate meaningful action, with what is meaningful being largely an individual perception; temporality – the stage of the life cycle when a disease impacts and the effects it has on established routines and future aspirations; spatial dimensions – that is the spaces we occupy and the need to feel we belong somewhere both in terms of a physical space that we might call 'home' and a set of personal relationships. Straddling case and person knowledge is 'patient' knowledge, that is the effects of a disease on a particular 'body' and the knowledge that is needed to understand the type of support mechanisms that an individual can draw upon (Liaschenko 1997).

Clearly professionals in our interviews can lay claim to case knowledge and they also seem to believe that with sufficient information and continuity of relationships they can attain 'person' knowledge. Carers on the other hand have only a limited amount of 'case' knowledge, but clearly feel that they have the type of person knowledge to which professionals cannot hope to aspire. Applying Liaschenko's analysis it seems that what professionals claim as person knowledge is more likely to be 'patient' knowledge, and that for truly individualized care to be given then the intimate knowledge of the family carer has to be both fully acknowledged and valued. In this way 'best care' can only ever really be achieved through the 'blending' of case (cosmopolitan) knowledge with person (local) knowledge to achieve a genuine synthesis of two groups of experts.

For this to occur there has to be greater recognition of the fact that constructive relationships are the key to high-quality care and that in addition to the ability to provide quality technical care, paid carers must acquire the skills to initiate and sustain relationships and negotiate closeness and involvement (Piercey and Woolley 1999). This mandates a strengths-based approach to working with family carers and a realization that even experienced professionals require differing skills to help unravel the multifaceted and complicated contexts that are family care (Berg-Weger *et al.* 2001) (see also Lundh and Nolan, Chapter 6, this volume).

Intuitively and historically the possession of 'expertise' has been the domain of professionals; indeed, this is the foundation upon which professions rest. More recently, both politically and philosophically, there have been moves to go beyond paternalism and to recognize that lay knowledge is at least as important as professional knowledge. Only when this shift has occurred will genuine partnerships emerge (Barnes 1999). The question remains as to whether professionals, even obviously well-meaning and motivated ones, are ready for such a cognitive shift, or whether they will continue to see 'expert' family carers as a threat (Allen 2000a). Changing this perception represents one of the greatest barriers to forging relationships that promote best care for people with dementia.

## 5

# Partnerships with families over the life course

## Gordon Grant and Bridget Whittell

### Introduction

For some families, caregiving is invoked at a very early stage in the life course, continuing for many years, even in some cases until the death of the caregiver. This is not uncommon in families supporting children or adults with learning disabilities. For such families, caregiving is not so much episodic but a lifetime commitment. Over such extended periods parents of children with disabilities experience many changes in their struggles with identity as parents (Todd and Shearn 1996a); in the structure and functioning of their support networks (McGrath and Grant 1993; Bigby 1997a); in their use of effective coping strategies (Grant and Whittell 2000); in balancing caregiving with other family needs and expectations as well as external responsibilities such as employment (Warfield 2001), and hence in their capacity to lead enriched lives outside the compass of their caregiving. Running in parallel with the physical, psychological, intellectual and social development of their child over the life course, parents are also exposed for a very long time to the small incremental steps their child takes towards reaching adult status with all the ambiguities this can bring (Simpson 2000).

Over the life course, therefore, parents in particular, but also siblings, grandparents and other relatives, face many changes in what is going on around them. These are often referred to as transitions (May 2000) or, where some lasting effect in transitions is envisaged, as 'turning points' (Rutter 1996). Some of these changes may be predictable, others less so, but the precise occurrence of these, their timing in life stage, sequencing, duration or even interaction between them, remains a substantial challenge for life course research in general (Mills 2000), and for families with children or adults with learning disabilities in particular.

Given this background, we briefly review how family caregiving is textured, structured or constrained by life course considerations. Initially, therefore, we raise some questions and issues about the nature of the life course itself. Then, drawing from a study completed by the authors in 1998 about the coping strategies of families with children or adults with learning disabilities, we revisit some of the findings in light of contemporary policy thinking about family support. In an attempt to illustrate life course continuities and discontinuities that are judged by families and key workers to be important, we then introduce some case studies, drawing attention to partnership arrangements with frontline health and social care professionals.

## The life course

For Heinz and Kruger (2001), the life course is 'a major institution of integration and tension between individual and society that provides the social and temporal contexts for biographical planning and stock-taking as well as for ways of adapting to changes in public and private time and space' (p. 29). With modernization spreading all around the world, these authors argue that life course arrangements are becoming more dynamic, less predictable, but more self-directed. In such contexts agency, and with it the linked notions of choice and control, is central to any understanding of the relationship between social change and biography. According to Heinz and Kruger (2001), 'the trend towards destandardization and increasing individualization of the life course has been leading to more individual diversity in the timing of transitions, duration of institutional participation and sequencing of transitions' (p. 41). This means that with modernization the traditional assumptions that tend to be made about the life course – transitions to adulthood, employment, marriage, children and parenting, grandparenthood – may not hold. Moreover, these life domains may be rather less predictable and not follow a more traditional sequence. Even family structures themselves (Silva and Smart 2000) may be represented in much more diverse forms than conventionally experienced. How we look to the future and the roles we expect of different institutions like the family or public services will be shaped by such forces.

The life course also involves journeys along different time trajectories, each making their own demands on families. Of relevance here is what Mills (2000) refers to as cultural time, referring to the subjective conception, use and meaning ascribed to temporality within different cultures, from social time which includes norms, values and rules about the time at which life events are expected to occur. In other words there are normative expectations about when or under what circumstances certain life events are expected to occur – obtaining a first job, leaving home, getting married, for example. For families with disabled children or adults these normative expectations may not be fulfilled, or, if they are, then possibly not 'in time' when compared to their peers. This points to the importance of Mills's conception of social time. However, we know very little about whether these social time considerations hold for different cultures.

Zerubavel (1981) differentiates private time (which is designed to prevent or discourage the formation of human contact and to separate people from one another) from public time (which is designed to achieve the opposite). This is a central issue for families with children or adults with learning disabilities at home as most caregiving takes place in the privacy of home, and much of it is deliberately carried out in such a way as to make it invisible to the recipient and to health and social care professionals (Grant *et al.* 1998; Grant and Whittell 2001), though for different reasons. We say more about this later. How families negotiate their way between private time and public time is a centrally important question here that goes to the heart of the roles that health and social care professionals play in their lives over the life course.

Finally, Mills (2000) defines forms of time in relation to different institutional calendars, claiming that these are often neglected or underestimated. Among these are religious, family, educational, work/production, and gender-based calendars. These calendars, or clocks, are of course ticking away in parallel, acting as shaping factors in decision making across the life course.

## The life course, family caregiving and learning disability

Before introducing our own study there are one or two further observations to be made about the life course with particular reference to families supporting children or adults with learning disabilities.

There is some evidence of what Rutter (1996) was talking about when he referred to 'turning points' in people's lives where some sort of enduring psychological shift had taken place. In relation to the everyday experiences of parents, Scorgie and Sobsey (2000) for example have identified a range of transformational outcomes associated with their caregiving. They refer to these as *personal transformations* in relation to the acquisition of roles or traits, *relational transformations* in regard to family relationships, advocacy relationships, friendship networks and attitudes towards people in general, and *perspectival transformations* that concern changes in how people view life. Several points are of direct relevance here. First, such outcomes may not be so evident in research in which investigators examine only short-term responses to events or circumstances people face in everyday life. Secondly, citing Palus (1993), they suggest that though challenging events and circumstances may produce negative results initially, disclosure of disability being perhaps an obvious example, positive outcomes are usually slower to be realized, more enduring and of a higher order (e.g. a change in values or the ability to form satisfying relationships). We may add, thirdly, that a good deal of the family research literature in this field is still orientated towards family pathology, stress and stress responses (Helff and Glidden 1998). This not unnaturally reinforces a focus on problems, challenges and short-term imperatives rather than long-term adaptations and patterns of resilience by families.

Although the early stages of the parental career may be described in terms of 'biographical disruption' (Bury 1982) consequent upon disclosure of disability, a realignment of identity, an immersion in the world of invisible caregiving and the possible loss or curtailment of other social roles, much can be done through principled and evidence-based disclosure practice, genetic counselling, early counselling and family support services to mitigate negative adjustment and reinforce positive parenting (Pilnick *et al.* 2000; Robinson 2000).

Understanding the interplay between the ticking of the biological and psychological development clocks of the person with a learning disability as opposed to the life cycle clocks of parents and other family members appears to be crucial to gauging when, how and under what circumstances support services might engage families. Careful research by Todd and Shearn (1996b) has shown, for example, that services failed to acknowledge or understand how parents experienced time in its manifold trajectories, and that over time little was done to help parents to raise their aspirations for a 'typical' life:

> Additionally, since parents exerted little control over the timing of services they were allocated, they, therefore, struggled to lead lives that permitted a rich or diverse range of social participation, which they saw as typical for their peers. Thus, parents could be characterized as living 'out of time' not only in the sense of having deviated from the normative timing of family careers, but also in the sense that their non-parental lives were lived outside of the conventional times of adult society.
>
> (Todd and Shearn 1996b: 390)

In short, parents were not recognized as having identities outside their roles as parents. They were parents first and people second.

Equally, in the study we are going to say more about shortly, we have drawn attention to the undue reliance by professional workers on mothers as key informants about all the family circumstances and caregiving needs, leaving fathers as rather 'shadowy' characters whose needs, experiences, contributions to caregiving and interests outside caregiving appear to be even less well understood than those of mothers, to the point that they were even neglected (Grant and Whittell 2000). What this suggests is that there is as yet little appreciation by professionals of the dynamics and interdependencies within the life world of families supporting the person with a learning disability.

In much of the family caregiving research in this field only limited use has been made thus far of the concepts of clocks and calendars applied to the life course. By and large researchers have relied on temporal categorizations based on the chronological age or developmental stage of the child (Baker *et al.* 1997, for example), or on rather arbitrary age-based groupings of parents as we ourselves have done (Grant and Whittell 2001). We think this rather limited view will need to change.

## The family coping study

Fieldwork for the study was carried out over an 18-month period within two unitary authorities in Wales, ending in 1998. Further details about the localities, the study sample and methodology are available elsewhere (Grant and Whittell 1999, 2000, 2001) but some background information is pertinent here.

The study was established primarily to assess how families evaluated their strategies for coping, and to examine factors related to the diversity of effective coping strategies. It was also concerned with assessing how frontline professionals intervened in the lives of families, and with identifying if there were uniting principles guiding that practice, as influenced by organizational and policy factors. There was already an extensive literature about the coping behaviour of families, but little of this was related to ideas about what coping strategies actually worked. Further, there was even less evidence about what professionals did to recognize and reinforce effective coping by families.

Two sets of theoretical influences shaped the construction and design of the study. The first of these was coping theory that recognized the importance of cognitive appraisal processes in mediating responses to potentially challenging events and circumstances (Lazarus and Folkman 1984). The large body of literature that has followed Lazarus and Folkman's seminal work has pointed to the importance of internal resources (skills, experience, aptitudes, analytic capacities) and external resources (finance, support networks, services, for example) as mediating factors in coping. It has also validated the underlying thesis that the appraisal process is critical here, demonstrating that it extends not only to subjective evaluations of challenges and threats but also to an individual's capacity to respond (Orr *et al.* 1991; Quine and Pahl 1991, among others). The second set of theoretical influences can be attributed to the work of Antonovsky (1987) whose 'salutogenic' thesis was founded on the notion that, when challenged by circumstances that threaten normative expectations, people generally seek to 'make sense' of the situation. Without this, coping becomes difficult and even meaningless. Antonovsky also recognizes the importance of a person's ability to comprehend challenges and to manage them, but he asserts that without being able to manage the meaning of situations a person's sense of coherence will be out of balance.

A third influence, part theoretical and part empirical, emerged from the first two. This concerned the fact that, despite apparent adversities, discontinuities in their lives, episodic threats and stresses, and cumulative fatigue from caregiving, some families still managed to rise above everything or else 'bounce back', suggesting a capacity for buoyancy and resilience (Hawley and DeHaan 1996). We ourselves had observed that families commonly report uplifts and rewards from caregiving even under conditions of severe challenge and adversity (Grant *et al.* 1998), as have others (Stainton and Besser 1998; Scorgie and Sobsey 2000), suggesting that positive attributions of caregiving, no matter how apparently small or mundane these might appear to third parties, have some sort of role in sustaining people through life's vicissitudes. This is something that is being increasingly recognized in the wider literature on coping (Folkman 1997).

We used a mix of stratified and purposive sampling in generating our sample of 27 families. They were drawn to cover the entire life span: six were supporting young children aged 4 or less, six were supporting youngsters aged between 5 and 19 years, five were supporting adult relatives aged 20–34 years, a further five were supporting relatives aged 35–49 years, and a final five were supporting relatives aged 50 or more. We endeavoured to interview all adult family carers in the household. This resulted in 41 interviewees, 26 women and 15 men. Seventeen of the 27 families were headed by couples, and the remaining 10 were lone carer families, nine of whom were women. Eight of the lone carers were single or widowed. One of the remaining two lone carers was a sister and the other a cousin.

Interviews were semi-structured, tape-recorded and transcribed. Themes covered caregiving history, caregiving challenges, coping strategies using CAMI (Nolan *et al.* 1995), family strengths, general health, and service use. Following interviews with each family member we obtained their permission to interview their respective care managers or key workers though we do not report on data from those interviews here. Not all families had care managers and relationships with some of them were based on infrequent episodic contact. Accordingly these interviews covered themes about awareness of family coping strategies, assessment of family caregiving demands and outcomes, and approaches to intervention.

## What coping strategies were useful?

Family carers used a variety of problem-solving, cognitive and stress alleviation coping strategies, consistent with what has been reported in the literature (Quine and Pahl 1991; Nolan *et al.* 1996a). Although some strategies were widely used by some families, the usefulness of other coping strategies appeared to depend more on life stage, family structure and the caregiver's gender. Women identified a slightly higher proportion of useful coping strategies than men. They also used more instrumental problem-solving strategies than men, and displayed greater self-belief and self-confidence in their self-assessed capacity to handle situations. Men were more likely to defer to the caregiving experience and expertise of their partners.

Parents with disabled pre-school children were least confident about their experience and expertise as carers and had less self-belief in their ability to handle situations compared to other parents, reflecting perhaps their 'novice' status as carers. Family carers of school-aged children placed greater importance on problem-solving methods such as having a regular routine, trying options until one is found that works, and working to a clear set of priorities. Older family carers on the other hand appeared more resigned to their role and indicated more acceptance of the way things were now, but wished they had been more assertive in the past to get what they needed.

Here we detected in outline some life course shifts in coping, albeit based on crude age-based categorizations. Family carers with the youngest children were least experienced and lacked self-confidence compared to peers with older children. They relied much more on stress alleviation strategies like having a good cry, eating, drinking or smoking, or getting rid of excess energy through exercise compared to other families. Families with school-aged children by comparison were more prepared to test out different coping options, in this way extending their coping repertoires until they found something that worked. This group of parents perhaps faced the greatest normative challenges of all with their children reaching towards physical and biological maturity but not intellectual and social maturity like their peers. In this respect these parents were undoubtedly facing the most acute dissonance in relation to the management of social time: caregiving demands were high; managing requirements for privacy were difficult so there were tensions in maintaining a 'proper' balance between public and private time (Zerubavel 1981) especially when 'inappropriate' or 'challenging' behaviours of sons or daughters were displayed in public, or were considered to be at risk of so being played out; and opportunities to live a life outside caregiving were few or restricted. Family carers of older relatives had worked through this status passage and were more philosophical, relying on their own beliefs, values and sense of faith to get them through things. They were more adept at reframing the meaning of situations than younger families and in this sense were better able to retain a sense of coherence (Antonovsky 1987) in their lives even though some recognized their own dependency on having or keeping their son or daughter at home.

Lone family carers across the life span were among the most vulnerable for a variety of reasons. They were highly reliant on cognitive coping strategies, often because problem solving was not possible. In other words, they sometimes just had to grin and bear it when their son or daughter was too challenging or if their own energy resources were too depleted to respond in a more proactive way. Though some lone carers had siblings or relatives on whom they could depend it was telling to note that they tended not to judge help from these sources as helpful. They often lacked confidantes and as a result had to rely much more on their own resources, a dependency that was further reinforced by still rather fragmented family support services that were considered to pay lip service to the in-home and respite/short-term break needs of these families.

From case study evidence we now review whether relationships between these families and their frontline health and social care workers resembled features connotative of partnership working. Instead of reviewing any substantive theoretical perspectives about partnership working at this point we prefer instead to offer a brief commentary about the policy context in which the study took place, and how this has since moved on.

As already mentioned, the study took place in Wales. It was part of a commissioned programme of research examining the implementation and outcome of the All Wales Strategy (AWS) for the Development of Services for Mentally Handicapped People (Welsh Office 1983). The AWS was premised on participatory principles. For families it was expected that they would be involved in the preparation, implementation and monitoring of individual plans together with their disabled relative, and that these plans should not be the product of professional assessment alone. The day-to-day monitoring of the quality and development of services was to be seen as a responsibility shared between individual service providers, people with learning disabilities and families. Further, formal and informal arrangements for consulting with people with learning disabilities and their families were to be established to facilitate the strategic planning of services, the methods involved being left for local determination. Hence partnership working with families was expected at different levels and in relation to different functions, with fine detail to be worked out locally. No overarching model of partnership working was put forward. How well this was executed is discussed elsewhere (Felce *et al.* 1998).

More recent UK policy pronouncements about people with learning disabilities and their families have reinforced and expanded the vision set out by the AWS. In Wales the Learning Disability Advisory Group's report *Fulfilling the Promises* set out proposals for a framework for services for people with learning disabilities that commits to partnership work with people with learning disabilities and families. At the time of writing the report's proposals are under consideration by the National Assembly for Wales (NAW 2001). In England the White Paper *Valuing People* (DoH 2001c) has made far-reaching proposals designed to promote rights, independence, choice and inclusion for people with learning disabilities, but it too has underlined the importance of partnership working. A few details from each of these important documents helps to set the scene.

*Fulfilling the promises*

> From the beginning, the child and their family need to be at the centre of all decisions about their needs. This should enable families to be well informed and to feel in control of their lives. It follows that parents should be treated as equal partners in any planning processes.
>
> (p. 63)

> It is anticipated that person-centred individual planning will become the established process for considering individual need and appropriate delivery of support throughout the life span.
>
> (p. 66)

> Effective planning arrangements will require fully developed, collaborative partnerships which entitle service users and carers to make meaningful contributions into service provision and development.
>
> (p. 61)

*Valuing people*

> Carers face many problems and challenges. They need: more and better information; better assessment of their own needs; improved access to support services such as day services and short break services (respite care) particularly for those with more severe disabilities; to be treated as valued partners by local agencies, not as barriers to their son's or daughter's independence.
>
> (para 5.2, p. 53)

> The challenge is to ensure that carers: receive the right support to help them in their caring role; obtain relevant information about services; know who to approach for advice and help; are respected and treated as individuals in their own right; make their voices heard at national and local level.
>
> (para. 5.3, p. 54)

These are tall orders. In the case studies that follow we do not seek to use them as devices for evaluating these policy aspirations as it is our view that conceptual and operational details of partnership work are still being played out. One only has to look to the literature on person-centred planning, and even official guidance about PCP (Routledge and Sanderson 2002), to appreciate the rich diversity of models that have been developed, but little of which yet have a basis in outcome evaluation terms. Hence we know what can be done in working with people, but not yet in terms of what works well and makes a difference to the lives of people with learning disabilities and their families. Partnership working sounds sensible and attractive but it still appears to lack a solid evidence base. Hopefully the case studies that follow will shed some further light on this issue.

## Case studies

Three from our sample of 27 families have been selected to represent families at different points in the life course. For the purpose of this chapter we have focused on how families talked about their caregiving and the kinds of relationships they had with frontline service providers in health and social care services, including their care managers and key workers. Names have been changed to preserve anonymity.

### Fiona, Mel, Ian and John

Fiona was nearly 4 years old and was born with Down's syndrome. Fiona was Mel and Ian's first child. John, their second child was less than 2 years old. Mel and Ian were part of a large extended family. Mutual helping between siblings and between generations was the norm. Fiona and her family had received lots of help from community health and social care services and from hospitals. Fiona had been attending a nursery and integrated playgroup and she was being seen by a health visitor and speech therapist on a regular basis.

Mel's experience of Fiona's birth was traumatizing for several reasons:

*Mel*: She was born by emergency Caesarean and taken to [name of town]. I only saw her face for a couple of minutes and then she was gone, and because I had had a Caesarean I couldn't see her until nearly a week later . . . I walked into the room and there were six incubators and I didn't know which one was my daughter, and then I spent three days with them telling me she was fine, there was nothing wrong, and then on the third day they told me there was something wrong. I rejected her at first didn't I? [to husband]. I didn't want to know, but then I felt sorry for her. I don't really know how to describe it . . . With having a caesarean it didn't feel like she was mine. It was really strange . . . I just wanted to walk out and go but I didn't. I went back and this tiny little thing who was only the weight of a bag of sugar, so helpless.

The impact of being given contradictory information by doctors created serious short-term adjustment problems for Mel and Ian:

*Mel*: Well that came afterwards when they sat us down. They said she wouldn't be able to do this and wouldn't be able to do that. Then they said that she was fine, but then they said, 'Well, she still won't be able to do this and she still won't be able to do that', and we argued, didn't we? He [Ian] wanted her going in a home, and just kept thinking no, she's my daughter, my daughter. And it was only after her first birthday that anything sort of got back to normal, if you can call it normal.

Mel had been told on her own without Ian being present about Fiona's disability, even though the doctors knew that Ian was rushing to get to the hospital at the time. The combination of having expectations raised and dashed by being given contradictory information, and then by experiencing disclosure without the supportive presence of her husband, destroyed the key element of trust between the family and the helping professions:

> *Mel:*   I spoke to one of the paediatricians and I told him that it should never be done like that, and he agreed . . . I felt then that they had been behind my back and I didn't trust them for the rest of the time that Fiona was in hospital which was seven weeks. I found it quite hard for quite a while to trust anybody you know.

However, this also became a turning point for Mel in that she started to adopt a much more assertive style in her dealings with people about Fiona:

> *Interviewer:*   You lost your confidence in them for a while after that?
> *Mel:*           Yes. It's the same now. Even with me, when I go in and see a doctor myself, I just say, 'Tell me. I don't want any of this waffling', or whatever.
> *Interviewer:*   Just tell me straight away what there is to say?
> *Mel:*           It totally changed me. It made me more outgoing and more 'I want this doing and I want it doing now.'

Over time, however, both Mel and Ian came through their grieving, but triggering events even like the negative one described here acted as a platform for adopting a re-evaluated position on coping with situations. Mel's mother played an important role at this time in breaking the news to other family members and friends, so that by the time Mel returned home everyone was most supportive and her worst fears about Fiona's rejection never materialized. This aided Mel's adjustment enormously.

Mel and Ian have largely left the diagnosis, the label, the fears and the anger behind, and have since come to regard Mel as a person with her own emerging identity who contributes things to family life and who, in their view, has proved the doctors wrong:

> *Mel:*   She's loving. She brightens up your day. Most people say that. She's like a little ray of sunshine, a pain in the neck like, but . . . I think personally it has made us better people.
> *Ian:*   For somebody who was supposed to be an absolute cabbage from what we were told first to what she is, she is a miracle.
> *Interviewer:*   Proved them all wrong?
> *Ian:*   Yes, totally wrong.

*Comment*

Mel and Ian's initial experiences of engaging health services, immediately following Fiona's birth, were of a preoccupation with Fiona to the exclusion of Ian. Their normative expectations about being together at the moment of the disclosure of disability were ignored, and hence their sense of social time (Mills 2000) was immediately thrown out of kilter. But then even this was compounded by vacillating clinical opinions which meant that their social time horizons were having to be adjusted and readjusted in rapid succession. Mel and Ian's story also provides some further evidence about ways in which negative encounters or circumstances can trigger an enduring psychological shift or transition (Rutter 1996). In their case it seemed to signal a more mistrustful but assertive stance with all the helping professions for years to come. Finally, despite Fiona's tender age, we also witness the parental discourse shifting from Fiona as an object, a thing (bag of sugar) to a young human being contributing to family life and with a personality invoking love and reciprocities.

*Darren, Jane, Phil, Joe and Molly*

Darren was 17 years of age and lived at home with his mum, Jane, and his two bothers Phil and Joe, and sister Molly. Jane was divorced. Her ex-husband rarely saw the family. All Jane's children were in their teens.

Jane has never had a 'proper' diagnosis of Darren's problems from anyone, even though it has been obvious that he has had learning difficulties for many years. He has attended a local special school but for the last seven years Jane has been trying to come up with an explanation for Darren's very challenging behaviours. Though she had come to the view that Darren had Attention Deficit Hyperactivity Disorder (ADHD) this had not been confirmed by doctors, not least because both she and they have been reluctant to put a label on him. Meanwhile coping with Darren keeps Jane in a state of constant alert, as is obvious from her summing up of the main challenges of everyday care:

> Jane: Just to keep him out of danger really. Even now he trips on his own shadow. I have to constantly tell him – he does a lot for himself now – I drum it into him to put the cold water in first when you run a bath. I have a mop for the floor . . . He used to have the water high up. He is so active. It just takes a second . . .

The implied reference to clear and present danger was something that permeated all the arrangements for Darren's support and care at home, with the inevitable consequences for Jane:

> Interviewer: So you don't have enough private time for yourself. How do you deal with that?
>
> Jane: I don't have any time when he is around really, not even to bath in. I couldn't stay there for 20 minutes and shave my

> legs etc. because there's nobody here to watch him . . . You can't relax properly.
>
> *Interviewer:*  You can never be on your own time, just for you?
>
> *Jane:*  No, except for when he was in hospital and I realized what normal living was like. I hadn't had that you see.
>
> *Interviewer:*  Sorry?
>
> *Jane:*  Normal living. To be able to sleep; to be able to use the bathroom when wanted; to be able to have tea when I wanted rather than sticking to the same routine with tea at five. Sticking to what he knows because what he knows is easier for him and it just makes it easier for everyone then, because if you take him out of something, he doesn't understand.

In this regard Jane and her family had become captives to Darren's needs with routines fixed to provide a necessary structure to aid both their coping and Darren's understanding of normative arrangements governing everyday life. Finding time to address all her children's needs was far from easy. Phil was in constant trouble with the police. Joe and Molly had more 'typical' lifestyles but they were described as having 'little patience' with Darren. Material circumstances made coping more difficult too. The family had no car and even travelling on the bus with Darren was hazardous because of his agitated state:

> *Jane:*  He wants to go off talking to people and moving from seat to seat.
>
> *Interviewer:*  He's too agitated and active?
>
> *Jane:*  Yes, and he pulls cords on the trains so it's very, very hard taking him on public transport. I only take him on public transport in emergencies.

Jane had had no holiday for years and little in the way of short-term breaks for Darren. However, in between the first and second interviews with Jane a place had been offered to Darren in a nearby community home, and this had been taken up. It made the world of difference:

> *Jane:*  But I realize now that I've had the break that I couldn't do it all the time again now. I couldn't do it. I don't know where I got the energy from or the patience.

Jane's care manager, a community nurse, had been instrumental in sorting things in this way and in helping the family, and Darren, to move on. From Jane's point of view it was he who made the difference in helping her to navigate this important turning point, giving her the opportunity to give her other children more attention and to give herself what had been a missing commodity in her life to date, time for herself.

Outwardly Darren looked 'normal' so, according to Jane, people expected him to 'act normal'. When he failed to do so Jane frequently found herself the butt of criticism from neighbours and strangers, blaming her for not bringing Darren up right. It was virtually impossible for her to avoid this constantly critical gaze.

## Comment

Jane had been a captive to time throughout her adult life. With four children to bring up, almost single-handedly, she had had little private time for herself. Darren's needs, however, had dominated the whole household such that a 'normal' lifestyle had become impossible. The constant demands made it hard for Jane to relax, sleep or enjoy things outside caregiving. Life was a battleground littered by multitudes of provoking agents from which she got no respite. It was a question of living from day to day, helped by structures and routines of her own making to create a predictable and safe environment for Darren. Darren's more recent move to a community home had changed all that, opening up the prospects of a return to an ordinary lifestyle. This once again illustrates another 'turning point' (Rutter 1996) in the life of the family, albeit one occasioned by the onset of a crisis.

## Cherie, Liz and Bob

Cherie still lived with her parents despite being 38 years of age. Her parents, Bob and Liz, were in their seventies and late sixties respectively. Liz and Bob were also grandparents. Their son, Frank, was married with a young son of his own but Frank had moved away and was described as having 'lost touch' with his sister and parents. Liz and Bob had lived in the area for several years and had a good network of friends and neighbours who empathized with their circumstances and offered practical help from time to time, including in-home help for Cherie on occasions when Liz and Bob had to be away from home for short periods. Cherie attended a local day centre and once weekly a short-term breaks home, providing her with opportunities to engage in different activities and socialize with a range of familiar people while also affording her parents some respite.

Cherie could only speak a few words, an outward expression of being someone with an autistic spectrum disorder. Communication was difficult. According to Liz:

It makes you frustrated with her ... the speech ... with there not being the contact. She doesn't give you the love ... And yet there's flickers of it occasionally, I do know that. You know what I mean. In fact it's like getting blood from a stone to get her to talk. So when that time comes when she probably has about 10 days of talking it's lovely, even though it all gets mixed up. It makes me feel so much better.

Cherie's talk was depicted by Liz as not having changed since she was a baby. Like many of their older parental peers, Liz and Bob found wrestling with a problem like this not only taxing, with occasional 'breakthroughs', but also in the end insoluble. Throughout their life they had replayed over and again that moment of realization when they were forced to accept Cherie's difficulties:

*Interviewer*:  So what impact did it have when you found that Cherie had problems?

*Liz*:  Devastating. I am still upset now. But what can you do? We keep trying but nobody seems to know, except it could be this vaccine damage. One doctor mentioned it, but you're left in the dark.

Even with Cherie's attendance at the day centre and respite home, and despite being retired, Liz and Bob still felt the social restrictions of their continued caregiving:

*Liz*:  I don't suppose we do have enough private time really, but we don't mind.

Liz and Bob described themselves as being 'resigned' to carrying on with caring for Cherie out of sheer love for her, but they were reminded almost every day that their private problem was also an unavoidably public one. A good example of this was the strategy for managing the public presentation of Cherie's communication difficulties:

*Liz*:  You try to explain to people. The taxi driver said the other day, 'Good morning Cherie', and she just stared, and I felt surely he'd understand. You cannot keep on, can you? We cannot make it an issue every day. You have to try to act normal, which we do . . .

Liz and Bob were at a time of life when it was difficult to avoid thoughts about the future for Cherie, especially after they were no longer there for her. So, although they were constantly being reminded of the past, the future was making claims on their hearts and minds too:

*Bob*:  We are in it together. I have a wife who doesn't show her emotions very much, just gets on with it. We have cried many a time, not so much lately because there's no sense in crying, but years ago we used to break down when we knew there was no hope, but not just lately because you get harder and say, 'Well, the problem now is what will happen when we are not here', because when you are gone you cannot do anything about it. We don't quarrel about it, just get on with it and be as happy as we can. I get a bit down, but I snap out of it.

Cherie, Liz and Bob had had a care manager for years and had a good relationship with him. Liz and Bob looked upon him as being approachable and as someone whom they could talk to openly and in confidence about their own needs as carers. The same could not be said of their relationship with the general practice:

> *Liz*: I think the only person who has been unhelpful is the doctor. Once Cherie was having problems with headaches and the young fellow said, 'What's the matter with her?' because they don't know. They should look, but that's everybody with doctors. Instead of having all your notes he was just clueless. Is she on the change or something like that?

On a more recent occasion Liz described an encounter with the general practice in which access for Cherie to the practice nurse had to be brokered by the GP. It concerned pills prescribed by the doctor for menopausal problems, which had had side effects about which they had not been informed. All Liz had wanted to do was speak to the practice nurse about this over the phone but the practice protocol demanded a visit first to see the doctor, which meant a lot of waiting around, making Cherie tense. Dealing even with apparently predictable health issues therefore was frustratingly complex.

*Comment*

Liz and Bob seemed to be living in three time dimensions at the same time – the past, the present and the future. Important aspects of the past such as the conditions giving rise to Cherie's autistic spectrum disorder were far from resolved and were still being replayed after all these years. Their consciousness of future demands for Cherie's support and care had become even more pressing, and at the time of interview were also unresolved. Though having partly accommodated restrictions on the use of their private time, they were still having to deal with confrontations between the management of private and public time (Zerubavel 1981), especially when seeking opportunities for Cherie's social inclusion. But even engaging the health service with Cherie proved to be unnecessarily time-consuming and complicated, and there was a lack of recognition of and sensitivity to the age-related health demands of her 'biological' clock. Like many other older parents Liz and Bob were seeking a life 'as normal' as possible, but accepting the restrictions that came with it. Their lifestyle could indeed be depicted as a struggle with time (Todd and Shearn 1996b).

## Discussion

From the case studies it can be seen that families have everyday experiences reflecting their position in the life course. It seems that, no matter how hard services and frontline professional workers tried to make life easier for these families, discontinuities and biographical disruptions (Bury 1982) were still common. Put another way, we could say that the calendars of services, health services in particular, and the life course time-tables of families were out of synch.

In the case of Fiona, Mel, Ian and John, services not only failed to syn-chronize the disclosure of Fiona's disability with Mel and Ian but managed to convey contradictory information to them about Fiona's disability over a period of days. With Jane and her family, there was a failure to acknowledge the lack of private time and personal resources available to Jane and her other children and a need for more timely intervention to ease the problem. With Cherie, Liz and Bob the demands of Cherie's biological clock seemed beyond the understanding of the GP and in any case Cherie's participation in the consultation was all but avoided. Liz and Bob meanwhile were struggling in managing private and public time (Zerubavel 1981) and in accommodating caregiving's past, present and future demands.

The case studies illustrate how families experience their caregiving on a number of different but parallel time trajectories. Accommodating these appears to be difficult but something that can in the end be managed, up to a point. Services, however, seemed to have even greater difficulties recognizing these trajectories and what they meant to families. Inter-ventions therefore were too often adjudged by families to be untimely or unhelpful. In the case of Fiona it was very evident how the disclosure experience destroyed an essential element of trust, affecting Mel and Ian for a considerable time, but in the end provoking them into adopting a very different and more assertive style of coping with things. The long-term effects of such 'turning points' (Rutter 1996) on future coping styles are not well understood. However, even in their case we can see that over time, albeit less than four years, they were able to disprove negative clinical prognoses. Each case in its own way also provides further evidence of transformational outcomes associated with caregiving (Scorgie and Sobsey 2000), reflecting ways in which families made sense of their cir-cumstances (Antonovsky 1987). Because these 'salutogenic' outcomes were typically slow to be realized and often buried within the minutiae of caregiving experiences, captured within the hearts or mindsets of parents, they were less obvious to professional workers and therefore rarely acted upon by them.

It would be fair to say that none of the case study families felt 'in con-trol' of their lives. Neither were they receiving the right support to help them in their caring role at their different life stages. In these regards visionary policy expectations published in the last two years (DoH 2001c; NAW 2001) are still far from being realized.

Interview data from the wider sample of families provided further evidence about the relationship between position in the life course and the types of coping strategies that were adopted by families. The findings reinforce the case studies in that they suggest that the idea of 'transition' needs to be applied right across the life course, and not just to the undeni-ably important transition between the child and adult world that appears to permeate learning disability policy thinking (DoH 2001c). For families there are twists and turns at every stage. A more concerted commitment to unravel the relationship between the life course, biography and family caregiving arrangements might help professionals to develop more sensitive models of partnership working.

## Acknowledgements

The research was carried out with the help of a grant from the Welsh Office/Department of Health for which we are grateful. We would also like to thank the families who participated in this study. Views expressed in the chapter are those of the authors and should not be taken to represent the position of the research commissioning bodies.

# 6

## 'I wasn't aware of that': creating dialogue between family and professional carers

Ulla Lundh and Mike Nolan

### Introduction

According to Johansson (2001), 'One of the cornerstones of the postwar Swedish welfare system has been that former family responsibilities should be taken over by the state' (p. 2). Consequently there has been little expectation that the family would provide care for its frail older members. Recently, however, a combination of factors, including economic recession, has resulted in the 'rediscovery' of the family as the major providers of support for people who need help to remain in their own homes (Johansson 2001). The Swedish government has therefore instigated several reforms intended to improve services for older people (Socialdepartementet 1998), including greater recognition of the need to support family carers (Socialstyrelsen 1998). Indeed, the provision of appropriate and timely support and information for family carers is now a policy priority (Vårdalstylesen 1999), with a total of some 300 million Swedish crowns being allocated by the Swedish government to develop support services for carers over a three-year period (Socialstyrelsen 1999). If such developments are to be of maximum benefit it is essential to be clear as to the form such support should take and when is the most appropriate time to provide it (Johansson 2001).

This chapter reports the results of a study funded by the Swedish National Board of Health and Welfare, the aim of which was to explore carers' perceived needs and consider the implications for the development of support services. Furthermore, as professionals in Sweden have not traditionally engaged families as partners, the study also highlighted the impact of such a model of working on professionals' views of the circumstances of family carers. Prior to undertaking the empirical component of the study, a detailed review of the relevant international literature was conducted so as to highlight trends in service developments for carers that might inform the Swedish situation (see Lundh and Nolan 2001). In setting this chapter in context a brief overview of this review is provided here.

## Why support family carers?

Although there is now widespread recognition of the need to support family carers, appropriate services have often been relatively slow to develop (Twigg and Atkin 1994; Nolan *et al.* 1996a; Askham 1998; Banks 1999), and while carers are now a policy priority throughout the developed world most services still focus on the needs of the cared-for person (Heaton *et al.* 1999; Lothian and McKee 2000). If this situation is to improve two key questions need to be addressed:

- What are the aims and purposes of supporting family carers and what types of interventions are needed?
- How can family and professional carers work together most effectively in providing best care?

Generally speaking, services to support family carers have been designed primarily to 'keep carers caring' (Nolan *et al.* 1996a), by reducing caregiver stress, maintaining the caring relationship and thereby preventing institutionalization (Collins *et al.* 1994; Zarit *et al.* 1999; Borgermans *et al.* 2001). Recently there have been calls for a more holistic approach and a broader conceptualization of the type of outcomes that can be expected and the range of services that need to be provided (Banks 1999; Qureshi *et al.* 2000). Central to these debates is the development of partnerships between family and professional carers (Banks 1999; DoH 1999; Qureshi *et al.* 2000; Borgermans *et al.* 2001) so that carers are empowered to make decisions and to take greater control of their lives (Schmall 1995; Brandon and Jack 1997; Askham 1998). Underpinning such a partnership is a broader definition of carer support such as that provided by Askham (1998) who concluded that carer support can be defined as any action which helps a carer to:

- decide to take up, or not to take up, a caring role;
- continue in a caring role;
- end a caring role.

Such a model clearly recognizes the temporal dimensions of caregiving and highlights the need for flexible and sensitive services which are responsive to the needs of carers as they vary over time. With regard to the outcomes of interventions Qureshi *et al.* (2000) contend that these fall into one of four domains:

- to maintain or enhance the quality of life of the cared-for person;
- to maintain or enhance the quality of life of the carer and to recognize that although caring is important it is also essential to have a life outside caring;
- to recognize and support the role of carers so that they feel informed, prepared, equipped and trained as appropriate;
- to deliver services in a way that makes carers feel valued as individuals, which recognizes their expertise and allows them to have a say in the way services are provided, and to ensure that services are consistent with existing caregiving routines.

Creating partnerships with carers will require a considerable reorientation of professional practice, with a move away from the 'unshakeable conviction' in the superiority of professional knowledge (Brandon and Jack 1997) and an acknowledgement that carers are also 'experts' in their own situation (Nolan *et al.* 1996a). However, accepting 'carers as experts' does not mean that professionals do not also have valuable knowledge and expertise. Rather the 'carers as experts' approach sees the carer as *an* expert rather than *the* expert (Lundh and Nolan 2001), and it is essential to recognize that carers, professionals and, importantly, cared-for persons all have a key role to play.

If more fruitful partnerships are to develop Borgermans *et al.* (2001) call for a family- and person-centred approach to assessment based on a common language and framework, the purpose of which is to identify a carer's need for support and to plan an individualized programme of help that builds upon existing strengths and resources. They define assessment as 'an interactive, personalized, contextual and determined helping relationship aimed at the provision of effective support of both the family carer and the cared-for person within the resources available' (Borgermans *et al.* 2001: 9).

The person-centred approach which they promote is based upon the following premises:

- Both the carer and the cared-for person have equal consideration.
- Assessment must include the perspectives of all the major stakeholder groups including carer, client, professional and agency.
- Assessment should be individual and multi-dimensional, recognizing that needs will change over time.
- Consideration of the nature and quality of the relationship between carer and cared-for person is essential.
- Value judgements about a carer's ability and willingness to care must be avoided.
- Good assessment requires the creation of a genuine partnership which recognizes and values multiple sources of expertise.

Others have also recently asserted that assessment must be based on individual need, with the outcomes of interventions being defined at least in part from a carer's perspective (Qureshi *et al.* 2000). A consideration of the international literature suggested an emerging consensus about the principles underpinning the assessment of family carers, and the study sought to explore the potential impact of such a process within a Swedish context.

## Background and method

Starting in 2000 the National Board of Health and Welfare in Sweden allocated 10 million US dollars (100 millions SKr) for each of the following three years to the 289 Swedish municipalities for developing support services for family carers. To be eligible for this money each municipality had to appoint coordinators in their area. In the present study six out of 13 coordinators in the county of Östergötland were asked to nominate professionals working in their area to act as data collectors for the project. Twenty-two individuals with varying backgrounds including nurses, professionals from the home help service, an occupational therapist, and a lay worker from the church were nominated. The main purpose of the study was to identify as many family carers as possible in each municipality, including those who were not already known to the home help service or district nurses and then to interview them to gain a better understanding of their caring situations so as to help inform future service development. To recruit carers, information about the project was distributed via newspaper articles and leaflets were left in public places such as pharmacies, healthcare centres, libraries and so on. Individuals who came forward were given oral and written information about the interview and were informed of their right to withdraw from the study whenever they wanted.

In order to gather information about the caregiving situation a structured questionnaire was used, comprising the three carer assessment indices devised by Nolan *et al.* (1998) (Carers' Assessment of Difficulties Index – CADI, Carers' Assessment of Satisfactions Index – CASI, Carers' Assessment of Managing Index – CAMI), together with additional questions identified by the home care service. The three instruments designed by Nolan *et al.* (1998) provide insights into: situations which carers see as stressful; how carers deal with stress in their caring situations; and their views on the satisfactions they experience from caring. These instruments were developed following extensive reviews of the literature and in-depth interviews with carers. They have been widely tested in Great Britain, Europe, North America and Australasia. They had been forward and backward, translated in Swedish and validated in previous studies (see Lundh 1999).

In the current study these indices were complemented by additional questions considered to be useful by the home care sector. In total 245 interviews were conducted, with each interview taking between 1½ and 3 hours. Data were loaded for computer analysis using SPSS Windows.

## Focus group interviews

When data collection was completed three focus group interviews were undertaken with 14 of the 22 interviewers in order to explore their perceptions of the assessment process and to consider the impact of the interviews on their view of carers' needs. Each focus group was tape-recorded and took about 1½ hours. Analysis of these data provided fascinating additional insights into the impact of the assessment process and how it influenced the way professionals viewed family carers. These data have a number of implications for interventions and also the relationships between professional and family carers, which will be considered later.

## Results

Before presenting these two sets of results attention is turned briefly to the sample characteristics. The majority of the carers were women (77 per cent), with 64 per cent caring for a spouse (n = 157), 21 per cent for a parent (n = 51) and 15 per cent for others (n = 37). Most respondents lived in the same household as the cared-for person (68 per cent) and of those who did not the majority (76 per cent) lived within five kilometres. In most cases the caring relationship was prolonged, ranging from less than one year to 66 years (mean = 6 years). Twenty-seven per cent of carers had gainful employment outside the home, mostly part-time (73 per cent). The age of the cared-for person varied from 10 to 95 years (mean = 76) with 22 per cent suffering from severe memory loss and most requiring help with several activities of daily living.

Carers were generally providing care to an older frail group of relatives who had considerable support needs, particularly with domestic tasks and to a lesser extent with washing/showering, toileting, dressing and grooming. However, despite the physical demands of caring and its restrictive nature, carers in the sample were more likely to identify satisfactions than they were difficulties and from their own perspective they had developed several very effective ways of coping. Knowledge such as this is essential if individually tailored and relevant packages of care are to be devised.

For the present purposes the quantitative results are summarized in five tables which respectively feature: the most frequent difficulties encountered by the respondents, together with their appraisal of how stressful each difficulty is (Table 6.1); the major sources of satisfaction (Table 6.2); and the most used and helpful coping strategies (Tables 6.3, 6.4 and 6.5). For brevity only frequently occurring sources of difficulty (reported by over 50 per cent of respondents), sources of satisfaction (reported by over 80 per cent of respondents), and ways of coping (reported by over 70 per cent of respondents) are included. This should not be taken to mean that difficulties, satisfactions or coping strategies reported less frequently are unimportant, rather that they have less to say about the types of services that might be needed by the majority of carers. While first and foremost the carer indices were designed to help create a dialogue between carers and professionals in order to facilitate an in-depth understanding of each unique caregiving situation, the aggregate data are more useful in informing decisions about the broad range of services that are needed, always remembering that these must be sufficiently flexible and able to adapt to carers' unique circumstances.

## The most frequent and most stressful difficulties of caring and their implications for service design and delivery

Table 6.1 presents the most frequent and most stressful difficulties of caring (as reported by over 50 per cent of respondents) categorized by: the restrictive nature of caring; the physical demands of caring; the difficulties caring can cause in relationships and the emotional effects of caring. Column 1 contains the percentage of the 245 respondents

**Table 6.1** Most frequent difficulties and how stressful they are

|  | % experiencing | % seeing as stressful |
|---|---|---|
| *Difficulties relating to the restrictive nature of caregiving (n = 245)* | | |
| Not having enough private time for myself | 76 | 84 |
| Not being able to take a break or holiday | 73 | 84 |
| Having a restricted social life | 65 | 83 |
| Not being able to see friends as I'd like | 59 | 81 |
| *Difficulties relating to the physical demands of caregiving* | | |
| Feeling physically tired | 68 | 85 |
| Having to give a lot of physical care | 68 | 65 |
| Caring for someone with mobility problems | 66 | 79 |
| *Difficulties with caring relationships* | | |
| Feeling the cared-for person plays me up | 61 | 77 |
| Feeling the cared-for person demands too much of me | 57 | 72 |
| Caring putting a strain on family relationships | 56 | 77 |
| *Emotional impact of caring* | | |
| Feeling out of control of the situation | 57 | 75 |
| Being unable to relax because of worrying about caring | 51 | 77 |

who reported having to deal with this aspect of caregiving and column 2 indicates the percentage of those reporting each difficulty who found it to be stressful (either causing a great deal of, or some, stress). So, for example, the most frequently reported difficulty was 'not having enough private time for myself' (reported by 76 per cent or 186 respondents). Of these 186 respondents 84 per cent (or 158) found this aspect of caring to be stressful.

As Table 6.1 demonstrates, the most frequently experienced and the most stressful aspects of caring for this sample related to the restrictions it places on carers' lives in terms of: not having enough private time for themselves; not being able to take a break or a holiday; having a restricted social life and not being able to see friends as often as they would like.

Such restrictions were experienced frequently and were seen as being stressful by over eight out of ten carers who experienced them. These data highlight the importance of services such as respite care which allow carers to enjoy other aspects of their lives (including employment where appropriate). Some indication of the things carers might look for in a good-quality break can be gleaned from the satisfactions data and this is discussed in more detail shortly.

Table 6.1 also indicates that the physical aspects of care, as might be expected, exert a toll. Feeling physically tired, having to provide large amounts of physical care, and caring for someone with mobility problems are all seen as stressful. This reinforces the importance of more 'traditional' services which provide assistance with direct caregiving. However, as with respite, these services need to be reliable and consistent if they are to be of maximum benefit, and the quality of any 'hands-on' care provided must be to the satisfaction of family carers if it is to be accepted.

More diffuse, but still stressful aspects of caring can cause difficulties in the relationship between the carer and the cared-for person or between the carer and his/her wider family. Difficulties in the relationship between carer and cared-for person are major causes of stress in caring, particularly where there are differences in the expectations of the carer and cared-for person (Nolan *et al.* 1996a).

The limited empirical work on the interactions between carer and cared-for person suggests that when each party is sensitive to the needs of the other then interactions are likely to be positive and proactive rather than angry and demanding (Cox and Dooley 1996). Conversely, in situations where carers feel that the demands of the cared-for person are unreasonable, or are inconsistent with their own beliefs, then fragile and possibly abusive relationships are more likely (Phillips and Rempusheski 1986; Steinmetz 1988; Nolan 1993). In such circumstances efforts to 'enrich' relationships can be helpful and this is an area in which there is considerable potential to design more innovative and imaginative services. Such interventions need not be complex and, as we will illustrate later, simply 'creating a space for dialogue' by giving carers 'permission' to discuss difficult and sensitive issues can often be sufficient.

The importance of attending to the emotional consequences of caring (such as feeling out of control or unable to relax) are also apparent in our data. Carers like to feel that they are 'doing caring well' (Schumacher *et al.* 1998) and that they are confident and competent to care (Brereton and Nolan 2000). However, many carers learn their skills by trial and error, and much could be done to help them to develop the skills they require in a more structured fashion (see Nolan *et al.* 1996a).

These data indicate that the difficulties of caregiving are diverse and complex and extend far beyond the physical act of caring (as important as this might be). This must be borne in mind when eligibility for services is considered, which too often is based primarily on the amount of care given. An undue emphasis on the 'tangible' aspects of care may well result in the most stressed carers being denied support (Levesque *et al.* 1995; Nolan *et al.* 1996a).

Moreover, assessment of need should not focus only on the difficulties of caring, as a complete picture will not be gained unless caregiving satisfactions and coping strategies are also included.

## Sources of satisfactions in caring and their implications for supporting family carers

Until recently relatively little attention has been given to the satisfactions of caring. However, it is now more widely accepted that carers experience many types of satisfaction and that satisfactions are at least as prevalent as sources of burden (Grant and Nolan 1993; Nolan *et al.* 1996a; Grant *et al.* 1998; Lundh 1999; Nolan and Lundh 1999). This was clearly the case in the present sample. Table 6.2 provides an indication of the major sources of satisfaction experienced by our respondents (this comprises statements that at least 80 per cent of respondents found a great deal or some satisfaction). To help with interpretation the sources of satisfaction have been divided into two main categories: those relating primarily to the cared-for person and those relating primarily to the carer.

As will be seen from Table 6.2, almost half of the items on CASI (14/30) applied and were perceived as satisfying by at least 80 per cent of the respondents, at levels much higher than those reporting sources of burden or difficulty. Importantly, those items that were seen to apply frequently were also identified as providing satisfaction in almost every instance. This gives an indication of the pivotal role of satisfactions to an understanding of the experience of family care. It is also important to note that while Table 6.2 includes only those sources of satisfaction seen to apply by over 80 per cent of respondents, only 1 of the 30 items in CASI applied to less than 50 per cent of the respondents (caring helps to stop me feeling guilty), giving yet another indication of the extensive nature of satisfactions in caring.

**Table 6.2** Major sources of satisfaction

| | Applies % | Satisfying % |
|---|---|---|
| *Satisfaction related to the cared-for person* | | |
| Seeing cared-for person clean, comfortable and well turned out | 97 | 100 |
| Being able to maintain cared-for person's dignity | 95 | 99 |
| Helping cared-for person overcome difficulties | 96 | 99 |
| Tending to cared-for person's needs | 92 | 100 |
| Getting pleasure from seeing cared-for person happy | 88 | 97 |
| Feeling you gave the best care | 85 | 95 |
| Keeping cared-for person out of an institution | 83 | 94 |
| *Satisfaction related to the carer* | | |
| Feeling wanted and needed | 97 | 96 |
| Knowing you've done your best | 93 | 94 |
| Enjoying helping people | 93 | 98 |
| Caring being an expression of love | 88 | 96 |
| Feeling appreciated by the cared-for person | 84 | 94 |
| Being able to test yourself out in caring | 83 | 98 |
| Feeling appreciated by family and friends | 82 | 98 |

Recognizing such sources of satisfaction can be useful in:

• identifying carers who may be in need of more support;
• thinking about the type of support that might be needed;
• thinking about ways of judging the quality of the support provided.

If attention is turned to the latter area first, several studies indicated that the uptake of services to support carers is often low. Respite care (or short breaks) provides a case in point. The need for a break from caring is well established but despite this carers can be reluctant to use such services (Briggs and Askham 1999; Moriarty 1999; Pickard 1999). One of the main reasons for this is that they have concerns about the quality of care that the cared-for person receives. Table 6.2 provides a good indication of the likely sources of such concern. It is quite clear that the majority of respondents feel that, because of their intimate knowledge of the cared-for person, they are able to give the 'best' care (86 per cent). Indeed, the desire to give 'best' care is one of the major motivations in caring (Brereton and Nolan 2000; Qureshi *et al.* 2000). Some of the main dimensions of 'best care' become apparent from Table 6.2. Obviously it is crucial that the cared-for person has his/her needs tended to and is clean and comfortable, but this alone is not sufficient. Care also has to be delivered in a way that maintains the dignity of that person and provides him/her with opportunities to overcome difficulties and to experience pleasure and happiness. Carers' desire in this regard must be accounted for when support services are designed.

The second area in which an appreciation of the satisfactions of caring can inform the design and delivery of services to support family carers is to stimulate thinking about the types of intervention needed. As the major focus of research in family care has been on burden it is not surprising that most interventions have also concentrated on reducing stress (Zarit *et al.* 1999). Far less attention has been given to the therapeutic benefits of increasing satisfactions in caring, despite the fact that it has been recognized for some time that the 'silver lining effect', that is seeing the positive side of situations, can be a very powerful way of coping (Summers *et al.* 1989, see also later under ways of coping with caring).

There has been some work in this area with, for example, Cartwright *et al.* (1994) arguing that attempts to 'enrich' caring relationships by devising ways in which carers and cared-for persons can either maintain their 'customary routines' (that is helping them to continue with activities which give shared pleasure) or identify 'innovative routine breakers' (that is finding new ways of gaining shared pleasure) can be an effective way of improving caring relationships.

Similarly, it can be therapeutic simply to help carers to identify the types of satisfactions that they experience, and reflecting upon such aspects can be very important, as they are easily lost in the 'long haul' of daily care (Rolland 1994).

Despite these potentially very positive sources of satisfaction, it is vital to recognize that they are not experienced by all carers, and that realization of this can raise delicate and sensitive issues (Keady 1999; Qureshi *et al.* 2000, also see later under focus group discussion). This brings us to the third area in which a consideration of satisfactions might be useful, that is in identifying carers in need of further support.

It has been recognized for some time that carers who experience mutuality (that is reward and meaning) in caregiving (Hirschfield 1981, 1983) are less likely to give up care. It has also been demonstrated that carers who find satisfaction in what they do are likely to be less stressed, often significantly so (Archbold *et al.* 1992). On this basis it has been argued that a lack of mutuality in caring relationships (affection, gratification and meaning) should be taken very 'seriously' as an indicator of 'potentially fragile' caring situations (Archbold *et al.* 1992). We would suggest that a consideration of the satisfactions of caring is essential and helps to focus on quality of care and quality of relationships, in addition to providing a potentially important coping resource. It may also help in the identification of carers who are in currently fragile situations, and for whom it is better to seek alternative arrangements.

## Helping carers to cope

The third component of the assessment of the caregiving situation used in the study considered the strategies and tactics that carers adopted to cope with their difficulties. Generally speaking there are three broad coping strategies, each of which potentially involves a variety of 'tactics'. First, there is problem solving, and if a problem can be resolved then this is the best strategy to adopt. However, many of the difficulties that carers face cannot be solved and in such circumstances the use of problem solving will not only be ineffective but is also likely to increase stress. Sometimes, if difficulties cannot be addressed directly it is possible to reframe them so that, while the problem itself does not change, it is no longer seen to be as stressful. Finally, if it is neither possible to solve a problem nor to see it in a different light then there are various ways of dealing with, or reducing, the resultant stress, for example relaxation techniques.

In order to aid interpretation the data from CAMI have been organized as above (i.e. problem solving/seeing things differently/stress reduction) with items being included in Tables 6.3 and 6.4 if they are used frequently (by over 70 per cent of respondents) and also seen as helpful. What emerges from these data is a picture of a proactive group of respondents who use, and find helpful, a wide variety of coping strategies with over half of the items on CAMI (21/38) being used and seen as helpful by over 70 per cent of the respondents.

The three broad types of coping strategy and the more specific tactics described above are considered separately beginning with problem-solving tactics (see Table 6.3).

Table 6.3 illustrates that for this group of carers problem-solving strategies are not only used frequently but are seen as being particularly helpful, with all of the strategies used being seen as helpful by over 90 per cent of respondents. The most used (94 per cent of respondents) and useful strategy (by 99 per cent of those who use it) is 'relying on your own expertise'. This provides further evidence, if any were needed, of the very deep sense of expertise that carers hold (Harvath *et al.* 1994; Nolan *et al.* 1996a; Allen 2000a), and reinforces the importance of professional carers

**Table 6.3** Ways of managing caring

|  | Used % | Found helpful % |
|---|---|---|
| *Problem solving* | | |
| Relying on your own expertise | 94 | 99 |
| Establishing priorities and sticking to them | 85 | 97 |
| Keeping the cared-for person active | 81 | 93 |
| Talking over problems with someone you trust | 81 | 99 |
| Preventing problems before they happen | 80 | 92 |
| Keeping one step ahead by planning in advance | 80 | 96 |
| Thinking about how to overcome your problems | 80 | 92 |
| Establishing a routine and sticking to it | 79 | 94 |
| Trying out a number of solutions until one works | 78 | 96 |

actively tapping into such expertise and building upon it. Carers in this sample were also proactive in terms of establishing priorities, planning in advance, and thinking about a range of potential solutions. These data reinforce the value of carers developing a structured approach, which is confirmed by the importance that carers attach to establishing and sticking to a routine. This is an important consideration for designing services, as interventions which do not take account of carers' existing patterns of activity may well be rejected.

Last, but by no means least, carers find it helpful to talk over difficulties with someone they trust. Although many carers may already have a confidant within the family there is recent evidence from Sweden to suggest that carers are often reluctant to reveal the full extent of their caring responsibilities to their children for fear of burdening them (Ericson *et al.* 2001). Moreover, for spouse carers their usual confidant (i.e. their spouse) may now be the source of some of their difficulties. The value of a sympathetic confidant should therefore not be underestimated and this is something to which we will return when the focus group data are discussed.

Table 6.4 suggests that in addition to the extensive use of problem-solving strategies, carers also rely heavily on tactics which involve looking at caring in a difficult light.

From the above data it seems that cognitive tactics are, if anything, used somewhat more frequently than problem-solving approaches, and are generally perceived as equally useful. Once again the range of tactics used is impressive and involves things such as:

- acceptance and stoicism (accepting the situation as it is, taking life one day at a time, gritting your teeth and getting on with it);
- humour and positive appraisal (seeing the funny side of things, looking at the positives in a situation, realizing there is someone worse off than you, remembering all the good times with the cared-for person);

**Table 6.4** Seeing things differently

|  | Use % | Find helpful % |
| --- | --- | --- |
| Accepting the situation as it is | 93 | 76 |
| Believing in yourself and your abilities | 92 | 96 |
| Taking life one day at a time | 92 | 92 |
| Remembering all the good times with the cared-for person | 90 | 97 |
| Realizing the cared-for person is not to blame | 89 | 92 |
| Seeing the funny side of things | 88 | 97 |
| Looking at the positive things in a situation | 85 | 97 |
| Gritting your teeth and getting on with it | 84 | 80 |
| Realizing there is someone worse off than you | 81 | 87 |
| Realizing no one is to blame | 76 | 91 |

- a non-blame culture (realizing that the cared-for person is not to blame, realizing that no one is to blame);
- self-belief (which further reinforces the emphasis on carer expertise noted in Table 6.3).

Such cognitive tactics are often portrayed in the coping literature as being less helpful than problem solving. However, it is apparent from the present sample that carers see them as being very helpful. Such findings are not confined to the present study and have been reported in other studies that have used CAMI (see Nolan *et al.* 1996a; Lundh 1999). It is therefore important to recognize that acceptance and stoicism do not necessarily equate with apathy or fatalism and that humour and positive appraisal are not the same as unrealistic optimism and fantasy. Rather, if used appropriately, they allow for a realistic but not unduly pessimistic appraisal of the caring situation.

However, it is important that any coping strategy used is the most appropriate one to deal with the difficulties that carers face and it is here that a comparison of the type of difficulties (as indicated by CADI) and the ways of coping (as indicated by CAMI) is helpful. Therefore, if the majority of difficulties that a carer faces are amenable to change then the development of the relevant problem-solving tactics should be encouraged. By the same token, if most of their difficulties cannot be changed then a cognitive or stress reduction strategy is more likely to be helpful. It is here that advice from professional carers can be particularly valuable, providing that they have in-depth knowledge of the caring situation.

Table 6.5 illustrates that compared to problem-solving or cognitively orientated approaches, stress reduction techniques are not used as frequently, but that when they are used they are seen as very helpful. For this reason those tactics which were used less often but still seen as useful have been included in this table.

Being able to take your mind off things and to maintain interests outside caring are used far more frequently than other stress reduction tactics and this further reinforces the value of flexible and high-quality 'short breaks'. Interestingly, attending a self-help group or using relaxation/meditation are not used very often (especially the latter) but when they are used they

**Table 6.5** Stress reduction

|  | Use % | Find helpful % |
|---|---|---|
| Taking your mind off things by watching TV, reading and so on | 91 | 97 |
| Maintaining interests outside caring | 74 | 96 |
| Getting rid of excess energy by walking, swimming etc. | 60 | 95 |
| Attending a self-help group | 43 | 95 |
| Using relaxation or meditation | 24 | 92 |

are almost invariably perceived as very helpful. Although a matter of conjecture it is possible that a lack of opportunity or limited awareness of these services inhibits their use, and this is another area that might be usefully explored in terms of services to support family carers.

The above data suggest that the sort of in-depth assessment made possible by using instruments such as CADI, CASI and CAMI provides a level of understanding that may not otherwise be possible. Moreover, the information obtained can feed into service planning at a locality level as well as providing the basis for constructing a personalized package of care. Our emphasis here has been mainly on the way in which the information gained can help inform debates about service planning and this has been reflected in the way the results have been presented. However, the focus group data also provide some telling insights about the effects of an in-depth assessment on the way caring is perceived.

## Focus group interviews

As the provision of services specifically for carers, as opposed to older people, is a relatively new phenomenon, especially in Sweden, it is important that initiatives are developed systematically and draw on the lessons learned from previous research and experience. An important starting point is to raise awareness of the situation of family carers and to gain as much information as possible about their needs and circumstances in order to devise the most appropriate and timely forms of support. This was the primary aim of the present study, and the results described above add to informed debate in a number of important ways. However, it was also considered useful to gain insights into the impact that gathering the data had on the interviewers themselves, as this might have implications for the development of good assessment practice, and the formation of genuine partnerships between family and professional carers.

The data collection instruments used in the study (CADI, CASI, CAMI) were developed primarily to facilitate discussion and interaction between family and professional carers in order to help both parties to gain as complete a picture of the caregiving situation as possible, and to share perspectives in moving towards new insights and understandings for both professional and family carers.

In order to make some judgements about the extent to which the above aims are met when using CADI, CASI and CAMI, data were collected by focus group interviews with 14 of the 22 researchers so as to understand better their experiences of the interview process and to explore the impact that this may have had. It is important to reiterate that the data in the present study were collected as part of a research project and did not constitute an assessment *per se*. On the other hand, all the people who collected data were professionals, many of whom had several years' experience of working with older people and their families. They were therefore able to provide valuable commentary on the likely impact of the indices if they were used as part of an assessment. Given their background and experience some of the comments from the interviewers are all the more revealing.

Other studies using the same overall approach to the assessment of need in family carers and based upon CADI, CASI and CAMI have suggested that the process does have a considerable impact on both professionals and carers, including:

*Professionals*

- raising their awareness of the caregiving situation;
- challenging a number of their existing perceptions/expectations;
- encouraging a more in-depth assessment;
- producing new or modified packages of care.

*Family carers*

- providing new insights into why they were caring and what they have achieved;
- helping carers to express feelings or emotions that they had been 'bottling up' for a long time;
- making it easier to discuss the difficulties they were facing;
- providing a boost to morale by highlighting some of the satisfactions of caring;
- giving them a greater source of recognition;
- helping them to accept support.

(Qureshi *et al.* 2000)

However, as Qureshi *et al.* (2000) point out, a detailed assessment also raises difficult issues which require sensitive handling, especially for carers who identify no satisfactions. In such cases the assessment can be stressful for both professionals, who could be confronted with problems for which they had no solutions, and carers, who are faced with the bleakness of their situation. Our data revealed several similar issues.

First, the interviews with carers focused greater attention on their needs, which had previously often been neglected by service providers:

> Earlier we have only concentrated on the cared-for person, you have hardly ever asked the relative. He/she has only been there and you take for granted that they take part in all this without even asking them how they feel, what they miss or what they wish.

Some interviewers suggested that despite carers' best efforts to highlight their own need for support, these were often overlooked:

> I meet relatives who wish to tell and give a picture, but staff are not interested, they are not receptive to this. I know relatives who have

been writing a life story about their mother or father who is demented and can't themselves. There is . . . sort of no interest (from staff) to read it.

Moreover, in addition to raising awareness, it was also clear that the type of assessment underpinning the study could be of considerable value to care managers, not only in identifying need but also in planning for services:

I think there is a need for this kind of questionnaire for case managers, home managers or others. So you gather information of the situation for the relatives and how they feel in a constructive way, possibly for documentation, and possibly also to develop a care plan for the relative.

In addition to raising awareness the assessment process must also provide a vehicle for dialogue which allows both parties to gain new insights into their own preconceptions and also highlight the other party's perspective. The focus groups provided some powerful indicators that the interview process had challenged and enhanced the interviewers' perceptions of the nature of family caregiving and also caused them to reflect upon their own roles. This occurred at a number of levels.

First, it gave the interviewers new and potentially profound insights into the world of family care. Such insights often left a deep impression, increasing interviewers' understanding of what motivates carers and of the skills they possess:

I have been visiting the homes doing several of the interviews. And I have seen things I never thought existed in the private home – fantastic such relatives we have! And how quiet they are despite their achievement. Incredible, I think, and it has enriched my knowledge.

One of the most telling and largely unexpected insights related to the satisfactions of caring. Indeed, some interviewers recounted how they had been unaware of these despite a career working in the area:

To see the satisfaction has opened new perspectives for me. And I get this through these structured questions. Although I have been working almost 35 years in old aged care I have not been used to hearing so much of the positive side, it is mostly the burden, what is difficult, what they need help with.

The above quotations eloquently capture the enhanced awareness and new insights that the interviews provided and some interviewers considered it important that this knowledge was more widely appreciated:

I sometimes wished ordinary staff had listened to what respondents told and maybe had come to a totally different understanding.

However, new insights are of relatively little use unless changes to practice result. This was not the purpose of the present study and therefore it is not possible to draw firm conclusions in this area. However, the focus groups did suggest considerable potential for change as the interviewers reflected upon their customary ways of working and taken-for-granted assumptions about family care:

> I have always been working on a ward earlier and felt there are those who take over when I finish, and now when I leave these small houses I feel I have to do a follow up somehow. They . . . many have told me, 'We don't get much help, but now we have you.'

> And you may hear this comment: 'Well, he has a healthy wife at home . . . it will sort itself out' and that; I feel I have got a new perspective – it will not sort itself out.

Although these data highlight the positive effects of the interview process, detailed assessments are not without costs, both in terms of the time that they take and the emotional impact they may have on the interviewers themselves:

> The talks have been wide also and time-consuming and it has been many long and difficult talks.

> One day I made three interviews and I had very much feelings inside that I didn't know how to deal with. It was such . . . well such a lot of feelings that I had.

These quotes highlight the importance of practitioners receiving adequate preparation and training for the challenges raised by working with family carers in this way. However, despite these difficulties the overall impression among the interviewers was that the benefits of the interview outweighed the drawbacks:

> It has taught me a lot personally.

> One feels a little tired afterwards, but it has been enriching. Not only sad in my opinion but . . . no it has been . . . in a way it has been good.

It was not possible to gain a first-hand account of the benefits, or otherwise, of the interviews from carers themselves, but another important part of the focus groups was to explore with the interviewers their perceptions of the likely impact on carers.

First, and significantly, it was clear that the interview provided many carers with a powerful source of recognition and affirmation, in contrast to the neglect they had previously experienced:

> Many perceive themselves as . . . well, custodians for their relatives, and that they don't receive any help from the municipality or county, and they feel they are forgotten and abandoned.

In some instances the interviews themselves provided sufficient recognition:

> And one woman started to cry when I only informed her about the study we were doing: 'Oh dear, how wonderful. Forgive me for crying, but at last someone is willing to listen to me.' I stayed with her for almost three hours.

The interview process not only helped to highlight carers' needs but also confirmed that they were people of value and importance:

> They thought that someone listened to *them*. *They* were in focus and not the cared-for person [original emphasis].

> I think the confirmation the carers got through this interview is fantastic. That someone at last sees the carers.

The interview also seemed to give carers 'permission' to talk about difficult and delicate issues. The importance of being able to share concerns with a confidant was highlighted in the quantitative data, but this can be difficult for spouses as their previous confidant might now be the source of the problem, and they are often reluctant to unburden themselves to their children:

> I also think many don't tell their children. It is something I have noticed anyway, that children actually don't know how the situation is at home.

The interview therefore provided a legitimate opportunity to raise issues of concern, and also helped carers to reflect upon their situation:

> I believe that many of the questions are of the kind they have not earlier considered. Now they have got some help to sort them out.

> That they could talk about their feelings and how they . . . even if they could not dress in words bitterness, annoyance and sorrow, and there was also some satisfaction. But I think this is something you normally do not talk openly about.

The creation of a non-judgemental and non-threatening atmosphere was crucial to the success of this approach:

> And they were encouraged to talk about their feelings, both angry and sad, it was permitted and they were not perceived as worse.

However, creating an opportunity to talk openly and with candour did raise a number of delicate and often relatively taboo issues:

> I think the questions are very good . . . In my opinion people are afraid to talk about unpleasant matters, things that might give offence or matters not acceptable so to say. It is not acceptable to

dislike the spouse. It is not acceptable to get bored, and wish to jettison everything and just escape.

Sexuality and personal relationships were often brought up when I did my interviews, with question 12, 'My relation to the person I care for is no longer meaningful' – that was where these questions often were brought up.

Dealing with such issues had an emotional impact on the professionals and this was also the case with the carers. Indeed, in some cases it could result in a realization of the bleakness of their situation:

The most difficult reactions I met when we talked about this area with 'satisfaction in care', then this came, no it doesn't give any satisfaction. No it doesn't give anything. This was where I met the most difficult reactions.

The most difficult questions were those about problems and difficulties. And this question . . . 'My relation to the one I care for is not meaningful any more', this was such a difficult, emotionally difficult question to answer. Then you reach the innermost.

Although discussing such issues is difficult they are nevertheless important to explore, as in some cases the relationship may have reached a point where alternative arrangements might have to be sought. However, despite the obviously sensitive nature of many of the questions the balance within the interview was considered appropriate:

It was good that they were divided into, say, sad questions first and then happy questions. It was possible to see when it was too sad; I have said, 'We'll soon come to positive parts' and it has been very important as counterbalance.

Furthermore, the overall impression was that the interview was a positive, and indeed a potentially therapeutic experience:

I have not interviewed anyone who thought it was negative; on the contrary.

Although there was a lot of tears and also anger I felt when leaving they were a lot happier than when I arrived. And that felt nice.

Indeed, further endorsement for the interviews came from carers themselves, as a number of those interviewed had recounted their experiences to friends and subsequently some of the interviewers were approached directly by other carers who also wanted to be interviewed:

The rumour was spread (about the interview) and someone came like this, 'I have heard that you have interviewed these persons . . . Yes, and it was a good interview'. So I believe in this.

Another relative gave me a tip about another so to say. But I told her that I could not call and that she had to talk to her. And the person called later and told me she wanted an interview. That was fun.

As will be apparent, the focus groups provided a rich additional source of data, which clearly highlight the new insights and challenges raised by the interview process itself. These findings mirror closely those of Qureshi *et al.* (2000) and confirm the potential for a detailed assessment to have a number of potential benefits for both practitioners and carers.

For practitioners it is apparent that the interviews raised their awareness of the circumstances of family carers and also challenged a number of often long-held preconceptions. And while no data were collected from carers themselves the data from the interviewers highlighted the potential for a detailed assessment to recognize and validate the role of carers, while giving 'permission' to discuss previously difficult or taboo subjects and thereby help carers to vent previously suppressed or 'bottled-up' feelings. Moreover, despite the sometimes emotional nature of the interviews the interviewers considered that the overall effect was positive and helped carers to feel that they were people of value and worth. This suggests that simply allowing carers to talk about their situation can be both cathartic and therapeutic.

## Conclusions

There can be no doubt that the last decade has seen significant advances, both conceptual and practical, in the assessment of carers' need, not only in the UK but across Europe (see, for example, Nolan *et al.* 1994, 1998; Nolan and Philp 1999; Qureshi *et al.* 2000; Borgermans *et al.* 2001). In the UK this has been accompanied by legislation intended to provide carers with a statutory right to the assessment of need. Despite this, several studies suggest that in reality many of these advances have yet to be introduced into routine practice (Fruin 1998; Henwood 1998; Warner and Wexler 1998; Banks 1999).

The study on which this chapter is based was intended to explore carer need in a country where previously it had received relatively little attention, Sweden. The insights provided have been widely used to inform debate in Sweden (see Lundh and Nolan 2001), but we would also suggest that their relevance extends to any context where there is a genuine attempt to create partnerships between family and formal caregiving systems. It is our hope that this will add to further debate and discussion as to the best way in which such partnerships can be forged.

# 7

# Caring for people with dementia: working together to enhance caregiver coping and support

## Mike Nolan, Prue Ingram and Roger Watson

### Introduction

As global ageing continues governments throughout the world are pursuing a policy of community care both in order to allow older people to remain at home whenever possible and to reduce costs to the state (Davies 1995). The success of such a policy rests almost entirely on the support that older people receive from their families and other informal sources; it is estimated that 80 per cent of the help older people need is provided by the family (Walker 1995). Growing political awareness of the vital contribution of family carers has resulted in renewed interest in services to support their efforts (Chappell 1996) and consequently carers have now moved from the margins of social policy to occupy 'centre stage' (Johnson 1998).

Moreover, the last decade has also seen the emergence of a new language of social policy based on promoting partnerships between service users, family and professional carers (Bernard and Phillips 2000), aiming to ensure that services more closely reflect the needs of older individuals and their families (Moriarty 1999). Although it is easy in principle to subscribe to such a philosophy, enacting it is far more complex and, as Qureshi *et al.* (2000) suggest, is likely to require a 'paradigmatic leap' in the way we conceptualize and deliver services. Clearly we cannot support people appropriately if we do not fully appreciate their needs (Chappell 1996), for in the absence of a detailed understanding the 'interactive, personalized, contextual and determined helping relationship' that is being promoted (Borgermans *et al.* 2001) is unlikely to emerge. Nowhere are these challenges more acutely felt than in the field of dementia care where, notwithstanding recent developments in drug-related treatments, it is argued that for the foreseeable future therapeutic efforts will still be best directed at developing and refining services to support people with dementia (PWD) and their carers (Pearlin *et al.* 2001).

This raises important tensions between the ways in which services are conceptualized, designed, developed and evaluated by researchers, policy makers and practitioners and how they are received and experienced by PWD and their carers. As Post (2001) contends, a key question becomes who sets the agenda and identifies the most salient issues. In contributing to this debate this chapter considers services designed to support family carers and, drawing on data collected from a survey of the Alzheimer's Association (Victoria, Australia), it suggests how more empowering models of working with family carers can be developed. Subsequently it briefly considers some of the implications of the results for further developments in research, policy and practice.

## Supporting family carers: what's the rationale?

The literature on family care has grown significantly over the last three decades (Pearlin *et al.* 2001) but, despite this, much of our current understanding is still based on a stress/coping paradigm (Nolan *et al.* 1996a; Schulz and Williamson 1997; Schofield *et al.* 1998; Montgomery and Williams 2001). Not surprisingly, therefore, this approach has been particularly influential in the design of support services, and reducing carer stress and burden has become a 'major tenet of gerontological policy and practice' (Zarit *et al.* 1999). Although some contend that efforts to reduce caregiver burden should remain as the primary aim of interventions (Clyburn *et al.* 2000), others voice concern that the dominance of such an approach 'pathologizes' caring (Twigg and Atkin 1994) and that greater attention should be given to promoting a sense of satisfaction and expertise among carers as specific and legitimate therapeutic goals (Nolan *et al.* 1996a; Qureshi *et al.* 2000).

Furthermore, despite the extensive research on interventions designed to reduce caregiver burden there is remarkably little evidence for the effectiveness of current service models (Zarit *et al.* 1999; Thompson and Briggs 2000; Cooke *et al.* 2001; Pusey and Richards 2001). This may lead some to the rather fatalistic conclusion that there is little we can do to support carers or encourage others to promote ever more 'sophisticated' controlled trials, with larger samples and more statistical power (Thompson and Briggs 2000; Beck 2001; Cooke *et al.* 2001; Pusey and Richards 2001). Rather, in concert with others, we would argue that we need to reappraise the way we define service goals and attempt to 'measure' success, and consider whether in fact current approaches are the most appropriate (Moriarty 1999; Bond 2000). This should herald a move away from the present reliance on relatively crude interventions that fail to capture the nuances of caregiving (Quayhagen and Quayhagen 1996) towards models which account for the complex nature of care

(Moriarty 1999). Adopting this more critical stance highlights the importance of challenging the received wisdom about the intended outcomes of caregiver support.

The whole issue of defining and measuring the outcomes of interventions is a vexed one, particularly if attention is turned to more subtle and diverse domains, such as quality of life. All too often the important dimensions of existing 'measures' have been specified largely by researchers and academics, and comprise objective and more easily measurable items (Farquhar 1995; O'Boyle 1997; Haas 1999; Reed and Clarke 1999). Even if subjective criteria are included these usually reflect the views of researchers (Day and Jankey 1996) rather than those of older people or carers themselves (Chesson *et al.* 1996). This is a significant limitation as there are often 'striking discrepancies' between the views of researchers and professionals and those of disabled people (O'Boyle 1997; Livingston *et al.* 1998; Reed and Clarke 1999), with both groups holding significantly different perspectives (Peters 1995). As a consequence it has been suggested that many existing measures 'lose the human-being' (Kivnick and Murray 1997), and this has led to calls to move beyond 'statistical sophistication' (Bowling 1995) and a professional perspective (Nolan 1998) in order that 'outcomes' are more relevant and appropriate to those in receipt of help and support (Qureshi *et al.* 2000; Nolan 2001).

Informed debate has been hampered by the fact that the goals of carer support services have remained largely implicit and have been defined primarily in instrumental terms (Twigg and Atkin 1994; Nolan *et al.* 1996a; Banks 1999). As noted earlier, it is well recognized that one of the main motivations for supporting carers has been to reduce their burden or stress (Schulz and Williamson 1997; Schofield *et al.* 1998; Zarit *et al.* 1999; Montgomery and Williams 2001), and this has resulted in the development of a limited range of services (see Zarit *et al.* 1999 for a review). However, the reason *why* a reduction in caregiver stress/burden is considered so important has not been clearly articulated. At one level this may seem intuitively obvious, with the implicit motivation being to reduce suffering. Conversely, it has been suggested that the often unspoken aim is to 'keep carers caring'. In other words, carers are viewed largely as resources, with services primarily intended to maintain them in their role (Twigg and Atkin 1994; Nolan *et al.* 1996a).

Recently, however, there have been calls for a more holistic approach in which support for carers is defined as any intervention which assists them to:

- take up (or not take up) a caregiving role;
- continue in a caregiving role;
- give up a caregiving role.

(Askham 1998)

Accepting such an approach clearly mandates both a broader range of potential interventions (see Table 7.1 for some recent suggestions) and,

**Table 7.1** Typology of carer support

| Askham 1998 | Schmall 1995 | Schumacher et al. 1998 |
|---|---|---|
| • Training and preparation | • Knowledge of medical condition | • Knowledge and skills about condition |
| • Equipment and technical support | • Coping skills | • Provide technical care safely |
| • Empowered to use services | • Family/relationship issues | • Meet needs safely |
| • Information | • Communication with cared-for people | • Attend to social care |
| • Direct help | • Community services | • Attend to personal care |
| • Respite care | • Dealing with emotions | |
| • Financial support | • Long-term planning | |
| • Relaxation services | | |

crucially, consideration of a much more extensive and diverse set of outcomes. Calls for a more expansive model are not new (see for example Collins *et al.* 1994; Nolan *et al.* 1996a; Whitehouse and Maslow 1997; Borgermans *et al.* 2001) but there has recently been far greater recognition of the potential limitations of existing approaches. For example, Aneshensel *et al.* (1995), in one of the largest studies of caregiving in dementia, suggested that outcomes must reflect the likely impact of interventions and that no matter how elegant they may be theoretically, aggregate indicators tell us very little about success, or otherwise, at an individual level. Indeed, as accounting for diversity seems to be the key to a better understanding of family caregiving (Aneshensel *et al.* 1995; Schofield *et al.* 1998; Clyburn *et al.* 2000), simply summarizing the scores on a measure of carer stress or burden can be greatly misleading, and averaging these scores across large samples of carers compounds the problem. Following a recent review, Zarit *et al.* (1999) conclude that we need to rethink the way in which outcomes are defined so that they are more logically related to the intervention. Furthermore, if the detection of change is 'critically dependent' upon selecting the right outcome (Braithwaite 2000), and if the outcomes of caregiving can only be fully understood following an 'individual's appraisal' (Clyburn *et al.* 2000), then it should be a matter of some concern that many existing studies manifestly fail to reflect the outcomes that carers themselves see as being the most important (Qureshi *et al.* 2000; Thompson and Briggs 2000).

If more sensitive methods of judging the success of carer support are to emerge there is a need to develop outcomes that are easily interpreted and seen as relevant by all the parties concerned, including carers (Thompson and Briggs 2000). Indeed, if we are to create genuine partnerships it would seem essential that carers themselves are the final arbiters of what counts as 'success'. This means that we must engage carers more fully in a dialogue about what they see as important. In developing a framework of what carers view as valued outcomes, Qureshi *et al.* (2000) identified four sets of concerns that carers see as important. These are:

- to enhance the quality of life of the cared-for person;
- to enhance the quality of life of carers;
- recognition and support in their caring role;
- support provided in a way which values and respects carers, recognizes their expertise and allows them to 'have a say'.

In the present context the third set of outcomes is particularly relevant and this includes enabling carers to:

- define the limits of their role, including their level of involvement and the nature of the tasks they undertake;
- feel skilled, confident and knowledgeable;
- experience a sense of satisfaction and involvement in caring;
- have a sense of shared responsibility and of being emotionally supported;
- manage the physical/practical demands of caring.

(Qureshi *et al.* 2000)

Although it could be argued that some of the above outcomes are addressed in current interventions, for example help with the physical and practical elements of caring, no comprehensive carer-focused model has been described in routine practice. In the UK, for example, carers have a statutory right to an assessment of need, and it is widely recognized that such an assessment is an essential prerequisite to the design of appropriate and sensitive interventions (Chappell 1996; Audit Commission 2000; Qureshi *et al.* 2000; Borgermans *et al.* 2001). However, several recent studies have demonstrated that assessment processes remain implicit and fragmented, with carers sometimes being assessed without even being aware of the fact (Fruin 1998; Henwood 1998; Warner and Wexler 1998; Arksey *et al.* 1999; Banks 1999). Indeed, it seems that a 'professionals as expert' model still predominates (Brandon and Jack 1997) and continues to exert a pervasive and often unconscious effect (Qureshi *et al.* 2000). What is lacking it seems is a set of principles to guide assessment practice.

Based on their extensive study of caregiving in dementia Aneshensel *et al.* (1995) delineate five fundamental premises that they believe should underpin clinical interventions with carers:

- There should be recognition that the multiple dimensions of caregiving interact in diverse and complex ways. Interventions should therefore be preceded by a multi-dimensional assessment that 'identifies the unique constellation of issues found within a particular family'.
- Subsequently goals should be based on 'the particular configuration of conditions that exist for each individual caregiver at a specific time in

his or her caregiving career, therefore goals for treatment should emerge from caregivers themselves'.

- On the basis of the above, broad and comprehensive interventions are needed.
- Multiple ways of defining success must be used which are resonant with individual circumstances.
- It should be recognized that the interests of the carer and the PWD may sometimes diverge.

The above principles are entirely congruent with the multifaceted nature of caregiving and the well-documented conclusion that individual appraisal is the key to understanding caregivers' responses (Schofield *et al.* 1998; Moriarty 1999; Clyburn *et al.* 2000). In essence the message is clear: caregiving can only be fully appreciated and adequately supported in its appropriate context (Dilworth-Anderson 2001; Montgomery and Williams 2001). This stands in marked contrast to the context stripping and standardization which underpins the so-called 'gold standard' of evidence, the randomized controlled trial which is currently promoted.

While Aneshensel *et al.*'s (1995) work relates specifically to dementia, Qureshi *et al.* (2000) have recently proposed a very similar set of 'key principles', which they see as being essential to an integrated outcomes approach with carers more generally. Foremost among these principles are that:

- the definition and recording of outcomes should be carer-centred, specific and relevant to the individual concerned;
- the evaluation of outcomes should begin with clarity about the outcomes intended;
- reaching a common understanding of intended outcomes requires a thorough and sensitive assessment;
- the carer should be actively engaged as an 'expert' in the process of identifying and reviewing outcomes.

Having highlighted many of the tensions inherent in attempts to design and evaluate carer support services, this chapter now utilizes data collected from a sample of carers in Victoria, Australia to illustrate how carers themselves define and evaluate their self-perceived coping efforts.

## The importance of coping

Although there are numerous definitions of coping (see for example Pearlin and Schooler 1978; Lazarus and Folkman 1984; Lazarus 1993) and there is still considerable debate about its relationship to concepts such as managing (Boss 1988; Burr *et al.* 1994) or mastery, competence and self-efficacy (see for example Schumacher *et al.* 1998), coping here is viewed in the broad sense defined by Turnbull and Turnbull (1993) as being 'the things people do (acting or thinking) to increase a sense of well-being in their lives and to avoid being harmed by (potentially) stressful events'.

Under this broad rubric, 'coping' has received considerable attention in the caregiving literature, with many authors arguing that helping carers to improve their various coping skills is a potentially very powerful form of intervention (Milne *et al.* 1993; Aneshensel *et al.* 1995; Schmall 1995; Maslow and Whitehouse 1997; Rapp *et al.* 1998; Szabo and Strang 1999). Certainly a feeling of mastery, competence and of being able to deal with difficult situations and thereby perceive that you are 'doing a good job' is closely associated with a positive self-concept in carers (Aneshensel *et al.* 1995; Schumacher *et al.* 1998; Szabo and Strang 1999). However, if we are to be true to the principles enunciated above (Aneshensel *et al.* 1995; Qureshi *et al.* 2000), it seems essential that the effectiveness, or otherwise, of various 'coping' strategies are primarily appraised from a carer's perspective.

The Carers' Assessment of Managing Index (CAMI) (Nolan *et al.* 1995, 1996a, 1998) was designed expressly for this purpose. It comprises 38 statements, derived primarily from carers themselves (see the above references for a fuller account of its development), and for each statement carers are asked to indicate if they use a particular 'tactic' and, if they do, to appraise its utility (not helpful, quite helpful, very helpful). The purpose is not to sum responses into an overall 'score' which indicates how well an individual is 'coping', but rather to produce a 'profile' that captures, as Aneshensel *et al.* (1995) recommend, the caregiving experience in the context of a particular set of circumstances.

CAMI has been used in several surveys in order to provide an indication of the broad categories of coping that carers see as most useful and to explore potential differences between varying caregiving situations (see for example Nolan *et al.* 1996a; Lundh 1999; Grant and Whittell 2000, 2001; Lundh and Nolan 2001; and this volume). Here we draw upon data collected from the Alzheimer's Association, Victoria, Australia. In collecting these data CAMI was distributed, together with other questions seeking demographic details, details of the caregiving situation, the type and amount of help needed and an indication of various potentially difficult behaviours. The questionnaire was sent out over a two-month period through carer support groups, through counselling and education sessions, with newsletters, and posted on the website. Reply paid envelopes were provided with all questionnaires. The majority of surveys were returned by people participating in carer support groups.

One hundred and fifty-six questionnaires were returned and entered for data analysis. Because the exact numbers of questionnaires distributed is unknown it is not possible to calculate a meaningful response rate. Moreover, as the sample was self-selecting we make no claims about the generalizability of the data. Indeed, this is not our purpose as the data are intended primarily to be illustrative of the types of coping tactics that carers employ and see as useful. However, in order to provide some

**Table 7.2** Demographic profile of sample (n = 156)

|  |  | % |
| --- | --- | --- |
| Gender of carer | Male | 30 |
|  | Female | 70 |
| Gender of cared-for person | Male | 42 |
|  | Female | 58 |
| Relationship of cared-for person to carer | Spouse/partner | 64 |
|  | Parent/parent-in-law | 34 |
|  | Other relative | 3 |
| Living arrangement | Share house | 82 |
|  | Under 1 km away | 4 |
|  | 1–2 km away | 2 |
|  | Over 2 km away | 13 |

context, brief details of the demographics of the sample are provided in Table 7.2.

As can be seen, the carers in the sample were primarily spouses or children generally supporting someone who lived in the same household. Several studies suggest that the major sources of difficulties in caring for someone with dementia relate primarily to the behaviour of the PWD rather than the amount of care that is provided, and among the sample the most prevalent potentially problematic behaviours included: disorientation to time (92 per cent); difficulty holding a normal conversation (88 per cent); upsetting behaviour (83 per cent); uncooperative behaviour (80 per cent); wandering within the home environment (58 per cent); following the carer around (56 per cent).

Despite these diverse and potentially stressful behaviours the carers in the sample adopted (and perceived as useful) an impressive range of coping tactics, the most prevalent of which are summarized in Table 7.3. For ease of interpretation the coping tactics have been divided into three broad categories: those concerned with problem solving; those concerned with cognitive approaches by which carers reappraise their situation, and those tactics which help carers to minimize any potential stress (Zarit and Leitsch 2001). As Lazarus (1993) notes, it is essential to have a broad range of coping tactics, and although problem-solving approaches are often promoted as being the most useful, Lazarus argues that all strategies are potentially helpful and the important issue is to utilize the most appropriate tactic to address a specific problem. For example, problem-solving tactics are only helpful when a situation is amenable to change and if carers continually try and 'fix what cannot be fixed', then more rather than less stress is likely to result. As Zarit and Leitsch (2001) argue, achievable goals can only be meaningfully set in relation to what is modifiable. The central question here is, which tactics do carers themselves see as being the most effective?

**Table 7.3** Coping tactics used and seen as helpful (n = 156)

|  | % |
|---|---|
| *Problem-solving tactics* | |
| Thinking about and overcoming the problem | 90 |
| Preventing problems before they happen | 88 |
| Relying on your own expertise | 84 |
| Planning in advance | 81 |
| Getting as much help as possible from the family | 79 |
| Trying out solutions until one works | 76 |
| Being firm with the cared-for person and pointing out what you expect | 75 |
| Getting as much professional help as possible | 72 |
| Finding out as much information as possible | 72 |
| *Cognitive tactics* | |
| Realizing there's someone worse off than you | 82 |
| Look for the positives in the situation | 76 |
| Realize things are better now than they used to be | 74 |
| See the funny side of things | 72 |
| Grit your teeth and get on with it | 72 |
| Draw on strong personal or religious beliefs | 71 |
| Realize the person you care for is not to blame | 70 |
| Take life one day at a time | 70 |
| Remember all the good times you had with the person you care for | 70 |
| *Stress reduction tactics* | |
| Take your mind off things by watching TV, reading, or similar | 91 |
| Have a good cry | 90 |
| Use relaxation techniques | 73 |
| Get rid of excess energy by walking, swimming etc | 61 |

It is quite apparent from Table 7.3 that carers in the present sample use and see as helpful a wide variety of coping tactics spanning the above three broad domains. Clearly carers are proactive in terms of problem solving, thinking about and planning a preventative approach, involving mobilizing help from family (where available), eliciting support from professionals, and finding out as much information as possible. Carers in this sample also held a very strong sense of their own expertise and, as will be highlighted below, recognition of this expertise is essential.

However, there is also evidence to suggest that the majority of carers (eight out of ten) often adopt a process of trial and error, trying out a number of solutions until they alight upon one that works. Although this may ultimately be successful it is doubtful whether it is the most efficient strategy and it may, for example, be possible for professionals to assist carers to identify effective solutions more rapidly.

While cognitive strategies are often portrayed in the literature as not being as helpful as problem-solving approaches, in the present sample carers used even more cognitive tactics than problem-solving efforts, and the data clearly demonstrate that the ability of carers to perceive care-giving in a different light is an essential coping approach. A number of these cognitive tactics relate to making positive comparisons (realizing someone is worse off, looking for the positives, realizing things are now better, seeing the funny side of things); a non-blame culture (realizing the cared-for person is not to blame); and stoicism and drawing on strongly held beliefs. The importance of a good prior relationship with the cared-for person is also apparent.

Although less extensive and diverse, stress reduction tactics also constitute a crucial resource for carers, enabling them to take their mind off things, or release emotions. Similarly, using relaxation techniques and getting rid of excess energy are strongly endorsed.

The above data paint a picture of a highly resourceful and proactive group of carers who, over time, have built up an extensive repertoire of coping skills that they both employ on a regular basis and see as helpful. This is consistent with other studies that have used CAMI, not only with carers of people with dementia (Nolan *et al.* 1996a), but also in more general caregiving populations (Lundh 1999; Lundh and Nolan 2001; and this volume), and among those supporting people with learning disabilities (Grant and Whittell 2000, 2001). In the present sample there were very few statistical differences between the use and perceived helpfulness of various coping tactics by, for example, the gender or relationship of the carer, with little indication that women used a more extensive range of strategies than do men, as was found in the studies cited above.

In addition to the quantitative data considered above, carers were also invited to provide further qualitative data in response to open questions about what more could be done to assist people in their situation. Over half of the sample took this opportunity and identified a range of items that they considered would be helpful.

A number, rather wistfully, hoped for a cure for dementia but the majority articulated rather more immediate and achievable wishes. Prominent among these was the desire for a better understanding of the needs and circumstances of carers, both within society as a whole and particularly among professional carers. General practitioners came in for particular criticism, especially for failing to provide sufficient information and advice both about dementia itself and the type of support that was available:

> Greater understanding and acknowledgement generally in the non-caring community of the enormity of the constant burden and personal strain of caring for a dementia sufferer. Because the person can appear almost normal for brief periods, and for years deny that there is any problem, it seems that the carer is the one who suffers more that the one with the disorder.

Better communication with the doctor. Maybe a system of written communication as to problems being experienced. Doctors, social workers, nurses – do not understand the difficulty of trying to manage to keep the family going emotionally and physically, when the husband is denying he has a problem.

Why aren't doctors more aware of (a) support groups, e.g. Alzheimer's Association, (b) the need for carers to learn new skills and strategies, (c) the availability of drugs, e.g. Aricept for use in early stage. We'd been going to the doctor's for two years and he never mentioned support groups. Friends finally gave me contact numbers. I only heard of Aricept well down the track; I was told by doctors it was unavailable. Further down the track I found out from supporters, e.g. Alzheimer's Association, that it is available but at a cost. I'd have been willing to pay in the early days.

It seems that difficulties in obtaining adequate support from GPs transcend contexts and have also been noted in the UK (Audit Commission 2000). In such circumstances respondents bemoaned the limited opportunities they had to talk through the issues they faced:

I need to be able to talk with someone with expert knowledge and without my husband being there. I don't think it would be good for his morale if I talked about his dementia in front of him because he thinks he's the same as he was before he was diagnosed as having Parkinson's ten years ago!

Perhaps not surprisingly, as the greatest number of respondents were drawn from support groups, there was strong endorsement for the benefits of attending such groups:

I believe it is vital for all carers to be part of the 'carer network' through carer support groups, associations or other links. This is the best way to develop some expertise, obtain practical and emotional support and also contribute to helping others.

Clearly such respondents turned to support groups to obtain the expertise and support that they perceived as lacking in their interactions with professionals. However, one of the rather paradoxical results of the survey was that, despite the largest number of respondents being identified via support groups, 'talking over problems with someone you trust' was only reported by 18 per cent of people in this survey. This compares with 82 per cent in survey data from the UK (Nolan *et al.* 1996a) and 84 per cent in Sweden (Lundh 1999). Interpreting this finding is difficult as it might relate to the private or stoical nature of the Australian personality. On the other hand, given the relatively high membership of support groups, it might have been anticipated that they would provide a forum for such discussion. This would suggest the need for further exploration of the nature and purpose of support groups, as clearly some respondents felt that they did not fully meet their needs:

> A self-help group that really *listened* to me. I have no difficulty doing this for others, but when it's my turn it doesn't happen.

By far and away the most frequently requested additional form of support, voiced by over 30 per cent of the sample, was the need for more respite and short breaks. A variety of models were proposed including more day care provision, more in-house respite, and longer breaks whereby the PWD spent time away from the family home. Irrespective of the type of respite that was requested, respondents wanted it to be flexible, affordable, consistent and of high quality. In many cases respite was not necessarily used for the carers to have a break, but rather to complete household and other tasks:

> A bit more respite during the week, to allow for shopping, paying bills, getting medical scripts made up etc. Time to spend in garden and upkeep – mowing, pruning etc. . . even time to do housework without worrying about what the person with dementia is doing, and being called all the time. With government cutbacks, respite from home help once a fortnight is not enough. I'd like it once a week.

> Having someone to come into the home to fit slippers, shoes (on the PWD). Having my respite carers (in home) help a little when I am out, e.g. bring washing in off line, iron, do dishes. I have three different ladies and only one does this – while my mum sleeps. The others sit and read or knit. Respite carers should also be taught how to wash dishes properly. In the past when some have done this, I have to rewash them when I come home.

> I would appreciate someone coming into the house to 'mind' or visit with my husband occasionally, perhaps once a week or fort-night so that I could visit elsewhere – not as a 'package' but on a casual, as the need arose, basis. I would also appreciate it if he could be picked up from and brought home from day care, as I find having to take the car out onto the road twice a day a bit daunting – tiring sometimes – I use those days to catch up with paperwork etc., when he isn't home. Easier access to short-term respite would be a relief – it is so difficult to find any beds available for months ahead and these situations are often acute, the 'carer' suddenly can't care anymore, either through illness or just plain total fatigue.

> To be able to use the same respite carer always, one that my husband knows and likes, someone who understands his requirements without a half-hour briefing session before I can leave.

In several respects the provision of respite care acts as a barometer for the tensions that carers face when seeking support from public and voluntary services, for while respite care is often one of the most frequently requested services, uptake is frequently limited (Briggs and Askham 1999; Pickard 1999; Zarit *et al.* 1999).

This raises the intriguing question of *why?* (Zarit *et al.* 1999), with it now being quite apparent that simply providing a service is not of itself sufficient. Carers often make subtle judgements about the relative 'costs and benefits' of accepting help (Clarke 1999c; Montgomery and Kosloski 2000), and are likely to reject services which are not consistent with their own perceived needs (Braithwaite 2000), or which they do not see as being of suitable quality (Pickard 1999; Braithwaite 2000; Clyburn *et al.* 2000). Consistent with our data, several recent studies have indicated that what carers want is help that is consistent yet flexible and responsive, and which addresses the needs of the person they care for, respects their individuality, and promotes a good quality of life (Riorden and Bennett 1998; Zarit *et al.* 1999; Pickard *et al.* 2000; Banks and Roberts 2001).

The above considerations are particularly relevant in the context of respite care and it is now recognized that new models of respite care are required which are more flexible and responsive to need (Briggs and Askham 1999; Pickard 1999). Concurrently, there has also been a change in the perceived purpose of respite care away from simply reducing carer stress towards improving the quality of life of both carer and the cared-for person (Lightbody and Gilhooly 1997; Moriarty and Levin 1998; Weightman 1999).

As recent research has shown, the interactions between family and professional carers, especially in the context of respite care, and the extent to which professional carers seek actively to 'integrate' their caring efforts with those of the family is a crucial factor (Gilmour 2002). In 'integrated' care professionals value the carers' expertise and work with them in promoting best quality care (Gilmour 2002). Similar sentiments were voiced in the present study.

> . . . organizations etc. viewed complaints as a quality assurance measure and are not threatened by a carer who is reasonably well informed. It is important that service providers do work with carers, and value their input and form a collaborative partnership that is focused on the needs of client and support for the carer. Words need to be followed by appropriate action to achieve a positive outcome.

As this chapter has sought to emphasize, what constitutes a 'positive outcome' remains a major conceptual and practical challenge in the context of carer support services and it is to this issue that we now return.

## Discussion

It is important to reiterate at this point that the data presented in this paper are not generalizable as they are taken from a relatively small, non-representative, convenience sample. However, we do believe that they are extremely useful as a heuristic, highlighting important points that can helpfully feed into current debates about the goals and outcomes, indeed the whole *'raison d'être'* for supporting family carers.

Despite the 'explosion' of empirical studies into family care over the last two decades (Fortinsky 2001), and the extensive research into interventions designed to support carers (Zarit *et al.* 1999; Zarit and Leitsch 2001), we still have remarkably little 'evidence' for the effectiveness of services. This has fuelled considerable debate, both conceptual and methodological, about the underpinning rationale for research and practice (Zarit *et al.* 1999; Charlesworth 2001; Cooke *et al.* 2001; Fortinsky 2001; Montgomery and Williams 2001; Pusey and Richards 2001).

Such debates are of more than academic interest as, despite advances in drug therapies in dementia, it is considered that the family will remain 'centre stage' for several years to come, and that the most potent way of influencing the consequences of Alzheimer's disease will be to shape the support given to people with dementia and their carers (Pearlin *et al.* 2001). If such support is to be 'shaped' in the most effective way it will be essential that future research and service developments take cognizance of, and respond to, a number of emerging trends. Foremost among these are:

- The need to move away from a view of professionals or researchers as being the experts to a more emancipatory and empowering model. Post (2001) argues that we have to adopt an 'epistemology of humility' in which the agenda is set primarily by the 'constituency' (i.e. people with dementia and their carers) itself. In relation to the outcomes of services one of the key questions therefore becomes 'outcomes for *whom*?' (Schulz 2001). Ideally outcomes must be seen as meaningful by all major stakeholder groups, including people with dementia, carers and service providers (Thompson and Briggs 2000; Beck 2001; Schulz 2001).
- Practice should be predicated on a model of 'working with' people with dementia and their carers (Nolan and Keady 2001), which may well require a 'paradigmatic' leap in currently prevalent approaches (Qureshi *et al.* 2000).
- Far greater attention should be given to the 'context' of caregiving (Downs 2000; Dilworth-Anderson 2001; Montgomery and Williams 2001) in order that the goals of interventions can reflect the 'unique' features of caregiving dyads (Aneshensel *et al.* 1995; Zarit and Leitsch 2001). Only in this way will support be provided as part of an 'interactive, personalized, contextual, determined and helping relationship' (Borgermans *et al.* 2001).

- There should be a clearer conceptual link between interventions and their intended outcomes (Zarit *et al.* 1999; Zarit and Leitsch 2001) based on what is 'reasonable' and 'modifiable' (Zarit and Leitsch 2001) within a given context. We would argue that any definition of 'reasonable' should be determined via negotiation and agreement whenever possible.
- There is a need to agree a 'typology' of interventions that provides a common framework for discussion and debate. Schulz (2001) suggests that this should include:

  *who* is the primary target of interventions (caregiver, person with dementia, service provider);

  *what* is the target of the intervention: for example, what is the primary domain to be addressed, such as skills, knowledge and so on;

  *how* is the intervention to be delivered: for instance, group or individual, face-to-face or distant and so on.

  We would add a fourth dimension to this helpful list – *when* is support most appropriate, so that interventions are linked to need at particular points in time (Aneshensel *et al.* 1995; Nolan *et al.* 1996a; Qualls 2000; Zarit and Leitsch 2001).

The above premises provide a summary of many of the major trends informing debates about interventions designed to support people with dementia and their carers. The focus in this chapter has been on services intended to support family carers and we have used data based on carers' own evaluations of the efficiency of their coping efforts as a heuristic to illustrate the above points. We have also illustrated that one of the most requested services is more respite, yet the paradox remains that uptake is often limited.

Zarit and Leitsch (2001) suggest that there needs to be more informed debate between carers and service providers about the goals of interventions, as the success of services will depend in large measure upon the extent to which they are consistent with carers' expectations. A continued failure to engage in a meaningful dialogue with carers is, they argue, one of the main reasons why a significant minority of carers reject services even when they are available and affordable (Zarit and Leitsch 2001). This is also likely to be the case in terms of helping carers to cope.

Carers in the present sample, consistent with those in other studies using the same methodology (Nolan *et al.* 1996a; Lundh 1999; Grant and Whittell 2000, 2001), have a very strong sense of their own expertise, yet this is often not acknowledged by professionals (Nolan *et al.* 1996a; Qureshi *et al.* 2000). Indeed, in drawing comparisons between families and care managers about their assessment of how well carers cope, there is evidence that care managers systematically underestimate the range of coping strategies that families use, especially in the cognitive domain (Grant and Whittell 2001). As these authors note, 'If what works well for families is not recognized the risk of inappropriate interventions from services will remain high.'

However, it is important to recognize that the samples in all the above studies were not representative and may have contained a disproportionate number of carers who perceive themselves to be 'coping' well. Nevertheless, such carers often engaged in a series of 'trial and error' experiments before they alighted on the best strategy. Although some individual modification will be needed to tailor strategies to unique circumstances, a more proactive and innovative approach from researchers and practitioners could help to ensure that carers cope as effectively as possible, as quickly as possible. For example, interventions that assist carers to become 'socially resourceful' could increase their ability to ask for and mobilize help (Rapp *et al.* 1998). Moreover, given the central importance of the quality and history of dyadic relationships between the person with dementia and the caregiver, both in influencing the quality of life of the person with dementia and the 'experience of caring' (Whitlach 2001; Woods 2001), interventions that foster improved communication between the carer and the person with dementia are likely to prove very fruitful (Quayhagen and Quayhagen 1996). Such communication strategies may overcome the 'closed awareness contexts' that can develop in caregiving (Hutchinson *et al.* 1997) and which prove very destructive to the quality of the relationship between the carer and the person with dementia (Keady 1999). Indeed, it is clear that much could be done to assist carers to cope more effectively across all three domains of coping (Zarit and Leitsch 2001) as this is currently a somewhat underdeveloped area, particularly interventions which are based on carers' own assessment of their coping effectiveness or self-efficacy (Fortinsky 2001).

This of course requires that we ask carers for their assessment of their own coping and not our own. If nothing else the use of CAMI appears to facilitate this:

> I have attempted to complete a few similar survey questionnaires in the last couple of years. This one would be the best in terms of relevance of questions, i.e. implicit understanding of the problems. Well done, best wishes with the survey.

However, perhaps most crucially of all, we need to move towards a more inclusive vision of research and practice in dementia care which strives to unite and understand the perspectives of all those involved (Nolan *et al.* 2002a), a fact recognized most insightfully below:

> I would like to see organizations connected to dementia being more positive (not all doom and gloom) and focus on the couple involved more, rather than just the problems of the carer (which are huge but not insurmountable). Admittedly support is certainly needed in this area, but it appears to me that the affected person is neglected to a large extent.

If, as is suggested, successful interventions in dementia will for the fore-seeable future be intimately related to efforts to shape support for people with dementia and their carers (Pearlin *et al.* 2001) then we need, as a matter of some urgency, to subscribe to an 'epistemology of humility' (Post 2001) in which expertise is not the sole or primary preserve of researchers, policy makers and practitioners, but rather increasingly lies with people with dementia and their carers.

## Acknowledgements

The authors would like to acknowledge the contribution of Alzheimer's Association Victoria in supporting this study, and the carers for taking the time to respond to the questionnaires.

This chapter is an expanded version of an article published in *Dementia: The International Journal of Social Research and Practice* (Nolan, M.R., Ingram, P. and Watson, R. (2002) Working with family carers of people with dementia: 'negotiated' coping as an essential outcome, *Dementia: The International Journal of Social Research and Practice*, 1(1): 75–93), sections of which have been reproduced here with permission.

# 8

# Family care decision-making in later life: the future is now!

## Gwynnyth Llewellyn

### Introduction

The words that form the subtitle of this chapter come from a mother in her eighties. During a long interview talking about how she has looked after her adult son with intellectual disability she was asked, 'And, what about looking to the future?' She did not hesitate with her reply: 'The future? The future is now!'

This interview and others with parents of adult sons and daughters with intellectual disability was conducted as part of a narrative family care study designed to investigate the service pathways taken by these parents over time. In setting up this study, one of our aims was to understand how older parents negotiated and experienced their involvement with formal services. As is often the case in qualitative research, other topics became more prominent over the course of the study. Drawn by the parents' stories about their lives over time – their caregiving biography – we began to think more about their parent-caring career as a way to improve understanding of service involvement and family care decision making in later life.

In contrast to other family carers, parents of adults with intellectual disability cannot expect caring to come to an end. In all likelihood their adult sons and daughters will outlive them and this presents unique concerns about the future. Their caregiving career does not start and end at a particular stage of the life cycle. It begins with the birth of their child and ends when they die. This elongated caregiving career spans generations and encompasses periods of social change. For example, attitudes toward disabled people and the services available today are very different from the time when these older parents began their parenting careers, in some instances over 50 years ago. A remarkable feature of these parents' lives is that they rarely think of themselves as caregivers. Instead they see themselves as parents caring for a child. They talk about their sons and daughters, regardless of their adult status, as still being their children. They refer to their duty, no matter what their circumstances, as being to parent or 'look after' their child.

In policy and professional terms, however, these older parents are referred to as caregivers. They appear in policy documents labelled as carers who require information, financial resources and service support for their caregiving. Many older parents do receive carers' benefits, home help, respite care, and other formal carer services. Yet their status as carers remains ambivalent. In their own minds they are parents responsible for the welfare of their disabled children who are now well into adulthood. Their sense of independence and strong feelings of responsibility for their child often means that many do not use services that could potentially provide some relief from their parent-caring responsibilities. Our preference is to refer to these older parents not caregivers but rather as parent-carers. In doing so we acknowledge upfront how they regard themselves as parents first as well as recognizing the caregiving label ascribed to them by others.

At the same time that older parent-carers continue to look after their adult sons and daughters they face increasing challenges to their parenting. Many experience new or increasing health problems as they age. Many also face new or increasing caring responsibilities for others. They may have to begin caring for their own very elderly parents or a dependent spouse or other sons and daughters and their children's children. Some older parent-carers are themselves in need of care. For some, their disabled sons and daughters also face increasing physical and mental difficulties associated with their own ageing. This group of parent-carers is therefore increasingly vulnerable as they reach older age.

Noting the potential risks associated with ageing in this group of parent-carers, researchers and policy makers have called attention to an apparent lack of parental preparation for their adult son's or daughter's future. In response, programmes to assist older parent-carers, for example in writing a will, setting up a trust account, and allocating guardianship, can now be found in many services. Despite these developments, a tone of frustration can be heard in some accounts of older parent-carers' failure to plan 'adequately' for the future. Researchers have noted the anger and frustration workers can feel toward older parents about their failure to make plans, particularly if this is seen to 'interfere' with the growth and development of their adult son or daughter with intellectual disability (Smith and Tobin 1993; McCallion and Tobin 1995). Bigby (2000: 29) summarized the central themes in the literature thus: 'The reluctance of parents to make concrete plans, and the dilemmas and difficulties that confront parents and service providers if they do embark on the planning process.'

To outsiders the need to plan for the future seems obvious. With increasing age it appears self-evident that arrangements should be in place to ensure a safe and secure future when parents are no longer able to look after their son or daughter. As the mother's words at the beginning of this chapter indicate, older parent-carers also recognize that the future is now. However, acknowledging an ever-present and uncertain future does not necessarily translate into engaging in the type of organized future planning that service providers prefer. Many authors (for example Kahana *et al.* 1994; Nolan *et al.* 1996a) have noted that it is never an easy task to engage in planning to place a cared-for relative in out-of-home care. Planning for your child's future after a lifetime of care and for when you are no longer around must surely be a daunting task. The focus on service use and degree of burden in previous studies of older parent-carers may have overlooked the critical fact that caregiving takes place within intimate relationships that have accrued meanings over a lifetime. The tasks of care are set within these relationships and the purposes of both the caregiver and the care-recipient. To explore the meaning and the purposes or ends to which older parent-carers direct their efforts we need to turn to narratives about their caring relationships over time.

This chapter therefore draws on the findings of a study with over sixty older parents in Sydney, Australia that was conducted between 2000 and 2002. One aim of the study was to explore the pathways taken by parent-carers in raising their disabled children. We believe that a better under-standing of lifelong caring, framed by the socio-historical context, offers some insight into parent-carers' later life decisions about family care. These pathways also shed some light on how individual biography is shaped by and in turn influences the socio-historical context in which parents raise their children.

We are aware that our study presents only one perspective, that of the older parent-carers, and does not include the experiences of their adult sons and daughters with intellectual disability. For readers interested to pursue the adult child's perspective we suggest turning to the growing number of publications in which adults with intellectual disability speak out about their lives. The work of Traustadottir and Johnson (2000) pro-vides a recent example of the lives of women with intellectual disability. We now turn to the study design and follow this with a description of the older parent-carer biography derived from our study.

## The study

The study was designed to explore the lifelong caring of older parent-carers and the inter-relationships between caring biographies and service use. Our central research strategy was narrative life history, a qualitative technique particularly well suited to understanding the lives of those whose experience departs from normative expectations. Derived from social constructionist theory (Blumer 1969) and following Gergen (1994), we view narratives as products of social interchange. Conducting in-depth interviews with older parents therefore provides the opportunity for them to tell their stories (narratives) as they occur naturally in their everyday lives. Thus, studying older parent caregivers' narratives offers insights into the way they portray – and understand – themselves within their ongoing relationships.

For the purposes of this study we defined primary older parent-carer following Schofield *et al.* (1998) as a person 60 years and over taking the main responsibility in caring for an adult son or daughter with intellectual disability. Intellectual disability was defined as per the 1992 American Association on Mental Retardation, 9th Edition Definition, Classification and System of Supports (AAMR 1992) where the results of previous intelligence testing were available. Alternatively, assessment was based on a history of special education placement or identification as intellectually disabled by a specialist developmental disability service.

## Older parent-carer sample

Our sample of over sixty older parent-carers was drawn from the northern region of Sydney, a large metropolis of approximately four million people. This geographical area was chosen because of its high concentration of late middle age to elderly people. We recruited older parents to the study by multiple methods. We approached aged care and assessment teams, developmental disability teams, home help services, non-government disability and non-government aged care agencies, general practitioners and support groups. At each entry point older people fitting the study criteria were given information about the study, and if they were interested in participating their contact details were forwarded to the research team. Articles in the local media attracted additional parents by direct contact and word of mouth. In this way we attracted parents who were service and non-service users and both co-resident (living in the same household) and non-co-resident parent-carers as well as those who had recently placed their son or daughter in non-familial care.

## The interviews

Parent-carers were interviewed in their own home or at another location of their choosing. Interviews were conversational in style, providing the opportunity for older parent-carers to 'tell their story'. Interviews usually began with an open-ended question such as 'how are things going with you and your adult son (daughter) these days?' We sought in the interview to answer the following questions:

• What is the older parent's point of view about his/her lifelong caring role?

- What major life events have resulted in adaptational changes or stresses on their parent-caring relationship?
- How do older parents regard their health status and what changes in their health status would they regard as desirable?
- How do older parents negotiate and experience support with their immediate family, extended family, friends and the wider community including health and community care services?
- What is the point of view of older parents about the likely future for themselves and for their adult son or daughter? How do they regard the place of services in their parent-caring relationship and do they anticipate that this may change in the future? What events can they foresee that may lead to their seeking help or additional assistance?

To explore further the status of this older parent-carer group, participants also completed four standardized self-report tools addressing health status, support network, and carers' assessment of difficulties and managing strategies. The findings from the self-report instruments are reported elsewhere (Llewellyn *et al.* 2002). In this chapter the focus is on the interview material that pertains to the parent-caring biography and its influence on family care decision making in later life.

All participants were followed up by telephone approximately one month after the initial interview to provide an opportunity to clarify or expand on the original material and for the interviewer to seek additional material based on preliminary analysis of the interview transcripts. Approximately one-fifth (13) of the participants, all of whom were over the age of 70, were interviewed a second time to explore and expand our thematic analysis of the parent-caring biography in later life.

## Analysing the interview material

Textual analysis of transcribed interviews was conducted based on the narrative approach developed by Riessman (1993). A parent-caring biography was developed for each participant detailing his/her broader experience of parent-caring relationships and inter-relationships with family, friends, formal services and the wider community. Close attention was paid to critical events and decision points described by participants over their parent-caring career. A typical parent-caring biography was subsequently constructed. This draws attention to new phases and ongoing experiences as older parent-carers negotiate and renegotiate their parent and carer status over their lifetime.

A thematic analysis of this typical biography reveals three distinct experiences common to the paths taken by older parent-carers over their lifetimes. The first of these derives from the myriad of ways in which parents come to understand that their child is perceived as being less able and consequently less worthy by others. This evokes a strong protective response that 'sets the scene' for parents to follow their parenting 'instincts' in family care decision making over their lifetimes. The second area is the ongoing hurt and deep frustration experienced by parents when, in spite of their developing expertise, they remain outside those admitted to the inner circle of experts – the professionals. This disregard for their parenting knowledge, as well as their family goals and beliefs, heightens their strong perceptions of themselves as 'those who know best' for their child, irrespective of their child's age.

The final experience pervades all others. The lack of worthiness accorded their child and the disregard for their expertise are experienced against the background of changing and uncertain policy and practice directions. The pendulum has swung from one extreme to another over the course of their lifetimes. The segregation of disabled people as the only solution available in their child's early years is now soundly condemned as inclusive practices for people with intellectual disability assume 'gold standard' status. Parents come to understand themselves and their values as the only stable and responsible constant in their child's life.

In the next section we describe the typical older parent-caring biography. Following this we discuss the three distinct experiences that arise from this biography and draw on interview material with the older parent-carers to illustrate the likely influence of these experiences on parents' willingness (or otherwise) to engage with services and planning for the future. In our view, elaborating these experiences aids our understanding of the biographical background against which older parent-carers make decisions about family care in later life.

We do not claim that this typical biography is a 'factual' description of the details of the lives of all our participants. Rather it is an aggregation of experiences constructed to represent a common story that captures the fundamentals evident in the experiences of all. Further, although a reasonable size sample for a study of this kind, this sample of older parent-carers cannot claim to be representative of all older parent-carers in a statistical sense. However, the ages of the participants were fairly evenly spread across the sixties, seventies and eighties with an average age of 68.8 years. Over three-quarters of the sample were women who identified as the primary parent-carer, which is consistent with social role expectations and an increased life span for women. The majority of participants, 60.9 per cent, were married and living with their partners. Thirty-nine per cent were caring alone, due to divorce (10.9 per cent), or being a widow (21.9 per cent) or widower (6.3 per cent). Among the adult sons and daughters with intellectual disability, over half (57.8 per cent) had an additional condition such as cerebral palsy, epilepsy, or other physical disabilities. The eldest adult child with intellectual disability was 74, the youngest 21, with an average age of 38.4 years.

We were pleased to attract participants from a range of parent-caring relationships. Almost half of the parent-carers (48.4 per cent) still had their adult son or daughter with intellectual disability living full-time in the family home. Other arrangements included living in a residential facility or hostel (23.4 per cent), independent living with another disabled person or alone (15.6 per cent), living in a group home (9.4 per cent), and living half-time with their parents and half-time in a service facility (3.1 per cent). For those adults with intellectual disability now living away from home, around one-third (32.8 per cent) had moved out of home as young adults in their twenties; 14.1 per cent had been placed out of home during their school years (from 5 to 18 years of age), and one child had been placed prior to starting school.

Older parent-carers missing from this sample are those of Aboriginal and Torres Strait Islander descent and those from culturally and linguistically diverse backgrounds. Our recruitment strategies failed to reach and engage the interests of these older parent-carers which is a major omission awaiting redress at a later date. In sum, the following older parent-carer biography needs to be read in light of this participant sample and understood as a narrative which reflects the commonalities of older parent-carers' lives while recognizing it is not able to capture the particularities of each participant's individual life story.

## Older parent-carer biography

*Finding out and declaring parental responsibility*

Older parent-carers' biographies begin with finding out that their child has an impairment. This is devastating. The 'news', however, is rarely unexpected. Mothers in particular report a sixth sense that they knew something was wrong before their child was born, immediately afterwards, or in the early months. Mothers hold on to these worries and their fears even in the face of patronizing dismissal of their concerns by others and especially doctors. When finally their concerns are acknowledged by medical intervention, and sometimes but not always result in a diagnosis, there is relief tempered by disappointment, dismay, and concern for their child's future.

Until parents and others talk about their child's impairment, however, it does not become 'really real'. 'Public' recognition comes with admitting their child has an impairment and sharing this knowledge with others. While the initial public recognition of impairment is devastating, it is not the last. Other impairments may become evident, as the child grows older. There may be short, sharp bursts of realization of the extent of their child's disability as, for example, a younger sibling overtakes their older child's development. There can be a slowly developing awareness as their hope for their child's 'recovery' diminishes. Each time parents need to 'rethink' their views about their child.

Acknowledging and accepting their child's impairments is made much worse by others' negative reactions and rejection of their child. This causes unimaginable hurt. Others may suggest that their child be put away in an institution and forgotten about. Family members may deny there is anything wrong even in the face of obvious difficulties and the parents' distress. Services supposedly catering for disabled children may restrict access to particular groups of children and parents then find they are denied support because their child does not fit into one of these groups. All of these behaviours speak to rejection of *their child*.

With this recognition comes a declaration of parental responsibility: *their child* will be loved and cared for as one of their own. This declaration is often reinforced by the contrasting advice coming from others. While typically being advised to place their children in institutional care, none appreciated being given this 'opportunity'. Feeling angry and hurt at this suggestion, many developed feelings of resistance and defiance and became extremely determined to raise their child at home.

In a myriad of ways parents come to understand that their child is, in stark contrast to typically developing children, not wanted in their community and not cared about. Their child is disabled. Parents come to understand that while their child has an impairment, the experience of disability is located within societal structures and cultural beliefs and practices, not within their child. It is society that disables and, conversely, it is the parents that come to see the need to rise to the challenge of making a place for their child in their family and their community.

*Seeking help*

Not surprisingly, parents seek help to deal with the difficult and un-familiar situation of having a disabled child. Without exception, they struggle to get information or to locate somebody who will help their child and find some hope of a future more positive than the present. This usually takes the form of seeking out medical advice from general practitioners and paediatricians. For older parent-carers in the early days of their caring career, little help was available on how to parent their child. Professional input was limited to expressions of intent such as giving their child lots of love or how to manage particular medical conditions such as epileptic fits. Clinical advice focused on weight gain and sleep patterns proved little help for parents whose children's development patterns were idiosyncratic and out-of-the-ordinary to those focused on 'normal' developmental milestones.

Seeking help becomes an ongoing part of the lives of parents of dis-abled children. It occurs prior to a 'diagnosis' being made; it happens again when an impairment is confirmed, and it continues as the children grow older. Many parents spoke about finding a person who helped them 'turn the corner'. This person may be the first who 'actually listened' to the parent, or had useful knowledge, for example about the child's impairment or a service available, or simply (although this was so infrequent it can hardly be spoken about as a simple matter) accepted the child for who they were and in so doing partly redressed the pain of rejection.

Given the unfolding of a child's development over time, having an impairment recognized can take time. There were likely to be periods of great uncertainty for parents – will the child be better than they dared hoped? Is the likely outcome indeed worse? The ambiguity and uncertainty surrounding diagnosis and predictions for the future left many parents in a state of limbo. Some, frustrated by the perceived rejection of their child, decided to go it alone, rely on their own resources and have no more contact with formal services, often for some time. Others became 'locked into' a cycle of visits and check-ups and second, third and fourth opinions.

*Developing expertise*

At the same time as they confront this unfamiliar and rejecting situation of parenting their disabled child, parents begin to develop expert knowledge about their child. They come to understand their likes and dislikes, which activities pacify their child and what activities to avoid, and to understand their child's abilities and the tasks that they cannot or will not do. This expertise was also rejected. Parents come to understand that only those who had specific professional training were to be accorded expert status. Parents' 'lay' knowledge has a secondary status (if any at all) compared to the 'expert' knowledge of professionals. Parents' experiential knowledge is dismissed in the face of professional technocratic knowledge. The gulf between these two knowledge bases and the privileging of the 'professional' over the 'lay' was to be repeated over and over during the parents' lifetimes. Examples included school teachers who knew 'best' about how to teach the child ignoring the parents' expertise in teaching many skills and tasks at home prior to school and throughout their school life. Later again, residential staff 'knew best' about medication routines and, despite explicit instructions otherwise, changed medication without consulting parents or medical practitioners. Job agencies sought inappropriate placements in opposition to parents' views on their child's capabilities; accommodation services chose housemates on criteria that neglected individual personality and preferences known to parents after a lifetime of living with their disabled child.

Parents most distrusted the 'distanced' stand taken by workers. Parents knowing their children well were able to anticipate their needs and offer appropriate and dignified preventative action. Without intimacy, workers relied on solutions typically formulated after an event. Adding insult to injury, 'professionals' came and went while parents and children remained, getting on as best they knew how with their family lives. Parents felt bound to get to know yet another professional, to tell their family story again, to listen to yet another 'perfect' professional solution and, as they and their adult children grew older, deal with workers who were many years their junior. The disruption in their lives caused by short-term professional involvement is in strong contrast to the continuity of a lifetime of parent-caring. 'Decreasing' worker wisdom contrasts sharply with parents' accumulating and deepening knowledge of their child over time.

### Life challenges

Professionals speak of life stages; parents speak about life challenges. Each challenge is determined by the public identity of disabled people at the relevant life stages. Each challenge forces parents to revisit their parental identity and typically expands and reinforces their parental protective responses toward their disabled child. So, for example, in the early years the significant challenge was seeking out an education and finding a school willing to accept their child. At this time little thought was given to educating disabled children, as they were considered outside the mainstream of those worthy of education. Parents faced significant barriers to be overcome; the notion and knowledge of special education was just beginning four or five decades ago. For parents whose children were severely intellectually delayed there were no schools; they banded together and started their own, later establishing day activities when their children's school days were over. 'Spastic' children were able to find a place in a recently established non-government organization that demanded intensive parental involvement with the promise of whole of life care. 'Slow' children were able to go to local schools for a few years, becoming increasingly socially isolated from the life of the school and the community such that parents frequently sought out segregated schools.

Despite these drawbacks, in retrospect parents talked about the school years as being less problematic. Schooling, in essence, was the only professional service that offered parents and their children some continuity over time. School days provided a regular, organized, available, relatively safe, 'normal', socially acceptable, and generally stimulating environment for their son or daughter and much valued respite, particularly for mother, from constant supervision and care. The school experience gained some of its positive value in contrast to the following huge void of long, unoccupied, empty days for their son or daughter when school attendance finished.

Once school was over there was a dreadful hiatus. With nowhere to go, and nothing to do, young adult men and women sat at home with their mothers (and with those fathers who were by now retired). Daily isolation, loneliness and lack of stimulation created significant stresses for parents and their young adult sons and daughters at this time. This is a time when older parent-carers spent many hours desperately searching for any alternative. For some the only alternative was to place their son or daughter in residential care. Parents or friends or family on their behalf actively sought out or lobbied government departments about day programmes or sheltered workshops or, more recently, supported employment opportunities. For parents a major achievement was being put on a waiting list and then offered a place; part-time, or unsuitable hours, or far from home – these features did not matter compared to parents' desires to have their son or daughter involved in an activity outside the family home. At the same time parents sought out or were occasionally offered respite services. Although appreciated, particularly as time out for the parent, respite assumed far less importance in older parent-carers' lives than achieving and maintaining meaningful activity in their adult child's life.

*Changing policy and practice*

Behind older parent-carers' activities in seeking a reasonable quality of daily life for their now adult children, professional philosophies, government policy and service practices continued to take new directions. From a position of almost total rejection of people with severe intellectual disability, new community services promising social integration, recreation and employment began to spring up. The now well-established services for people with physical disability were no longer allowed to conduct 'whole of life' services and schooling, activity centres, workshops, employment and accommodation became separately organized and run. Service workers and organizations known and trusted over a long period of time began to disappear or were 'reinvented' as separate entities, often in new locations. Parents had to start over again with a new service, a new organization and new workers. Promises were made about providing a fulfilling life for their adult children and parents' expectations were raised. Many assessments of adult children were undertaken; family meetings and individualized planning occurred; there was a lot of strategic planning and whiteboard exercises. There was little action.

Government policy, in contrast to when their children were born, was now promoting independent community living. For all parents 'letting go' of their adult sons and daughters was a difficult and emotionally wrenching task. Some began working with services to set up small group or independent living situations for their child. Once achieved, the 'settling in' period in community living was prolonged for some: typically parents felt less control than they would like over what went on. They had many questions: What do workers do with their children? Does this fit with their family values and standards? Who is making decisions and how are these made? How stable are the arrangements and are these in their adult child's best interests? Will support be decreased as others demand more, or government policy and funding levels change yet again?

Other parents, after years of disappointment or disgust at 'the system', decided to keep their children at home, often 'soldiering on' and coming to understand that they are now carers as well as parents. They have decided that there is no alternative that can ensure their son or daughter's welfare, as they desire. Regardless of where their adult son or daughter now lives, parents express their strong, enduring sense of responsibility for their child's health and happiness. Almost universally an atmosphere of 'this is as good as it gets' pervades their discussions, coupled with ongoing concern for the future. This is a time when older parent-carers explain their parental responsibility as being ever vigilant in monitoring their adult child's welfare.

And, the future is now. Parents universally express their deep concerns, some more urgently, others less, about when they will no longer be able to take responsibility for their son or daughter through ill health or death. When their adult child is happy and healthy and all seems to be going well, concerns for the future are not always so pressing. Alternatively, when their son or daughter is ill or in declining physical or mental health there is increased concern and particularly about whether they will be 'thrown out' of their current accommodation and, if so, what next? Less extreme but equally worrisome is parents' concern about meaningful activity once their son or daughter is too old to work or attend a day centre. With little thought apparently given to retirement activities for disabled people, and particularly for those living in the community, parent concerns focus on their adult child's likely isolation, loneliness and depression.

Confronting their own disability or impending death, a few parents make financial and/or guardianship plans. Some enlist the help of others such as siblings with the promise of resources to assist care for their brother or sister in the future. Others hope, without overtly discussing this with their family, that siblings or other family members will fulfil their 'responsibilities'. Many continue to put aside thoughts of no longer being able to care for their son or daughter and wish them to die before their own death and thus avoid the painful task of confronting the finality of their parenting career.

## The future driven by experience of the past

Recognizing the inevitable time when older parents are no longer able to take care of their adult son or daughter with intellectual disability, service providers are assisting parents to plan for the future building on recommendations from empirical studies (for example Walker and Walker 1998a; Bigby 2000) and practice wisdom (for example Magrill *et al.* 1997). Yet many parents remain reluctant to deal 'realistically' with what they fear is the end of their parent-carer career (Engelhardt *et al.* 1987; Freedman and Freedman 1994). We did not set out to examine how many parents had made firm plans for the future or whether these plans remained firm over time. Rather, our interest lay in understanding the parent experiences that may reasonably be expected to influence why older parent-carers may feel ambivalent about, avoid, or totally reject planning for the future. In this section, we draw attention to three distinct experiences evident in this parent-caring biography and suggest how these may explain older parent-carers' approaches to family care decision making in later life.

*Parental protective response*

Older parent-carers in this study reacted strongly against attitudes of rejection, segregation and institutionalization of their young disabled children. At the same time they were subjected to the 'unworthiness' sentiment embedded within these negative community responses to childhood disability. Their overwhelmingly strong reaction to rejection speaks to an extraordinarily strong parental protective response evoked in these older parent-carers. Our view is that this protective response toward their child in the early years expands and consolidates over time to exert a pervasive influence on family care decision making in later life. There are many examples of this protective response coming into play in the parent-caring biography. We have selected just one to examine here. This is parents' responses to others' view about where disabled children (and later adults) should live.

When others reject their infant or young child by suggesting institutionalization parents spring to their child's defence. Protecting their children from removal from the family home begins early and in some families may continue over a lifetime as 'expert' others advise parents that their offspring and their families would be better off if their disabled child lived away from home. We are not suggesting here that children were, or are, forcibly removed by the authorities. We are suggesting, however, that when people in positions of power and authority such as medical professionals and service providers recommend a particular course of action, and when family, friends or the wider community condone this course of action, parents may need to summon abundant energy and strength to resist this agreed and socially condoned position.

Much has been written about the socio-cultural processes that generate negative attitudes about impairment and disability. More recently attention has been given to how these processes impact upon 'disabled people in diverse ways and can lodge themselves in their subjectivities, sometimes with profoundly exclusionary consequences by working on their sense of personhood and self-esteem' (Thomas 1999: 47–8). Mothers of children with disabilities have also noted how having a disabled child disables the family in ways which undermine their sense of family and family well-being (Read 2000; Llewellyn *et al.* in press). This is not a trivial issue in the development of a meaningful family life and parental identity.

Our view is that these older parent-carers suffered such exclusionary consequences, yet, driven by their strong protective response to their children being rejected, they developed an enhanced sense of parental responsibility. In turn, this fuelled their ongoing desire to retain parental control as protectors of their children. Later life, with the potential adverse changes associated with their own ageing, their children's ageing and the inevitable realization of life nearing its end, works to destabilize this deeply embedded sense of parental control. As parents reach this phase in their parent-caring career they are confronted by many events over which they feel little sense of control. Their diminishing energy, potential ill health, and possible additional caring responsibilities undermine their sense of parental control and drive the growing realization that some or all of this control over their adult son or daughter's life will need to be relinquished.

In contrast to their confident appraisals in earlier years, where they could rely on their parental expertise, they are now faced with an entirely new situation without prior experience to draw upon. This situation is full of anxiety because in essence it is about the remainder of their child's life. At the most fundamental level their anxiety focuses on their adult child receiving a similar standard of physical care to that which they have provided over a lifetime, a concern noted by many authors (for example Smith *et al.* 1994; Bigby 2000). The greater worry for older parent-carers, however, is the uncertainty about who *might* or *could* or *will* take their place in making sure their son or daughter is happy and busy and enjoying his/her life, a feature also noted by Brubaker and Brubaker (1993).

*Remaining outside the circle of experts*

The strong thread of parental control in the older parent-carers' biographies faces a serious challenge from others' denial of parental expertise. Not surprisingly, parent-carers talk about knowing their children best; over time they develop a deep and sustaining knowledge of their children's preferences, personalities and idiosyncrasies. When this knowledge is denied parents are deeply hurt. The parent-caring biography illustrates several settings where this is likely to occur. Don speaks to this hurt when he describes how, when his young adult daughter went to live in a group home,

> the staff suggested that they could get all these things happening with Lydia, like getting her teeth really clean regularly and getting her reliably toilet trained. We were very hurt – they now realize the difficulties; they haven't achieved anything that we didn't achieve ourselves and we did a better job in some areas like teeth cleaning and toileting.

There is now good evidence from several countries that a substantial proportion of older parents of adults with intellectual disability – in some cases at least half – do not use the family support services that are available to them (Delaney 1994; Twigg and Atkin 1994; Smith 1997; Janicki 1996; Pierce 1991 cited in Bigby 2000). A number of reasons have been advanced for this somewhat surprising finding given the potential vulnerability of older parent-carers with increasing age. Smith (1997) suggested from his study with 235 mothers aged between 58 and 96 years in the state of New York that one plausible explanation was that the mothers did not perceive a need for many of the services on offer. Taking into account that greater service use was found among those mothers who reported high levels of subjective burden suggests that other mothers felt able to manage their situation without resorting to formal service support. Greater service use was also found among mothers of younger offspring. Older mothers, who had raised their child from a time when so few community services were available and who were unlikely to consider using such services, could explain this. Hayden and Heller (1997), for example, have suggested that mothers of this generation without access to services had to develop coping strategies which, in turn, effectively negated their need to seek outside support. As the parent-caring biography illustrates, our participants felt they had no choice but to manage alone – without services, without support and, in many instances, without understanding of their situation.

Another likely explanation of why older parent-carers do not use services is that their child was born at a time when people with intellectual disability where hidden away in institutions or at home. Indeed, Twigg and Atkin (1994) found in a British study that feelings of personal responsibility for their child (now an adult), embarrassment and a desire to keep 'one's troubles to oneself' were common among older parents of adults with intellectual disability and that these feelings effectively kept older parent-carers away from seeking help from others. This generational cohort effect is reflected in our data. George, for example, speaks for many when he says,

> To be successful at looking after someone who has a disability, you need to have a culture, or background of 'if you want something done, do it yourself'. I grew up with that; my wife grew up with it. Her attitude was, if there's a job to be done you do it, and you do it yourself.

There is another salient point about this generation. The older participants had lived through the experience of World War II, some in the tragic circumstances of Central Europe. One mother speaks about surviving the Holocaust and how that shaped the way in which she approached life with her disabled daughter. She talks about learning as a young child to be very strategic, to think clearly and quickly, and never to react purely on impulse. She learned to weigh every option carefully and choose a response that was likely to have the best possible outcome. This careful and strategic thinking helped her to gather the information needed to help her daughter, and directed the way in which she responded to her daughter's needs.

Researchers have also reported consistently greater satisfaction by older parent-carers with caring and less stress than their younger counterparts (for example Smith and Tobin 1993; Hayden and Heller 1997). Several factors have been identified including mutuality in the caregiving relationship that develops between older parents and their adult children over time (Grant 1993; Hayden and Heller 1997). Of critical importance here is the satisfaction of older parent-carers with a job well done. The converse of this is that the area of greatest worry for many of the older parent-carers is the safety, health and well-being of their adult children when they are not directly under their care.

The essential point is that older parent-carers use their experiential expertise to anticipate and prevent deleterious situations. This is in contrast to the care offered by professional carers who are less familiar with the care recipient or who are new to caring and are therefore forced to rely on theoretical knowledge, not experience (Eraut 1994). Two examples from our data will suffice. The first comes from a widowed mother in her eighties who was very aware of maintaining a calm and quiet environment with no bright lights and loud television or radio to reduce the possibility of her son's recurring epileptic fits. Another comes from a 78-year-old mother whose daughter has cerebral palsy. She abstains from using perfumed solvents and avoids carpets as well as undertaking a regular intensive cleaning regime to decrease the likelihood of respiratory illnesses for her daughter with reduced mobility. Dissatisfaction with the standards maintained by residential care providers or fear of inadequate attention to basic health needs reinforces for many older parent-carers their view that they are the only ones who can provide appropriate and adequate care.

Across many types of caregiving, authors have reported that negative experiences with services can and do drive caregivers away, often for extended periods of time and beyond the time when re-engagement would be in the best interests of the caregiver and the cared-for person. There are many reasons given for this disengagement, including lack of respect for the caregiver, unsuitability of the services offered in terms of their content or the time and place where they are available, and perceived inattention to caregivers' needs. Robinson and Williams (1999) note, for example, that even when a system has been put in place to assess carers' needs, older parent-carers report that aspects of their lives concerning their health, housing, work and ability to continue caring are not even discussed during these assessments.

With the exception of writings by parents about their experiences of raising a child with a disability, there has been little attention given in the research literature to the invasion felt by families when medical and other professionals enter their lives. A poorly understood component of this invasion is how it permeates all aspects of families' everyday lives. In a practical sense, older parent-carers in this study reported being required to alter their preferred daily routines to fit the time schedules of service providers, often travelling long distances and waiting for extended periods to suit the professionals and not the families' convenience. At a personal level, older parent-carers reported feeling all aspects of their family lives open to scrutiny by an ever-changing parade of 'strangers'. Their intimate relationship with their partner, their family values, beliefs and goals for their children, their financial status and many other areas of family life were frequently examined. While recognizing that questioners may have offered the opportunity not to divulge information, parent-carers frequently reported feeling under 'pressure' to comply for fear of losing out on a potential service or backlash against their child. Parent-carers' protective responses, coupled with their belief in their ability to provide the best care for their adult children and their desire to do so within the privacy of their family lives, all help to shape their reluctance to look beyond their present situations to a likely uncertain future.

*Uncertain policy and practice directions*

A lifetime of parenting a disabled child leaves older parent-carers with superior knowledge of the 'changing fashions' in disability policy and service provision. In one lifetime all have experienced the full range of advice on what they should do and how this should be done with their (now adult) children. For example, in relation to where their children should live at birth or in their early years, the 'best' advice was to place their children in an institution and to go home and forget about them. Community attitudes reinforced rejection of disabled children by segregation in institutional care and special schooling at the same time as promoting a sense of protectiveness born out of pity for these 'poor unfortunate' children. Organizations founded by parents at this time worked hard to accumulate bricks and mortar to ensure secure 'birth to death' care for their disabled children. Within a decade or so, the tide had turned and including people with disabilities in the mainstream of society had become the watchword of policy makers and professionals. Now children were to be integrated and to take their place in their local school. Parent-carers were expected to give up the special support offered by segregated schooling and welcome this 'mainstreamed' opportunity. Parent organizations providing cradle-to-grave care found themselves out of step with policy directives and funding opportunities yet were forced by financial imperatives to take on board, however reluctantly, the fragmentation of their whole-of-life services.

This brief overview suggests that over time parent-carers face remarkably different options and pressures resulting from changes in policy and practice direction. More deeply felt, however, is the impact these changes have on parental identity and satisfaction. Here we return to our example of where disabled children 'should' live. Older parent-carers participating in this study considered that, in keeping their child at home in the early years, they had rejected public opinion and overcome the objections raised by others. They felt they had done a good job, a not always easy and sometimes quite difficult job. Not surprisingly, they felt an important and deep sense of satisfaction in doing so, and thus becoming a competent parent of a disabled child. This sense of parental competence was reinforced by others' changing opinions – parents came to be seen as those solely responsible for their child and as their child's protector ready and willing to provide whole-of-life care.

With little consultation or regard for their views, the tide of professional sentiment turned and parents became the guilty party if their adult child remained in the family home. Phrases such as 'over-protective parents' entered professional discourse and writers began urging parents to 'let go' of their adult disabled children. Comparisons were drawn between the expected ages of leaving home and independence for non-disabled adults and the so-called extended dependence of disabled adults upon their parents. Institutionalization was now regarded as very bad – and indeed in many situations no longer available – while living away from home was considered the preferred option. In an ironic twist, parents' behaviours now became framed as obstructionist and particularly so with regard to the rights of their adult disabled children. In earlier days they had kept their young children at home (then not advised, and now recommended). Now they were willing to continue their parental responsibilities and have their adult children remain at home with them – their desire to do so now criticized as interfering with their adult son or daughter's right to be independent. Against these deeply conflicting views experienced within one parent-caring lifetime career how certain can an uncertain future become for older parent-carers of adult sons and daughters with intellectual disability?

## Family decision making in later life

There is evidence from a number of studies that a significant proportion of older parent-carers, generally around one-half to two-thirds, do not make plans regarding future financial, residential or guardianship arrangements for their adult sons and daughters (Grant 1989; Heller and Factor 1991; Kaufmann *et al.* 1991; Prosser and Moss 1996; Freedman *et al.* 1997). Heller and Factor (1991), for example, found that less than one-third of the 100 family caregivers they sampled had taken any specific steps regarding future living arrangements, an issue of critical importance once the adult child is no longer able to live with his/her parents. Among the over two hundred mothers in the study by Smith *et al.* (1995), one in five had not even discussed plans for the future and another 13 per cent had only engaged in early discussions. These authors concluded, 'Unless permanency plans are made, adverse outcomes are likely to occur' (p. 497). This is of serious concern given that likely outcomes are the need for an emergency placement that may be unsuitable and uncertain financial and guardianship status for offspring who survive their parents when no future plans have been put in place.

The evidence to date suggests several factors are positively associated with planning (Essex *et al.* 1997) including behaviour problems of the adult with intellectual disability, high unmet needs of the parent-carer and small support networks. In addition, Smith *et al.* (1995) found perceptions of more adverse changes with age and reports of more help from other children without disabilities were associated with higher levels of planning for future living arrangements. The involvement of other children without disabilities may be influenced by the importance noted by several researchers (for example Seltzer *et al.* 1991) of practitioners engaging siblings to help ease the stress associated with the inevitable separation of older parents and their adult offspring. This may, however, not always be a desired outcome for the siblings or a desirable outcome for the older parent-carers and their disabled son or daughter. As younger children, siblings become drawn into their parents' caring responses, and are often entrusted with looking after their brother or sister with intellectual disability. In adulthood, this may translate into unstated parental expectations that siblings will share the care of their disabled brother or sister as their parents age, take over when one or both parents die, and thereby bypass formal support (Smith *et al.* 1995).

Overall the literature suggests that the older parent-carers most likely to engage in making future residential plans are those who are currently linked into the service system (Heller and Factor 1991; Wood and Skiles 1992; Smith *et al.* 1994). It could be that involvement with services decreases older parent-carers' apprehensiveness towards community residential placements or simply provides an opportunity for dealing with a difficult issue that at best evokes ambivalence and at worst is actively avoided (Richardson and Ritchie 1989). The parent-caring biography presented in this chapter suggests that experiences with services lead many older parent-carers to be wary of turning to others for assistance. Nor can we ignore the gratifications experienced by many older parent-carers as a reason why they are reluctant to seek service support. Their views on the rewards of caregiving contrast sharply with the widespread professional view that caregiving by its very nature is overwhelmingly stressful and experienced as a burden (for example Grant *et al.* 1998). Positive effects experienced over a lifetime of care may render this group of older parent-carers less likely to seek help outside their family relationships. However, it could also be that these older parent-carers are bound into relationships that mean they do not seek help when the balance of interest turns against continuing.

The desire of service providers that older parent-carers make concrete and detailed plans appears logical in the face of their increasing parental age. Making plans for adults with intellectual disability to live outside the family home also sits comfortably with current service philosophies about the meaning of adulthood, independence and quality of life for adults with intellectual disability. There is a strong financial imperative for policy makers and service providers to consider who will pay for the care of the adult with intellectual disability once their parents are no longer able to do so. In contrast, the interests of older parent-carers in the uncertain future are rooted in their strong parental identities established in response to earlier rejections of their children, their traditions of independence and personal responsibility and their experiences of having their parental expertise overlooked or denied. Simply put, for older parent-carers the question is *who* will look after my child and in the way that I have done?

In this chapter we explored the caring relationships of older parents of adults with intellectual disability and their involvement with the formal service system over time by way of a typical parent-caring biography. The unique features of their caregiving careers include a strong sense of parental identity and enhanced protective responses, denial of their achievements and the rewards of their parent-caring career and their concerns about consistent service provision in the future based on their past experiences. These characteristics present a challenge in terms of engaging older parent-carers in family care partnerships that effectively plan for the future.

In order to meet more effectively the needs of older parent-carers already engaged with services, Grant (2001) suggests replicating the family-orientated case management strategies that have been systematically evaluated with families with younger children with disabilities. The caregiving careers of older parent-carers of adult children with intellectual disability began – and continue – in a different time and place. Confronting the immediate presence of an uncertain future will need to be a central component of case management underpinned by recognition of older parent-carers' lifetime experiences brought to any talk of the future. Successful case management may well hinge on acceptance and affirmation of the unique characteristics of their caring careers in tandem with giving full rein to their strong parental identities. The task ahead is to develop and evaluate family care partnerships that create a more certain future acceptable to both older parent-carers and their adult sons and daughters with intellectual disability.

# 'Reaching the end' and 'a new beginning'

We anticipate that one of the most important future directions for caregiving research will include the focus on the impact of transitions involving the institutionalisation or death of the care recipient.

(Schulz and Williamson 1997: 122)

In many respects the stage of caregiving termed 'reaching the end' (Nolan et al. 1996a) is a misnomer as, other than the death of the cared-for person, caring rarely ends *per se*. Indeed, it is now abundantly clear that placing the cared-for person in a care home does not mean the 'end' of caring and that family carers remain involved in several ways. This section focuses on the nature of transitions from one type of care to another.

Bigby's chapter flows seamlessly from that of Llewellyn which ended the last section, as it too concerns people with learning disabilities and again draws on data from Australia. Here, however, Bigby focuses on the informal networks of older people with learning disabilities who are no longer supported by their parents. She highlights the central role played by one key 'support' person, usually a sibling or more distant relative or friend. However, she also describes the vulnerability of such informal networks and advocates that planning for caring transitions should begin early and be ongoing.

It is the absence of just such planning that is the central message of the next two chapters which address issues surrounding placing a relative in care in Australia and Sweden. Once again, remarkable similarities emerge which point to the difficult, stressful and often unplanned way in which the search for a care home is experienced. Pearson *et al.* provide a useful summary and overview of their study in Australia and a particularly important contribution of the ways in which implicit 'rules' shape discourse around entry to care. Within the academic literature the central message is 'home is best' and the vilification of institutional alternatives is reinforced by the media which portrays care homes as places to be 'feared and avoided'. Similarly the policy rhetoric presents seemingly strong economic arguments as to why community care is the way forward. However, as Pearson *et al.* tellingly note, the reality is that some alternative form of care will always be required and there is an urgent need for a discourse that provides a view of care homes as a 'positive choice'.

Sandberg *et al.* explore how such a 'positive' choice might come about and focus on the nature and quality of relationships between staff and families in care homes. They highlight the delicate way in which carers need to '(re)-construct roles and relationships' and discuss how this process is either helped or hindered by staff. They argue that if staff show 'empathic awareness' then carers and staff are far more likely to develop positive and mutually rewarding relationships.

It is the interface between staff, older people and families that also forms the substance of Davies's chapter. Based on interviews with family carers and case studies in three care homes, Davies develops a typology of three types of community that might exist. She terms these the 'controlled community', the 'cosmetic community' and the 'complete community'. She argues that such communities may not fully exist anywhere, in other words they should be viewed as 'ideal types', but believes that one community type or another tends to dominate in a given set of circumstances. Her description of the 'complete community' and the factors that shape it provide a powerful lens through which to view the quality of relationships, quality of life and quality of work environments in care homes.

In the final chapter in this section Lundh *et al.* return the focus to Sweden and describe how they piloted and evaluated an intervention designed to promote better working partnerships between staff and families in care homes. Their work demonstrates that with goodwill and hard work small but potentially significant improvements can be made providing that initiatives have the support of all the key players. However, in order to be sustained there is a need for ongoing commitment and support at all levels. Therefore, while they strike a positive chord, Lundh *et al.* conclude that 'the search for better partnerships has only just begun'. A fitting frame of mind in which to approach this final section of the book.

# 9

# The evolving informal support networks of older adults with learning disability

## Christine Bigby

### Background and scope

In recent decades significant advances have occurred in connection with the rights of people with learning disabilities to exercise choices and social inclusion. Nevertheless, in the UK, USA and Australia a majority of adults with learning disabilities continue to live with their parents until they are middle-aged, out of choice, due to family commitments, or simply because they lack alternatives (Seltzer and Krauss 1994; Beange and Taplin 1996; Walmsley 1996). The transition from parental care for this group is inevitable rather than a choice, as they are more likely than in previous eras to outlive their parents. What will happen when we die? can be a source of overwhelming anxiety for parents. Families and policy makers confront the issue of who will replace the myriad of roles that parents have fulfilled in the lives of their adult child with learning disability.

This chapter examines continuities and changes in the informal support networks of middle-aged adults with learning disability as they make the transition from parental care into a largely uncharted world. The term informal support lacks precision and, within the literature, is often used interchangeably with informal care, social support, support networks and social relationships. The distinguishing characteristic, however, is that informal support relationships are based on personal ties between individuals as individuals. These may stem from membership of a common kinship system in the case of family members, personal affinity as occurs between friends, or geographic propinquity or use of common spaces by neighbours or acquaintances. The concept of networks is a framework for the analysis of informal relationships, and a vehicle through which support is exchanged. A social network approach draws attention to the structure of relationships that exist between network members, the specific exchanges that take place and the roles they play in relation to one another.

Contrary to commonly expressed fears, it will be suggested that when parents can no longer manage to care, other family members or friends become more involved in the life of the person with a disability, taking on some aspects of what were previously parental roles (Bigby 2000). However, as people age their support networks retain dynamic qualities, reflecting both changing needs and life course adaptations. Nevertheless, demonstrated are the enduring and vital roles of family support in optimizing opportunities and reducing vulnerabilities in the later part of the life course for people with learning disability.

The latter part of the chapter considers the importance of 'key person succession plans' as a mechanism for facilitating the transition to non-parental care while ensuring continuity of roles played by informal support networks. Although more robust than often expected, the informal support networks of adults with learning disabilities are vulnerable to disruption and shrinkage as they age in the years that follow the transition from parental care. This leads to a discussion of how families, practitioners, planners and policy makers can support the maintenance of networks and create conditions that foster their development. This may involve looking beyond existing long-term family relationships towards the broader community.

## Informal support of adults living at home with elderly parents

The networks of adults with learning disabilities who remain at home with parents are smaller and less diverse, with a more central role fulfilled by parents, compared to those of adults who leave home in young adulthood (Krauss and Erickson 1988). Parents are pivotal; they not only take on major 'caring for' and 'caring about' tasks but also link their offspring to more distant family members and share common friends.

Networks of adults with learning disabilities who live at home with parents are characterized as family-embedded and community-insulated (Grant 1993) – dominated by family members but without significant linkages into the wider community through friendships or participation in community organizations. This insulation may be a parental strategy to protect the self-image of their adult child (Todd and Shearn 1996b). Family, primarily parents and siblings generally, account for three-quarters of all network members. Parents, usually mothers, provide the instrumental care required, with little practical assistance from others in the network or formal services. Siblings and more distant relatives take on supportive tasks, affirming the role of parents, and providing emotional support and companionship to the adult with learning disability (Krauss *et al.* 1992; Prosser and Moss 1996; Bigby 2000).

Relationships between adults and their siblings are variable and where a person has more than one sibling they have different kinds of ties and strengths of attachment with each. Zetlin (1986) found the spectrum of relationships between siblings extended from warm with frequent regular contact and provision of companionship to resentful with minimal contact. Krauss and her colleagues in their longitudinal study of adults with learning disabilities living at home highlight the significance of siblings' roles. They conclude, 'as adults siblings have sustained contact with and rather extensive knowledge about the contemporary needs of their brother or sister with mental retardation and have engaged in a variety of familial experiences that signal continuing and meaningful roles in adulthood' (Krauss *et al.* 1996: 30). Sibling relationships where one of the dyad has a learning disability are both similar to (characterized by a low level of instrumental assistance) and different from (the salience of their involvement with respect to mothers' well-being) patterns reported among typical adult siblings (Seltzer and Krauss 1994).

Support networks of adults with learning disability living at home are small, usually around five to seven members, and distinguished by long-term relationships and frequent contact. As adults often share the friends of their parents, network members tend to be from a similar or older generation than themselves. Studies indicate that almost 50 per cent of adults at home have no friends and those they have are shared with parents or are seen only in the context of attendance at a day programme (Bigby 2000).

Age, life course stage of other family members and family milieu are some of the factors that stand out as influencing the relationships of adults who remain at home with parents. As parents age, their networks are likely to diminish due to death and incapacity of their spouse and peers, which will impact on the support available to the adult with learning disability. During young adulthood, siblings are likely to leave home due to career demands or to form their own families, both of which are likely to reduce the intensity of their relationship with the adult with learning disability. However, siblings remain more involved in families that are cohesive and orientated to achievement and independence (Seltzer *et al.* 1991).

Reciprocal relationships are likely to develop between adults with learning disability and their primary carers as parents age, become frail or are widowed (Todd *et al.* 1993; Walmsley 1996). Strong bonds of mutual aid and a sense of interdependence may develop between an elderly carer and the adult with learning disability. By undertaking domestic chores, providing a watchful eye in case of falls, and contributing to the financial viability of the household their presence may ensure their parent can continue to live in their own home (Walmsley 1996).

## Study participants

The empirical findings that follow are based on the author's research in Australia that retrospectively tracked the life changes of a group of older people with learning disability since they had left parental care in middle age (Bigby 2000). Sixty-two older adults and members of their formal and informal support networks participated in the study. They were recruited after an intensive case finding exercise that ensured the group included people who were not using disability services as well as those who were. For each older person the primary informant was someone with whom they had a close, long-term relationship. They were mainly siblings but included friends, nieces, cousins, an aunt and service providers from aged care or disability service sectors. Fifty-one of the 62 older people were also interviewed.

All the older adults in the study had lived with their parents until at least the age of 40 years. The age at which they had left parental care varied from 40 to 73 years, and the average age of leaving had been 52 years. They were all born prior to 1940 and at the time of the study were aged between 55 and 87 years, with an average age of 65 years. The average age of parents when they relinquished care had been 86 years. At the time of the study adults had been away from parental care for between 1 and 46 years. Most of the adults had a mild to moderate level of intellectual disability that had been acknowledged since childhood. Most had led quite sheltered lives characterized by limited expectations and participation in community life. Many had only a few years' schooling and only a few had participated in paid employment. All except three of the adults were from Australian or Anglo-Celtic backgrounds. At the time of the study 25 per cent had age-related health problems that restricted their mobility and had reduced their functional abilities and another 25 per cent had more minor problems such as sensory losses. In-depth interviews sought detailed descriptions about all aspects of the person's life since they left parental care. This included the types of plans made by parents, how the transition from parental care had occurred, events in the life of the person since the transition and the nature of their supportive network. Qualitative data were analysed for common themes using the constant comparative method (Huberman and Miles 1994), with the aid of a 'search and retrieve' computer program, the Ethnograph.

## The transition from parental care

Unlike most other 'caring' relationships, that between an adult child with learning disability and their parent is likely to be disrupted by the death or incapacity of the main family carer. This represents a major life transition, precipitating a shift to non-parental care and an upheaval and rearrange-ment of informal support. However, the transition from parental care for the majority of people with learning disability is not a sudden crisis event; rather it is a gradual process as parent/s become more frail, and is typically managed informally by close kin often without recourse to formal services (Bigby 2000). In my study 10 per cent of transitions were pre-planned and implemented prior to parental incapacity, 8 per cent were sudden while 77 per cent occurred in a gradual manner as parental health deteriorated. This is contrary to the perception of community service providers, many of whom are inevitably involved only in crisis situations or when the informal support networks break down.

The process of transition for the majority of adults with learning disability occurs as a key member of their informal network gradually assumes day-to-day responsibility for their well-being, and begins to consider and negotiate longer term alternatives for care. This usually parallels changes in the situation of parent/s as they become increasingly frail and require more support from other family members. By foreseeing the need to renegotiate responsibility, the key person often protects parents from difficult decisions they wish to postpone. Key people deal with the current contingencies of care, investigate available options, and negotiate alternative care. Acting in this way as *de facto* case managers they are able to avert crises and inappropriate short-term solutions. For example:

> Brendan's mother's health had deteriorated and she was fast losing her sight. Her daughter investigated and organized alternative supported accommodation for Brendan that in turn made it possible for Brendan's mother to agree to move in with and be cared for by her daughter.

> When Joe's mother went into hospital for the first time his sister visited him daily to assist with cooking and other household tasks. At the same time she began to investigate services that might provide in-home support for Joe and his mother when she came home. She organized a home help service and meals on wheels, and involved several neighbours in monitoring the household. After several hospital admissions Joe's mother didn't come home and Joe was able to remain in the house with regular support from formal services, his sister and his neighbours.

The transition from parental care involves at minimum a change in who takes charge of day-to-day care for the person. It may also mean the death of a parent, and a residential move, with associated changes of locality and day programme. In my study 45 per cent of adults did not move house at the time of transition, 18 per cent moved to supported accommodation for people with disabilities and 21 per cent to an aged care facility.

As parents relinquish instrumental roles assumed by siblings and other relatives, the roles of informal network members change during this process of transition. In the present study, directly after transition another informal network member replaced the everyday care parents had provided for just over half of the adults. It was mainly siblings who replaced parents but these tasks were also taken on by more distant relatives such as an aunt or niece or a family friend such as a church minister. However, continued provision of everyday care is often short-lived as informal network members experience life course changes, such as ill health or the incapacity of their spouse. In the years that follow transition, primary care is increasingly taken over by formal services until by the time adults with learning disabilities reach 65 years the majority are likely to live in supported accommodation. An example of this trend is Josh:

> Josh lived at home with his parents on a farm until his father died, at which time both he and his mother went to live with his sister Freda and her husband. Josh's mother died several years later when Josh was 53 years old. Josh continued to live with his sister but both she and her husband began to have health problems. Eventually Freda found that she could not care for both Josh and her husband and arranged for Josh to move to a local older persons' hostel. Freda is still very involved in Josh's life and visits him every day as does one of her daughters.

A characteristic of the transition process and post-parental care phase is the split of two functions hitherto performed by parents; provision of primary day-to-day care and responsibility for oversight of the well-being of the adult with learning disability. While primary care is progressively transferred to formal services, oversight of well-being is generally retained informally, with a key person replacing parents.

## Informal networks in later life

Informal networks of older adults in the post-parental phase remain small with an average of six people in touch with the person at least twice a year. They continue to be dominated by family members, dense, i.e. people are known to each other, and made up chiefly of people from the same or an older generation as the person with learning disability. The roles played by various network members, particularly siblings, often change and intensify, although when individuals leave the parental home people often lose the incidental contact with extended family members who had close links with their parent rather than themselves. The distinguishing feature of post-parental informal networks is the existence of a 'key person' who has a strong role in oversight of well-being and partially replaces roles previously fulfilled by parents. Overall, however, the most common type of support received by older people from members of their informal network falls into the 'caring about' rather than 'caring for' category, and involves social contact in the form of visits or outings.

Research findings on the extent to which older people with intellectual disabilities have contact with family members vary a great deal. For example, my study found that 92 per cent of all the older people had at least twice yearly contact with a family member. In comparison an earlier Australian study found that only just under half of the older people they surveyed had contact with family members (Ashman *et al.* 1993). A similar proportion of older residents in UK long-stay hospitals were found to have contact with their family (Kearney *et al.* 1993). It would seem that earlier life experiences influence the strength of relationships in later life, and that people who have stayed at home with parents till middle age are likely to have stronger relationships with family members in later life than those who have left home at an earlier age (Skeie 1989; Bigby 1997a).

Ties with siblings are the most significant relationships as well as the closest for most older people with learning disability. Seventy-nine per cent of the older people in my study still had a live sibling, and 96 per cent of these people saw at least one of their siblings twice a year or more. As discussed below, siblings are most likely to act as key people, but where there is more than one sibling in contact or someone else plays a key role, the other siblings have mainly social contact with the older person. In a very few instances a sibling may be alienated from their brother or sister with learning disability and have little or no contact. In such cases there has usually been a long history of a poor relationship between them (Bigby 1997b).

## Key person role

More than three-quarters of the older people in my study received more concrete 'caring about' support such as advocacy, mediation and negotiation with service providers or monitoring service quality. This was usually provided by only one network member – a 'key person'. The existence of a key person who proactively oversees the well-being of the older person by managing their affairs and negotiating service provision is the most striking feature of the informal networks of older adults with learning disability in the post-parental phase of their lives. These key people are not spouses or children as is the case with older people in the general community, as these relationships are absent in the network of most older people with learning disability. Rather, key people are more distant relatives or friends. Key people have frequent contact with the older person, often sharing social activities as well as performing more instrumental tasks. They have a strong attachment, a long-term relationship, and are very committed to the person's well-being.

It is primarily siblings who are key people but they also include more distant relatives and friends. The 11 key people who were not siblings comprised, three very elderly parents, four church-related or family friends, two nieces, a cousin and an aunt. A close long-term relationship with the older person and a negotiated commitment to them, which will often have been foreshadowed in parental plans for the future, are the basis of key person relationships rather than genealogical ties alone. The relationship between Jean and her brother John is typical in this particular respect:

> When Jean's parents died she wanted to remain in the local community where she had lived all her life rather than moving nearer to her brother Harry, who lives on the other side of Melbourne. Harry organized for her to move into a private supported residential service and visited her regularly. When he became aware that the home had changed hands and the standards at the service were deteriorating he lodged a series of complaints about the care provided for Jean. Eventually, when things did not improve, he helped Jean to find an older person's hostel to move into. He visits Jean once a week and takes her out for a walk around the shops and a coffee. Harry negotiated her entry to the hostel and helps Jean manage her financial affairs. She has recently had problems with her eyes and he has organized medical appointments for her. Jean has another brother whom she sees on special occasions. Harry says he has always had a much closer relationship with Jean than his brother and it was agreed with his parents that he would 'look after' Jean when the time came.

Key people took on strong advocacy, monitoring and negotiation roles with formal services. Given the reliance of older people with learning disabilities on formal organizations for their day-to-day care this was a crucial role in several respects. The longer the time that individuals were away from parental care the more likely they were to have moved more than once, and to have lost any contact with specialist disability services. A clear trend existed in the post-parental phase of entry to specialist disability accommodation and then exit to mainstream aged care services. Many of these moves were contentious. Key network members vigorously contested such transfers when they considered them to be inappropriate. As a result many older people with learning disability lived in what were considered by their key person to be an inappropriate environment. Issues of concern were: fostering of dependence, lack of stimulation, other residents being substantially older and frailer than the adult with learning disability, and staff who lacked knowledge of disability or who were poorly attuned to their needs. Key network members were involved in advocating for better day-to-day care and support. The issues with which they were involved ranged from relatively minor issues such as helping people to put on their glasses to major issues such as provision of nursing care, stimulation and exercise. Where the quality of care was considered too low, key network members took a lead role in negotiating a change of accommodation.

Key people usually came from a different generation with different perspectives of what was possible for people with learning disability and took definite steps to seek out opportunities for social contacts and to broaden their horizons. Half of the adults with learning disability experienced considerable personal development in the years following their transition from parental care. This included matters of major importance like the development of new skills and social relationships, expansion of social and domestic activities and the increased exercise of autonomy and independence. Freedom from the constraints imposed by living with a frail parent, release from the protectiveness of parents and for the first time being perceived as an adult rather than a child provided the context for later developments. Further opportunities were presented by formal services, such as day programmes or specialist disability accommodation as well as by the helpful attitudes and efforts of key people. References to protective parental attitudes were not judgement or blaming but recognized the very different historical context and attitudes held about people with intellectual disabilities when they become parents.

## Relationships with other family members

Family members, other than those who fulfil a key person role, were siblings, sisters- and brothers-in-law, and more distant relatives. Their contact was 'friendly', neither as frequent nor involved as that of a key person and without the same sense of commitment. However, other family members did play significant roles in providing social contact, opportunities for outings and some instrumental tasks. The wives of brothers who are key people often took responsibility for helping with shopping for clothes or furnishings. Sons and daughters of key people, who are often potential future key people, act as 'back-up', replacing the roles of their parents during holidays or times of ill health. Contact with more distant relatives occurs at time of celebration, reflecting family traditions, and is usually reliant on an effective replacement for the kin keeper role that was previously the mother's role.

## Friends and acquaintances

Two-thirds of the older people in the study named at least one person as a friend. Relationships with friends were usually affective and contact with them was tied to a specific context such as a day programme or place of residence. The several exceptional people who socialized with friends 'after hours' had been actively encouraged and supported to do so by staff or their key person.

Accounts and perceptions of friendships differed between informants. Family and service providers were often unaware of friendships or dis-counted peer relationships by taking the view that, because of their poor social skills, an older person had no friends. In contrast, older people themselves were in little doubt about friendships, often naming friends about whom other informants were unaware. However, a UK study by Grant and his colleagues (1995) found that very few older people had friendships that involved intimacy or reciprocity.

The value of friendships between people with intellectual disabilities and of those with people without intellectual disabilities is a source of debate. It is argued by some that the relations between people with and those without disabilities are of more value as they provide avenues to inclusion, access to more valued roles and to instrumental tasks (Chappell 1994). However, Chappell argues that such a position devalues the social connections that arise from relationships of this kind, and ignores the aspects of solidarity, which have the potential to bring about social change. The fundamental question, however, should be whether friendships between peers with disabilities are based on common affiliations and choice and therefore quite different from enforced segregation solely on the basis of a shared disability. Ethnographic research that has tapped the views of older people with learning disabilities suggests that they often do not distinguish between friends on the basis of their disability but value friendships from both sources (Mahon and Mactavish 2000).

Many of the people who continued to live in the vicinity of their family home regarded one or more neighbours as friends. These neighbours were an important source of informal support, providing affective support and sometimes undertaking tasks such as taking the person shopping or contacting relatives on their behalf. However, only two of the 46 people who had moved locality retained contact with previous neighbours. Older people who lived in supported accommodation had contact with co-residents but rarely with other people in their neighbourhood.

Older people sometimes referred to unnamed groups of people as friends. For example, one person said, 'I go to the football every week, they all know me there.' This suggests that some older people also have a network of acquaintances that gives them a sense of identity and belonging to the community but, unlike friendships, places few expectations on them. The importance of acquaintances was also suggested in a UK study conducted by Grant and his colleagues that examined the place of older people with learning disability in the community. This study concluded, however, that despite the existence of acquaintances, older people did not appear to have strong relationships with their communities and they 'experienced degrees of physical, functional and organizational integration in their social lives but lacked personal, social and societal integration in a variety of ways' (Grant *et al.* 1995: 42).

## Vulnerability of informal networks

Older people with learning disabilities appear to be vulnerable to loss of contact with family and friends and to a reduction in network size as they outlive siblings and other relatives. For some of the older people in this study the key person, who replaced many of the roles undertaken by parents, died before they did. In some instances they were replaced by someone from the younger generation such as a niece or nephew. However, the older a person was the more likely they were not to have the key person replaced. Godfrey's experiences are typical of loss of network members experienced as people age and the eventual absence of a network member with a close relationship who can play a key role:

> Godfrey is the youngest of a family of three brothers and a sister. When Godfrey's parents died he went to live with his brother in the country and really enjoyed helping him on the farm. But after living there for five years his brother died and his sister-in-law sold the farm. Godfrey moved in with another brother and his family, but he too died a few years later. Godfrey's sister then organized for him to move into an aged persons' hostel close to her home. She visited him regularly and monitored the quality of care he received from the hostel, taking up issues with the staff when necessary. When Godfrey was 70 she too died. Her daughter who lives locally now visits Godfrey on special occasions but does not know him very well and now has her own family to care for. Godfrey still has occasional contact with his other brother but has not seen him for several years.

Long-term friendships were also at considerable risk from the death of older friends who had been shared with parents and from disruption as people moved accommodation or were 'retired' from day centres. The context-specific nature of friendships meant that when older people moved on they lost regular contact with friends. Maintenance of such ties requires recognition of their existence and positive strategies, neither of which were evident in the processes of residential or programme moves.

## Importance of informal networks

The development of strong networks of informal relationships is regarded as fundamental to the social, psychological and physical well-being of people, particularly older people. Social gerontology, for example, has accumulated considerable evidence as to the association between informal support and the well-being of older people. The multifaceted benefits are captured by Hooyman who states, 'In sum, social support for older people appears to be related to higher morale, less loneliness and worry, feelings of usefulness, a sense of individual respect within the community and a zest for life' (1983: 139). The protective aspects of informal network ties extend to mortality, health, survival and recovery following acute medical conditions (Mendes del Leon *et al.* 1999). Informal social relationships lie also at the heart of the movement for inclusion of people with disabilities.

Reinders (2002), for example, suggests that social citizenship requires not only the creation of space for formal roles but also the inclusion of people with disabilities in the informal sphere, which he terms 'civic friendship'. This depends on the formation of relationships between people with and without disabilities.

The value of informal relationships is magnified by the recognition that formal organizations cannot replicate all the tasks they perform. In middle age and beyond, formal services increasingly replace informal carers in providing direct care for people with learning disability while informal networks continue to fulfil the 'caring about' tasks, providing affective support, managing and mediating relations with formal services and providing significant advocacy. These latter functions are those not easily replicated by formal services but crucial to the quality of life of people who live in shared supported accommodation. For example, formal organizations find it difficult to take into account idiosyncratic needs and perform non-routine tasks. Nor can they adequately fulfil tasks that require long-term commitment, advocacy or an affective relationship such as emotional support, financial or personal affairs management and monitoring and negotiation of services quality (Litwak 1985). Services such as case management, statutory guardianship and the Public Advocate's Office only undertake fragments of tasks such as these and then only for limited periods. (The Office of the Public Advocate is an independent statutory office working to promote the interests, rights and dignity of Victorians with a disability. It provides advocacy, guardianship and investigative services, particularly in cases of abuse or exploitation of people with a disability.) Formal services cannot provide a continuing comprehensive oversight of an individual's well-being (Bigby 2000).

## Planning for and supporting robust informal networks

The inability of formal services to substitute for roles fulfilled by informal network members emphasizes the vulnerability of those people who lack strong networks and suggests the importance of actively acknowledging and supporting the maintenance of such ties and finding ways to foster their development. For this to occur attention must be paid to the everyday structures that govern people's lives to ensure they support and develop rather than rupture and ignore relationships (Bayley 1997).

Informal networks as demonstrated in this chapter are dynamic, determined by a combination of personal characteristics, social and economic context and the pattern of opportunities available. A useful concept is that of a 'convoy of social support' which suggests that the history of supportive networks is central to understanding present relationships, and that people move through life surrounded by a convoy of others who vary across time and situations (Antonucci and Akiyama 1987). This life course perspective suggests that the type of relationships developed in earlier years may be an important factor in those experienced in later life. This suggests that across the lifespan families and service providers must focus on assisting people with learning disability to develop and sustain meaningful and supportive informal relationships.

One mechanism that can support the continuation of robust informal networks into later life is parental planning for the future. The author's research suggests that the most successful plans made by parents are 'key person succession plans' (Bigby 1996). These plans are not formal and detailed but rather informally based. They are characterized by the planned transfer of responsibility for overseeing the well-being of the person with learning disability to a future 'key person'. Choice of this key person is based on strength of their prior relationship with the adult with a disability rather than simply family relationships. The tasks involved in such a role and specified in the plan vary from being prescribed to vague and open-ended. What these plans entail, however, is negotiation, explicitly or implicitly, of a long-term commitment by a key person to the older person's continued well-being. Plans of this nature are usually successfully implemented and go awry less often than more detailed residential plans. They are flexible and responsive, providing a mechanism, in the form of a key person, for dealing with the unforseen contingencies in the person's life. While they do not always achieve stability in the provision of primary care they do guarantee that an informal network member is available to negotiate, monitor and oversee the well-being of adults with learning disability and their relationship with the formal service system.

The nature of key person succession plans suggests that if parents are assisted with future planning other family members should also be sought out and involved in the process. People nominated as key people will often find discussions about the future less emotionally challenging than parents, and drawing them into discussion of plans may also facilitate the involvement of the person with learning disability themselves. Following the development of a future plan, formal services could assist in equipping potential key people with knowledge of the formal services system, later life opportunities, and the developmental potential of adults with learning disabilities.

Planning is not a one-off event but rather a continuing process. As key people nominated by parents are often the same generation as the older person it is important that they plan for the continued commitment of a younger generation key person. This role may be taken on by a nephew or a niece who has known the older person all their lives and established a strong relationship with them.

Service providers must recognize and respect the involvement of informal network members in the lives of older people with disabilities even if the nature of involvement is not the 'norm' one may expect from more distant relatives. For example, parents and children of older people are usually the most involved relatives of older people, but in the case of people with learning disabilities it is more likely to be siblings, nieces, nephews, cousins or even non-related family friends such as a minister.

On the other hand, while respect for the views of others involved in the person's life is crucial, formal services may at times have to deal with conflicting views as to what is in the best interests of the person with learning disability, or the type of decision the person themselves would make if able to do so. Formal service providers must always be alert to such tensions, be prepared to talk them through and if necessary to have recourse to more formal mechanisms if they believe that decisions taken on behalf of an older person by a key person are not in his/her best interests. Though such occurrences are few they do occur.

## Supplementing family support

The pool of family members committed to the well-being of an older adult with learning disability and the potential for replacing members lost due to death and incapacity is limited by both family size and intergenerational ties. The evidence clearly suggests that the size of family networks and their strength of support diminish as people age. It is therefore important to consider ways in which family support can be supplemented by fostering the development of other informal relationships. However, older people with learning disability are particularly dependent on externally provided support and opportunities to develop and maintain informal networks (Myers *et al.* 1998; Hawkins 1999).

Too often opportunities to develop personal relationships are mediated by the limiting factors of resources and the low expectations of others. Research in the UK by Walker and Walker (1998b) clearly demonstrates the ageist and discriminatory attitudes held by service providers about the potential of older people with disabilities that inevitably restrict opportunities for expansion of their social lives. Additionally the devaluation of relationships between people with disabilities may lead to unforeseen losses and social disruption of people's networks.

This suggests that families and staff in disability services must acknowledge the importance of all kinds of informal relationships and the continuing potential of older people for development and develop organizational and staff skills in fostering the development of these valued relationships. Staff require education about normal ageing processes and ageist attitudes together with training in practical strategies to foster relationships. Although formal agencies cannot replicate the tasks of informal relationships, formal programmes have demonstrated a capacity to build informal networks. Examples of innovative service models such as PLAN, circles of support, volunteer companions, citizen advocacy and community builders are found in many countries (Gold 1994; Jameson 1998; Etmanski 2000; Kultgen *et al.* 2000).

One approach to deliberate network building is the work of Planned Lifetime Advocacy Network (PLAN) in Canada. This parent-run organization supports the development of a 'personal network' around an individual with a disability. The aim is to build a web of relationships, not only between each member and the focus adult but between members, thus developing the network's collective identity and strength. Individuals are deliberately and carefully recruited and cultivated to provide support and advocacy for the adult. A paid facilitator oversees a three-stage establishment process – exploration, development and maintenance. The facilitator is a person who has knowledge and connections with the local community and compatibility with the person with a disability and their family rather than a human service professional. The first phase involves an exploration of the person, their interests, aspirations and capacities, and seeks out possible connections and contacts in the local community. A plan is made for network development that is implemented in the next phase. Members are recruited by the facilitator. Goals, strategies and commitment are made and the network fashioned in the development phase. The final phase is networks maintenance in which the facilitator supports regular meetings ensuring follow-through on commitments and adaptations to change are made. It is estimated that initial network formation takes up to 40 hours of facilitator time over an eight-month period with ongoing support taking about two to three hours a month. Keys to this type of network development are a vision of what is possible, the willingness to look beyond traditional social service systems and the ability to ask for support and involvement of others. Development of such networks is used as a means of planning for the future of the adult with a disability. A major challenge for parents may be stepping aside and making room for the involvement of others in the lives of their adult child.

Other examples of formal programmes that support the formation of relationships stem more from the community membership/inclusion perspective. They are based on the premise that participation in community-based activities or acquisition of valued social roles is not only an end in itself but a means to individual relationships. An example of this type of approach is the Community Membership Project in Indiana (Kultgen *et al.* 2000; Harlan-Simmons *et al.* 2001). This programme uses person-centred planning techniques to build up a picture of the person with a disability, his/her capacities, interests, aspirations, strengths and preferences. A paid 'community builder' gets to know the person in a range of different social contexts, at the same time exploring the local community for sites and activities where the person may play a valued role or contribute to community life. The community builder facilitates the introduction of the person to activities, and seeks out and develops natural contacts within them. The degree to which friendships develop depends on attentive listening, strategy, persistent support and sometimes luck. Community builders are risk takers, creative and flexible with an ability to take an unbounded approach. Approaches such as this require significant investment of time, intensive in the exploratory stage and less so but often continuing in the long term. This project estimated an investment of up to ten hours a week for each person.

Descriptions of programmes that seek to build and support informal relationships demonstrate the intensive and lengthy processes involved. It is not an easy task, but one that requires planning, commitment, resources and a positive outlook. Although people with learning disabilities often continue to have at least one strong and committed relationship with a family member, the absence of the younger generation in their networks makes them particularly vulnerable to social isolation, and undue control and decision making by formal service providers. Supporting and nurturing a range of informal relationships each of which in a different way contributes to the quality of care, social well-being and quality of life is a vital role for formal services across the life course and well into a person's later years when they are perhaps most vulnerable to loss of strong support from family members.

# 10

# Relatives' experiences of nursing home entry: meanings, practices and discourse

## Alan Pearson, Rhonda Nay and Bev Taylor

### Introduction

This chapter discusses the experiences of the relatives of older people who are admitted to a nursing home. Our discussion largely considers the Australian context, while drawing on the international literature, and we focus on two major areas. First, we broadly examine the literature on nursing home entry and demonstrate the need to research the experience of relatives and carers, and secondly, we briefly overview our study of relatives' experience of nursing home entry.

### Nursing home entry

*The nursing home*

The literature on nursing homes in Australia suggests that despite the introduction of Commonwealth legislation guiding residential care standards in 1989 (including the Charter and Agreement), aimed at nationally improving nursing home care (DHSH 1994; Australian Law Reform Commission 1995: 135, 155), negative perceptions of nursing homes are still widely held in the community (for example Groger 1994a; Pitkeathley 1995). In general, these perceptions relate to their institutional and economic structures. The literature often refers to a more general community disapproval of institutional care. Nursing homes are perceived as alienating places where clients go to die and concomitantly as places where individual rights are subsumed by institutional routines and regulations (Levine 1995). An article by Jill Pitkeathley, the Director of the United Kingdom's Carers' National Association, notes that there is a pervasive community view that '. . . it is better to be cared for at home'. According to Pitkeathley, this idea is '. . . deeply embedded in our national consciousness . . . [and] . . . probably stems from the workhouse era when people were only put into institutions when they were too poor, mad or unloved to stay at home . . .' (1995).

The literature on nursing homes has also frequently highlighted a public ambivalence that is often expressed towards nursing home owners and the cost of nursing home care more generally. In this scenario, nursing home owners are seen as profiting from an aged care industry (Anson 1995) that already costs the community and taxpayers too much (Montgomery and Kosloski 1994; Kosloski and Montgomery 1995. The Australian Law Reform Commission reports:

> From the early-1980s Commonwealth policy has moved away from funding aged care in institutions, particularly nursing homes, . . . [where this ] . . . change was driven by cost concerns and a recognition that institutionalized care is not the preferred option of most frail older people.
>
> (1995: 13)

The concern in the literature with attitudes towards nursing homes is, in most instances, coupled with demographic projections of the ageing population, and the subsequent problem of the social cost of care and forms this will take in the future (for example Lemov 1994; Montgomery and Kosloski 1994; Barusch 1995; Dellasega 1995). The dual concern with demography and nursing home admission is clearly apparent in the following passage by Dellasega and Mastrian:

> Although consensus on the nature of family adjustment post place-ment has not been reached, this is an important issue to consider. Continued growth of the population 65 years of age and over increases the likelihood that almost every person with an elderly relative will be confronted with the need to make some type of caregiving decision during his or her lifetime. Identifications of problems that family members experience during this process will help structure interventions that can promote a healthy family situation for both the elder and his or her relatives, both before and after institutionalization has occurred.
>
> (Dellasega and Mastrian 1995: 124)

It is these projections as they relate to an increase in the future of nursing home admission that articulate the more general concern with cultural perceptions of institutional forms of aged care. In the past nursing homes and nursing care of elderly people have been subjects of more thorough academic investigation. Some Australian examples include Howe (1990), who focused on nursing home policy, Nay (1993), who examined nursing home life, and Stevens (1995), who described attitudes to nursing aged people. None of these works have been interested in finding ways to connect these to nursing home admission. In clarifying the relationships between an ageing population, the increased use of nursing homes and negative public attitudes towards institutional care, what is needed then is an approach that can articulate possible connections.

*Relocation and its effect on relatives and carers*

It might be expected that entry into a nursing home, with an anticipated reduction in twenty-four-hour care, would result in a reduction in stress for carers. Evidence to date does not support this expectation. Although agreement on the nature of relatives' and affected families' adjustment to relocation has not been reached (Brown *et al.* 1990; Dellasega and Mastrian 1995), most studies to date suggest the transition and post-placement period is experienced as a major life stressor. Studies that have been identified, although inconclusive, indicate this is associated with guilt, anger, despair, resentment and general psychological distress (Matthiesen 1989; Schultz *et al.* 1993). Dellasega's (1991) study into the effects of institutionalization upon the carer reports that, although physical stress was reduced, psychological stress increased. A more recent article by Dellasega, co-authored with Mastrian (1995), observes that post-placement difficulties often stem from how family members perceive themselves in relation to their older relative, where social expectations on family members create pressures for continued caregiving (p. 24). Some writers note that family expectations are affected by the commonly held view that home care is the ideal form of care. According to this scenario, relinquishing the elder to nursing home care appears to represent failure[1] (for example Matthiesen 1989; Groger 1994b).

In a study of daughters' perspectives, Johnson (1990) found that placement of a relative was 'the hardest thing (they) had ever done'. Gwyther (cited in Stephens *et al.* 1991) found that after institutionalization, caregivers reported increased health problems, stress, psychiatric symptoms and psychotropic drug usage. In fact, death of the relative resulted in greater well-being than did institutionalization. A study by Zarit and Whitlatch (1993) supports these findings, results from their research indicating that one-half of caregivers show an increase in mental health symptoms after placement. They suggest that this is because post placement the burden of caregiving is shifted rather than eliminated; and while hands-on caregiving is no longer provided, often the complex feelings associated with relinquishing caregiving in the home, together with the strain of negotiating relationships with the nursing home staff, complicate parent–child or spousal relationships, already strained by chronic illness. Research by Lewis and Meredith reported by McLaughlin and

---

[1] Moody quoted in Groger notes that nursing home placement is the least preferred option because in our society this step is '. . . commonly seen as a sign of moral failure' (1994: 78).

Ritchie (1994) found that the post-care period included loss of identity and purpose; loneliness; a sense of lost opportunities and lost confidence; and long-term economic loss. All carers, they reported, experienced these problems to a greater or lesser extent.

In an attempt to address post-placement stress, several writers have suggested the transition from home to nursing home could be eased by promoting an understanding of relocation as yet another phase in the normal life cycle of the family. Nursing home entry in these studies is reconceptualized as a process rather than a single life event (Chenitz 1983; Schneewind 1990; Close 1995). The focus of these writers has been to suggest ways in which the transition may be made less traumatic. For instance, Close (1995) and Schneewind (1990) observe that the enactment of simple rituals that say goodbye to old contexts and assist in the acceptance of the new living environment prepare families for the relocation. Schneewind concludes:

> . . . as placement becomes commoner and more acceptable, the elderly and their relatives will find it easier to recognize that it does not spell the end to affection and nurturance. As professionals, we can help by fashioning *family rituals* for nursing home admission and by treating the post-placement family as a normal family going through yet another stage of restructuring.
>
> (Schneewind 1990: 135, our emphasis)

### Nursing homes and relatives

Several researchers have highlighted the need for nursing home staff to be made more aware of the needs of relatives so that they can work with relatives to reduce the stress of nursing home admission (for example Schneewind 1990; King *et al.* 1991; Bartlett 1994; Maccabee 1994; Tilse 1994; Dellasega and Mastrian 1995; Hamel 1995). The admission process however, usually focuses entirely upon the needs of the resident to the extent that the difficulties that relatives experience are largely ignored by nursing home staff (Duncan and Morgan 1994; Vinton and Mazza 1994; Tickle and Hull 1995). Johnson (1990) argues that nurses are frequently oblivious to carer stress. Kaplan and Ade-Ridder (1991) refer to caregivers as the 'hidden clients' of nursing home admission, a term that is gaining wider currency in the literature (for example Vinton and Mazza 1994).

In a study by Hamel (1995) it was found that guilt and grief in relatives is often manifested as anger that is then directed at nursing home staff. She advises, like the above writers, that staff need to be educated in how to recognize and deal with the needs of relatives and suggests that the pre-admission meeting, as it marks the '. . . beginning of an ongoing relationship, not only with the resident, but with the family . . .' (p. 60), provides an opportunity to address these issues.

Frequently writers report attitudinal barriers that obstruct good communication between relatives and nursing home staff. One such barrier, outlined by Safford (1989), is the view commonly held by staff that families have ceased to be interested in their relative once they have placed them into nursing home care. Contrary to this view, as Safford goes on to explain, is that studies have consistently produced evidence that relatives in most instances continue to care for their relative, and although their role is transformed, many emphasize the importance of their contribution in the nursing home context (Bowers 1988; Safford 1989; Tilse 1994; High and Rowles 1995). In particular High and Rowles (1995) found that families' involvement in decisions concerning the care of their relatives actually increased along with the length of time that the relative had been in nursing home care (p. 103). Tilse (1994) and Bowers (1988) note that in representing the interests of their relatives, carers often act in a role akin to advocates or case managers.

More generally the literature demonstrates that involvement with nursing home residents by relatives can have positive results for relatives and residents (Harel 1981; Greene and Monahan 1982; Montgomery 1982; Shuttlesworth *et al.* 1982; Rubin and Shuttlesworth 1983; Bowers 1988; Brody *et al.* 1990; Maccabee 1994). Nevertheless, debate continues over the types of involvement that result in positive outcomes and there is evidence to suggest relative involvement is not always welcomed by staff, or the type and extent of involvement is prescribed by staff to the dissatisfaction of relatives (Hasselkus 1988; Stephens *et al.* 1991; Tilse 1994; Tickle and Hull 1995). Some studies suggest caring be divided into technical and non-technical tasks, with relatives being relegated the non-technical tasks. Others argue a more useful approach is to explore the purpose of tasks and emphasize collaboration between staff and relatives rather than task division (Bowers 1988; Thompson 1990; Duncan and Morgan 1994). Bowers (1988), for example, identifies purposes such as protection, prevention, anticipation and supervision. Relatives in this study saw their role as monitoring staff care, teaching staff appropriate caring behaviours and generally protecting the resident. Relatives frequently felt that staff failed to provide appropriate care. Complaints related to such things as staff failing to dress the relative appropriately, controlling times for eating, sleeping, toileting etc. addressing the resident in demeaning fashion and staff being inadequately educated for the role. Relatives in Bowers's study explain their need to monitor care because of poor communication, the reluctance of staff to work with them and lack of staff continuity. Hasselkus (1988) also notes tension between staff and relatives over 'ownership of special knowledge'. Hasselkus concludes that shared perspectives are more important to successful collaboration between staff and relatives than task division. This contention is supported in Bowers's (1988) work in terms of families perceiving staff as failing to provide care which preserved family connectedness and the resident's dignity, hopes and control. Relatives in this study saw it as important that they 'individualized' the resident for staff. In addition, they related indirect strategies that were used to teach staff, fearing direct approaches may result in staff anger. Montgomery (1982) reports on a study of three nursing homes which had differing policies regarding relative involvement. In one home the relatives were expected to visit and provide non-technical support, in a second there was no specified role for relatives who were simply viewed as visitors, and in home three relatives were regarded as clients with their own special needs to be met by the home. The policies of home three were found to be associated with greatest relative well-being. Greene and Monahan (1982) associate frequent visits by relatives with improved well-being in residents.

Each of these studies, however, as they have mainly focused upon the subject of task division and collaboration, have excluded many other aspects of how relationships are structured and experienced in the nursing home context. Concepts of 'task division' and 'collaboration' operate to define a predetermined field of inquiry that excludes insight into other dimensions of nursing home relationships. The prescriptive nature of this debate is mainly structured by quantitative methodological approaches to the subject. Recently, there has been a shift towards qualitative ethnographic studies that are well suited to generating rich descriptions and relational models for interpreting how individuals are situated in cultural institutions. So far, however, there have been very few of these studies that have focused on nursing home admission.

Notably in the Australian context Tilse (1994) is the only reported study that utilizes an ethnographic approach to examine nursing home admission and explore relationships between relatives and staff. In her study of three facilities in south-east Queensland, Tilse observes that while there were varying degrees of recognition given to the needs of relatives in each context, on the whole the current policy emphasis is on the resident to the exclusion of relatives. She suggests relatives' needs tend to be marginal to the focus of these facilities. Tilse argues for further Australian studies in the area that attempt to combine an understanding of the experience of nursing home admission from the relatives' perspective with an understanding of how relationships are structured in the nursing home context. These insights, according to Tilse, should be used to inform future policy provisions that take relatives' needs into account. Nay (1996, 1997) explored relatives' experiences of nursing home entry as described by 18 relatives of nursing home residents in NSW. She identifies a number of themes that revealed this experience as 'the hardest thing' the participants had ever had to do. Further, the experience is characterized by tension: tension in relation to felt 'ownership' of the resident, between staff and relatives, and so on. It was clear from this small study that further research was required to increase understanding of nursing home admission for relatives.

# Researching relatives' experience of nursing home entry

*The measure or meaning of care?*

There is an extensive body of quantitative literature documenting the prevalence of carer stress in the community and, within this, a growing amount that is specifically concerned with carer stress as it relates to nursing homes. Most of this literature is concerned with identifying various carer groups (spouses, men and women, adult children, and sons and daughters) and defining and measuring the impact of carer stress in terms of psychological, physical and economic components. (Some more recent examples: Brody *et al.* 1990; Nygaard 1991; Laitinen 1992; McFall and Miller 1992; Riddick *et al.* 1992; Barber 1993; Grau *et al.* 1993; Zarit and Whitlatch 1993; Kammer 1994; Montgomery and Kosloski 1994; Barnes *et al.* 1995; Clarke and Finucane 1995; Fuller and Lillquist 1995; Gladstone 1995; Jette *et al.* 1995; Kosloski and Montgomery 1995; Mui 1995; White-Means and Chollet 1996). Different authors have emphasized or compared the inter-relationships of these categories of analysis and made differing claims about the extent to which identified groups have been affected. Quantitative analysis, in this sense, has mapped out and measured many of the salient social issues related to relatives and nursing home admission.

Some writers more recently have highlighted the need to design future research projects that effectively address social policy and community supports offered to the carers of older people. Their particular concern is with the alarming growth in literature on caregiver stress without any significant progress on alleviating the problem of this stress (Zarit *et al.* 1986). According to these commentators, there appears to be a gap between the academic literature on, and analytical understanding of, issues related to caring for elderly people and the formulation of effective policy to improve and devise services and clinical practices. Despite all the available studies, and the recognition that caring for older relatives can be highly stressful, there still appears to be very little understanding of the needs of relatives and how to address carer stress. After reviewing three books on family caregiving, the writer Karl Pillemer (1996) notes: 'One refrain throughout the chapters in the edited volumes appeared so frequently that it became repetitive: How little we know about ageing families, and especially caregiving, that would help us decide what to do for families in trouble' (p. 270). According to Pillemer, researchers need to re-evaluate seriously the research field (p. 271).

One redefinition of the field is possible through focusing on qualitative data and interpretive and critical research methodologies. Several writers have drawn attention to what they see as inherent limitations in quantitative research methods (cf Kaplan and Ade-Ridder 1991; Baker *et al.* 1992; Duncan and Morgan 1994; Tilse 1994; Dellasega and Mastrian 1995; Lewis *et al.* 1995). In particular, Kaplan and Ade-Ridder (1991) have argued that there is yet to be a study that adequately '. . . explain[s] *feelings experienced* by non-institutionalized spouses when their mate moves to a nursing home' (p. 83, our emphasis). It is therefore not surprising to them that while there is a general acknowledgement in the literature of the need to support caregivers, there still exists a lack of research and development of practical programmes. In their own attempt to address this problem their research adopts a qualitative model based on intensive interviews with the spouses of nursing home residents. Researchers in the genre of Kaplan and Ade-Ridder argue that qualitative models hold out greater possibilities of capturing and generating understandings that will be able effectively to address policy makers and those involved in the provision of care services.

The general consensus among those that advocate qualitative approaches is that quantitative approaches are unable to attend to the complexity and detail associated with the relatives' experience of the admission process. Quantitative approaches, they argue, apply generalized models and cross-sectional data analysis; they tend to homogenize experience and present, as one writer puts it, '. . . fixed static notions of caregiving . . .' (Abel 1995: 87). By contrast, in qualitative approaches, experience and voice are represented from the perspective of those studied. Through these approaches the enduring contingencies of living are not denied their complexity and in this way context is not generally subsumed into a positivistic measure. Moreover, because qualitative approaches draw relationships between data and interpret this material, they are flexible in design and adaptive. They allow, that is, for contradictions to emerge that through a dialectical process enrich our understanding of issues (cf Kaplan and Ade-Ridder 1991; Baker *et al.* 1992; Duncan and Morgan 1994; Tilse 1994; Dellasega and Mastrian 1995; Lewis *et al.* 1995: 126).[2] This point is clearly illustrated in the following passage from Jaber Gubrium's article called 'Qualitative research comes of age in gerontology':

> Meaning is not necessarily made on the spot but develops in relation to the retrospective and prospective attention given to it. We learn from the apparent contradictions we hear when, say, retirees report one thing at one time and later say the opposite. Or from the story of experience told by an adult daughter in a field setting that is conveyed in a different version by her frail mother.
>
> (Gubrium 1992)

Qualitative approaches in nursing represent a relatively new disciplinary approach and there is still much debate concerning the rigour of

---

[2] Dellasega and Mastrian note: 'The qualitative methodology was chosen because of the need to examine in an in-depth way the experiences and perceptions of family members. The advantages of a qualitative approach are flexibility of design, depth, and exploration of ambiguous concepts and processes . . .'

analysis (Gubrium 1992; Koch 1993; Koch 1996), and also the benefits of one method over another, for instance the benefits of an ethnographic approach over a phenomenological or grounded theory approach. As different approaches, however, they set out to achieve different things and, in reality, when the divergent perspectives are put together, they provide a multifaceted view of the subject of inquiry that deepens our understanding of it. In this sense they are not substitutes for each other due to some essential superiority of one method over another, but rather they represent a theoretical 'tool kit' of heuristic devices. And, depending on the task at hand, one methodology on one occasion may be a more useful tool than another. An important precautionary warning, however, has been issued by Baker *et al.* (1992) who are concerned with the problem of 'method slurring' in nursing research which refers to the tendency '. . . for nurses to blur distinctions between the various qualitative approaches and to combine their methodological prescriptions eclectically' (p. 1355). Using the example of grounded theory and phenomenology they outline the rudiments of each approach to demonstrate how they are discrete in application and method and, in this sense, different in what they set out to achieve.

Several researchers (such as Kaplan and Ade-Ridder 1991 above) have commented that there have been very few studies on the subject of nursing home admission that utilize qualitative approaches, and even fewer that specifically focus on the relatives' experience of this process (Kaplan and Ade-Ridder 1991; Bartlett 1994; Bartlett and Font 1994; Duncan and Morgan 1994; Tickle and Hull 1995). It is of particular importance in the Australian context that, of those studies that have been completed, most are from Northern America (for example Kaplan and Ade-Ridder 1991; Dellasega and Mastrian 1995; Lewis *et al.* 1995; Tickle and Hull 1995). Only three researchers have conducted studies into the experience of relatives in Australia (Tilse 1994; Nay 1996; Kellett 1997).

## An overview of the study of the meanings, practices and discourses surrounding relatives' experiences of nursing home entry in Australia

This three-year study (Pearson, Nay and Taylor) was funded by the National Health and Medical Research Council and set out to:

1 explore, describe and interpret the meanings relatives make out of their experiences of placing significant others in nursing homes;
2 explore, describe and interpret current nursing home practices, particularly in relation to the admission of new residents;
3 explore, describe and interpret the public discourse on nursing home care and admission of new residents;

4  integrate and critically analyse data from 1, 2 and 3 above and identify consistencies and inconsistencies between these three discourses;
5  generate understandings and insights to inform and assist people who will have this experience in the future;
6  generate publications and debate to inform and improve the practice of health professionals, particularly nurses working in nursing homes;
7  generate publications and debate to inform and influence policy makers.

*Study design and processes*

The study consisted of three phases of data collection and analysis. In the first phase, completed in 1996, an interpretive process was pursued, focusing on capturing the meanings of the experience of people who had recently been involved with the admission of a relative into a nursing home through the phenomenological analysis of experiential interviews. Concurrently, an interpretation of the meanings of ageing and nursing homes embedded in the public discourse was commenced.

The second phase, completed in 1998, was descriptive in nature, focusing on a detailed and substantial ethnographic case study of a nursing home and in-depth interviews of leaders in the field who played a major role in shaping the public discourse. The case study concentrated on the nursing home as a whole without paying specific attention to the admission of new residents, but included it as part of the nursing homes' everyday work. This phase also included a discussion of the descriptive results with relatives and leaders in the field in order to clarify and validate the interpretations and provide a degree of integration across the different spheres.

The third phase, completed in 2000, was one of integrative analysis based on the critique of the discourses emerging from phases one and two. The phenomenological data, ethnographic data, interpretations of public discourse and feedback from participants of the second phase were brought together as text for critical discourse analysis to integrate the different spheres. From this it was possible to identify, locate and critique the discourses emerging from a number of different, sometimes contradictory, perspectives which represent the current state of nursing home admission in Australia.

## Overview of the study findings

*Making meaning of individual experience*

Sixty participants were recruited from the North Coast of New South Wales and Adelaide, South Australia through advertisements placed in local newspapers. Relatives of nursing home residents were invited to express an interest in the study. Ethical processes were adhered to in order to maintain participants' privacy, confidentiality and anonymity.

Phenomenological data were gathered by encouraging relatives to tell stories of their experiences, within a relaxed interview that resembled a conversation. The audiotaped conversations were analysed to locate themes that expressed the essential nature of the experience. Themes and subthemes were identified which gave insights into the essence of what was being communicated about the experience. The analysis of the data occurred in two main stages: the analysis of individuals' experiences and the collation of common themes in relatives' experiences.

Relatives' experiences differed according to their respective contexts, lived experiences and accounts of their subjective feelings relating to the events that led up to, incorporated, and followed nursing home admission of the person involved. The accounts also show the complexity of people's specific experiences. The themes that have emerged from the data show that relatives experienced a range of responses and emotions in relation to nursing home entry of their family member.

Although it is important to retain the uniqueness of each relative's experience, it is also useful to ascertain the ways in which the experiences were similar. The usefulness of finding common themes lies in being able to make certain generalized statements about the ways in which nursing home admission of a family member was experienced by relatives. The interviews encouraged relatives to relate their experiences around four main stages of admission to a nursing home: events prior to admission; difficulties encountered in locating a suitable nursing home; the days on and immediately after admission, and subsequent experiences.

In all the accounts, participants told of the events leading to the decision to admit a family member to a nursing home. The main aspects arising from these accounts were the complex histories of illness and accidents; the increasing inability of the aged person to cope alone; the increasing inability of the family to support the aged person, and relatives' expressions of lack of support from other family members in managing the events leading to the admission.

Accounts exemplified the complex histories of illness, disabilities and accidents leading up to the decision to seek nursing home classification of the family member. None of the stories recounted a simple trajectory of events, because a certain level of incapacity and need for care is required for a person to be classified for nursing home admission. Almost without exception, the aged family member not only had diseases of ageing, but also suffered some other sort of difficulties, such as accidents and lack of social supports.

Many of the older people had been living alone until they got to a point at which they could no longer cope. Many of the stories showed how the family came to the realization that they could no longer support the aged person within the family network. Other stories showed that one or two relatives were left with the work to do in order to prepare for nursing home admission. Emotions varied, and they included feelings of anger, disappointment, resignation, resentment and annoyance.

Experiences included the difficulties in looking around for a nursing home, reasons for accepting the home placement, feelings attached to making the decision, and the haste in which decisions for placement needed to be made. With very few exceptions, relatives took a considerable amount of time and effort to try to find a suitable nursing home for their family member. Many people had to travel large distances across the city and view nursing homes at short notice. Some of the nursing homes would not allow visits to certain parts of the institution or insisted that the visit be made at specified times. Many relatives acknowledged the difficulty in finding an ideal place, especially as they needed to be placed on a waiting list, often at nursing homes that were not their preferred choices.

The main reasons for accepting a particular nursing home were convenience, feelings of desperation to have the family member placed as soon as possible, and initial positive impressions of the nursing home. There were many and varied feelings expressed in relation to making the final decision to place a family member in a nursing home. The feelings included relief, guilt, devastation, inevitability, remaining objective, and many more, but all the feelings were expressed as having a great deal of depth and personal significance to the relative experiencing them. Many of the research participants told of the haste with which they had to make a decision for placement of a family member in a particular nursing home. This meant that the family member and his or her possessions had to be gathered up quickly and dispatched to the nursing home, leaving little time for resolving residual anxieties and getting accustomed to the transition from one place to the other.

Experiences on the day of admission included the first impressions on entering the home to admit the family member there and memories of the admission process itself. First impressions of the nursing home varied from favourable to unfavourable. The participants recounted their impressions as part of their accounts of the experience of admission. For some relatives the admission process was positive, while for others it was not. Aspects of the experiences after the admission related mainly to the family member settling in, or not settling in, and to the relative accepting or not accepting that the family member needed to be in a nursing home.

### Practices that affect the nursing home admission

An ethnographic description of everyday practices in a nursing home was developed by research assistants who conducted fieldwork interviews and kept diaries of observed events and conversations in two homes. They did this while immersing themselves in the everyday happenings of the nursing home culture in order to reconstruct a rich description of the settings in which admissions took place. The aim was to correlate informa-tion as participant observers in the nursing home setting: making field notes, talking to people and working within the homes on various shifts.

The resulting ethnographic description of nursing home life identified a number of themes that characterized the cultural practices surrounding the admission event. Nurses, care workers, residents and relatives all adopted clearly defined roles within the nursing home.

Nurses were occupied mainly with instrumental, medically related tasks such as administering medications and treatments, completing documentation and responding to calls for advice from care workers when residents became ill or exhibited a change in their general condi-tion. Communication with residents was generally brief and relatively formal.

Care workers were the most visible actors within the nursing home. They performed most of the direct care and were the most frequent communicators with residents and relatives.

Residents were passive recipients of a system of care and routines that progressed around and apart from them throughout the day.

Relatives were 'outsiders' who rarely participated in, or fully understood, the patterns, norms and rituals of the nursing home day.

At the point of admission, the new resident struggled to make sense of the requirements of his or her new living place, and spent the first weeks watching and learning the rules. Relatives were given information, follow-ing a uniform formality, and invited to become involved in the facility by registered nurses. However, after a few days little communication between nurses and relatives occurred, and the care workers became the link between the relative and the resident. Some relatives easily identified with the nursing home's routines and became absorbed into the culture. Such relatives were often treated in a very friendly manner by the care workers and appeared to be regarded as 'good' relatives. Others, however, were dissatisfied with the way that care was given. They communicated less with care workers and frequently requested to see the nurse on duty to critique care practices and seek assurances that care planning and implementation would coincide with past practices and patterns of living.

Overall, the admission process focused on residents and the 'slotting in' of their requirements with the well-established practices of the nursing home. Relatives were treated courteously but were seen to be 'outsiders' by staff.

## The discourses that surround nursing home admission

The discourse analysis component of the study examined professional literature, Australian newspapers, government publications and radio and television broadcasts. Material was gathered through several means. Recent professional and academic literature (relevant articles published mainly in the last three years) was collected through searching the University of Adelaide and the University of South Australia library catalogues, as well as relevant bibliographic databases including: CINAHL; APAIS; MEDLINE; SOCIOFILE; AGELINE; PSYCLIT; and Current Contents. Further material was gathered through manually searching relevant journals. Government reports and relevant legislation were manually collated from the government libraries and shopfronts such as the South Australia Health Commission and State and Commonwealth Government bookshops.

Pamphlets and published information concerning health services for the aged and carers were selectively gathered through visiting local aged care organizations. Media reporting relevant to the study was retrospectively compiled for the years 1994–96 by searching a press search database covering all major Australian papers. Media reporting for both the electronic and printed media has been compiled on an ongoing basis through using the private consultancy group, Media Monitors. The emphasis was on the experience of nursing home admission for relatives rather than residents. The analysis was directed at identifying the unwritten 'rules' that largely determine accepted social norms and values, and whose views were represented in, or missing from, the discourse.

From the analysis the following rules were identified:

*From the scholarly literature*:
- 'home is best';
- there is a filial responsibility to provide care for the elderly;
- women will be carers;
- caring stress must be reduced to prevent premature nursing home admission;
- nursing home entry results in guilt and continued stress for the carers.

*From the public media*:
- the costs of a greying society must be curbed;
- filial responsibility is expected;
- filial responsibility must be encouraged by government support;
- those who can afford to pay their own way should be required to do so;
- the family home is highly valued and it should not be taken from old people to pay for care;
- nursing homes are to be feared and avoided;
- the frail aged must be cared for 'at home'.

*From government*:
- the cost of ageing must be curbed, managed and privatized;
- healthy ageing will reduce the drain on the public purse;
- families have primary responsibility to care for the aged;
- societal members must be self-responsible;
- supporting carers will reduce the drain on the public purse;
- old people have the right to care when it is needed;

- care provision should be determined by recipient need rather than provider need;
- efficiency and effectiveness will be rewarded.

It can be seen from this inventory that there were few differences in the dominant rules identified across the three texts. However, the voices identified were clearly those 'speaking about' more often than those 'spoken about'. Voices of the informal carers and the recipients of care were rarely identified in the discourse. It is important to note that discourse analysis is not directed towards the subjective experience of the interview informants; rather, its emphasis is on the authority and the position from which the informants are allowed to speak.

## Conclusion

In Australia, it has been estimated that approximately 25 per cent of people aged 65-plus will experience admission to a nursing home (Howe 1990; Rowland 1991). This figure is expected to rise as the Australian population ages and concomitantly the number of frail aged and those suffering dementia increases. Placement of a relative in a nursing home is generally frowned upon by society (Dellasega 1991). This is associated with the view of nursing homes as 'homes of hate' and the emphasis being placed upon home care as 'best' and nursing home care as a 'last resort' (Smallegan 1981). The decision to place a relative in a nursing home often occurs after a long and stressful period of home care (Nygaard 1991). For many older people, as their health declines, nursing homes in reality are equipped to offer better care than the home environment. To qualify for a nursing home, a person must require continuous nursing care (Australian Law Reform Commission 1995) or be chronically ill but not so sick as to require hospital care. It is of some concern therefore that cultural perceptions undermine the critical social value of nursing homes. Studies have been conducted into the experience of relocation for the aged person (for example Coffman 1981; Borup 1983; Young 1990; Mikhail 1992; Nussbaum 1993; Dickinson 1996) and there is a substantial literature on carers, especially in relation to carer stress in the community (for example Barnes *et al.* 1995; Mui 1995; White-Means and Chollet 1996). However, the majority of these are grounded, to a greater or lesser extent, in positivistic methodologies. There has been little literature to date that examines the lived world of carers and relatives. There is also very little that explores the culture of the nursing home and the relative's involvement in the admission process. Finally, there is no study to date that looks at the broader social level (the discursive level), involving the political, economic and cultural perceptions of nursing home admission where this is linked to the particular situation such as the subjective experience of the admission process itself.

Drawing on the literature and the findings of our study, it is reasonable to draw a number of conclusions:

- It is clear that there is a degree of urgency to develop strategies to ensure that society views nursing home/residential care as a positive care choice for a section of the older population. Nursing homes are a positive alternative to community care for many older people when there is a need for high-quality professional nursing.
- Relatives find the task of finding a suitable nursing home onerous and stressful. This could be made easier if shopfront-type bureaux are accessible to assist prospective residents and relatives to 'choose' a nursing home/residential aged care facility.
- The admission process is stressful for relatives if they are not included in the planning of care. A clear, detailed admission protocol that addresses both the needs of the new resident and of the relatives/significant others is fundamental to good practice.

# 11

# Placing a spouse in a care home for older people: (re)-constructing roles and relationships

## Jonas Sandberg, Ulla Lundh and Mike Nolan

Based on a Swedish study, this chapter describes the experience of placing a spouse in a care home. It adopts a temporal perspective beginning with the initial decision to seek care and extending to subsequent involvement in the life of the care home. In order to provide as complete a picture as possible the chapter presents the views of several key stakeholders (spouses, adult children, community staff, and staff in care homes) and highlights the ways in which their interactions determine whether placement is perceived as a positive experience or not. Before setting the chapter within a Swedish context, attention is briefly turned to the literature available when the study commenced.

## Background

Although, relative to other aspects of caregiving, there has been comparatively little research into the process of placing a relative into a care home, several studies do provide important insights into this difficult period. For example, it is known that due to the frailty of the older person at the time of placement it is often a family member who is most closely involved in the placement process. However, until recently, carers' perceptions of events precipitating the placement, how the move is experienced, and the nature of their subsequent adjustment, have not been the subject of systematic study (Aneshensel *et al.* 1995; Naleppa 1996; Dellasega and Nolan 1997). This deficit needs redressing as the move into care and placing a relative in a care home are major life events (McAuley *et al.* 1997; Morgan *et al.* 1997; Ross *et al.* 1997), yet there is often relatively little planning, as families frequently view placement as a last resort (Naleppa 1996; Victor 1997) and rarely discuss such a possibility in advance (Nolan *et al.* 1996b; McAuley *et al.* 1997; Lewycka 1998; Wright 1998).

There is also a growing recognition that the entry of an older person into care does not mark the end of caring but rather signals a new and still potentially stressful form of family involvement (Aneshensel *et al.* 1995; Dellasega and Nolan 1997; Nolan and Dellasega 1999). Most family members continue to visit regularly (MacDonald *et al.* 1996; Naleppa 1996; Ross *et al.* 1997; Wright 1998), but in so doing face a host of uncertainties about their new role and how to interact with staff (Aneshensel *et al.* 1995; Naleppa 1996; Dellasega and Nolan 1997). Because there has often been little contact with the home prior to the placement, role responsibilities have rarely been discussed. This can lead to misunderstandings between relatives and staff (Ehrenfeld *et al.* 1997; McDerment *et al.* 1997; Pillemar *et al.* 1998), as family carers work to 'preserve' the individuality of their relative and ensure that important rituals and routines are maintained (Bowers 1988), and that their expertise is used by staff as a basis for planning care (Bowers 1988; Kellett 1996). However, relatives who wish to play a more active role can be seen as 'interfering' by staff (Robinson and Thorne 1984; Darbyshire 1987), and as a consequence adversarial and competitive roles can develop unless care is taken (Ehrenfeld *et al.* 1997; Pillemar *et al.* 1998).

Unfortunately staff may have little awareness of relatives' desire to remain involved in care, with McDerment *et al.* (1997) suggesting that staff and relatives often appear to be occupying 'separate planets'. As these authors point out, relatives are more than simply visitors, and staff must ensure that the support needs of relatives do not go unrecognized during and after the placement process (Pillemar *et al.* 1998). In achieving this, staff must be aware of views of relatives and build these into the admission process (Ross *et al.* 1997).

## A Swedish context

In common with the rest of Europe (Davies 1995), Sweden is pursuing a policy of community care in order to enable older people to remain in their own homes for as long as possible (Hokenstadt and Johansson 1990; Johansson 1993; Berg and Sundström 1999). However, in contrast to welfare systems in the UK and the USA where families have always played a large, if often unrecognized, role in the provision of care for frail older people, one of the cornerstones of Swedish postwar policy has been the belief that families' responsibility to care for elderly family members should be assumed by the state (Johansson 2001).

Consequently there has traditionally been little reliance on the family to provide support to frail older relatives. However, over the last decade it has become apparent that, in the face of increasing numbers of frail older people, state provision alone is insufficient. Indeed, early in the

1990s it was recognized that the family were playing an important caring role (Thorslund 1991), with an estimate that if the home help service were to assume roles occupied by families then the state would need to double the existing numbers of staff (Thorslund and Parker 1994). More recently Johansson (2001) has calculated that state provision accounts for only three out of every ten hours of care that are needed. The Swedish government has therefore implemented several reforms intended to improve services for older people including more and better trained personnel (Socialdepartementet 1998). Moreover, as Johansson (2001) notes, the 1990s marked the 'rediscovery' of the family in Swedish welfare provision. Notwithstanding these developments there remains a gap between demands and resources, particularly relating to older people and their family, signalling a need for more conscious and carefully targeted allocation (Bergmark *et al.* 2000), based on the realization that although Sweden has well-developed welfare provision the majority of carers are, and will continue to be, family members (Socialstyrelsen 1998). This will require greater knowledge and understanding of the needs of Swedish carers.

However, until recently, carers' needs have received relatively little attention and research on family caring is scarce in Sweden. Ties between formal caring organizations and family care are weak and relatives' roles as carers are not sufficiently supported. Relatives often do not feel appreciated by society or professional carers, and lack sufficient information about possible sources of help and support (Almberg *et al.* 1997). Currently carers' opinions are seldom sought (Socialstyrelsen 1998) and, therefore, if more appropriate services are to develop it is important to explore the ways in which important decisions are made (Thorslund 1998). This is particularly true of difficult decisions, such as placing a relative in a care home.

Although the majority of older people in Sweden remain in the community, about 20 per cent of those aged 80–89 live in care homes (a generic term for accommodation including nursing homes, sheltered housing and group homes), with this figure rising to about 50 per cent at the age of 90+ (Socialstyrelsen 2001). Traditionally care homes in Sweden have been highly regarded and admission has not been as stigmatized as it is in many European countries (Jani-le Bris 1993). However, this position is now changing, with several high-profile media reports over the last few years focusing on issues to do with poor standards in care homes. Consequently, this has engendered increased public concern and eroded public confidence in care homes, a situation fuelling worries among families contemplating admitting a relative to a care home.

## The study

The study upon which this chapter is based sought to understand the placement process from a temporal perspective, ranging from the initial decision to seek care to the post-placement experience; from the perspectives not only of spouses, but also of others who play a potentially important role, such as adult children and professionals working both in the community and in care homes. The desire to gain a more holistic view of placement was the motivation for the study, the overall aim of which was to explore the experiences and processes involved in placing a spouse in a care home from a variety of perspectives (Sandberg 2001). The study comprised several rounds of data collection involving in-depth interviews with: spouses (Lundh *et al.* 2000; Sandberg *et al.* 2001); adult children (Sandberg *et al.* 2002a); professional carers working in the community (Sandberg *et al.* 2002b); and staff in care homes (Sandberg *et al.* 2002c). The ultimate aim was to generate new insights that might lead to improvements in the placement process and enhance subsequent adjustment for carers. Although the individual stakeholder accounts have been published elsewhere (see above), this chapter, for the first time, presents a synthesis of all the findings and considers their implications for service development. Prior to reaching this synthesis attention is turned briefly to the methodology adopted.

## Overview of method and sample

As there had been little previous research on the placement process in a Swedish context, a qualitative method was selected for the study, and because the aim was to provide new theoretical insights, which would also have direct practical application, a grounded theory methodology was chosen. The key attributes of grounded theory, namely fit, work, modifiability and relevance, made it ideally suited to developing theories with an action potential (Charmaz 2000). Two key processes, that is the constant comparative method and theoretical sampling, are central to grounded theory (Charmaz 2000) and informed data collection in the present study.

The study began by seeking the views of spouse carers (see Lundh *et al.* 2000; Sandberg *et al.* 2001), as these are the main 'live-in' carers in Sweden; it is very rare for parents to move in with their adult children. Spouses over the age of 65 who had placed a partner in a care home in the last six months were interviewed using a semi-structured schedule that was informed, but not prescribed, by the existing international literature. Initially 14 spouses (11 women, three men) were interviewed and, in order further to develop emerging themes in line with a constant comparative method, data were gathered from a further 12 spouses (eight women, four men). From those interviews it emerged that adult children played a significant role in the placement process and therefore 13 adult children (11 daughters, two sons) constituted the next sample for interview (Sandberg *et al.* 2002a). Both spouses and children stressed the role played by community staff, and the next round of interviews therefore focused on this group with data being collected from 15 individuals (four home care assessors, eight home care managers, two district nurses and one home help assistant) (Sandberg *et al.* 2002b). Lastly, it was apparent that the views of care home staff were essential and, in order to complete data collection, 16 staff were interviewed (two managers, seven nurses, four auxiliary nurses and three care assistants) (Sandberg *et al.* 2002a).

Data analyses from these various rounds of interviews occurred sequentially, with the first round of interviews being completed before the second were commenced. Main themes emerging from each set of interviews helped to inform subsequent data collection in an iterative fashion. An overview of the results of each set of interviews is now presented prior to a synthesis of the main findings.

## Overview of findings

The first study (Lundh *et al.* 2000) highlighted that placement is best understood as a temporal process, comprising four overlapping phases:

- Making the decision    – factors influencing the decision to seek admission to a care home.
- Making the move    – events surrounding the admission process itself.
- Adjusting to the move – describing carers' early efforts to establish relationships with the care home and to maintain relationships with their spouse.
- Reorientation    – carers' later efforts to adjust to the admission and to 'move on' with their lives.

The interviews suggested that the decision to seek placement was often delayed by carers who initially 'pretended' that it was not needed, only for the inevitability of placement to 'dawn' on them (Lundh *et al.* 2000). The placement process itself (making the move) was a highly emotional experience for spouses, involving the separation from an often lifelong partner. However, spouses were largely unprepared for the extent of their loss and, although adult children and others were supportive at this time, the help provided was usually of a practical rather than an emotional nature. After the placement spouses worked hard to maintain the identity of their partner, seeking continuity in their relationships with their spouse, while trying to reorient themselves both to a life outside the care home and to new caregiving roles. Overall the data highlighted the very limited 'preparation for separation' that spouses experienced (Lundh *et al.* 2000), reaffirming the reactive rather than proactive way in which place-ment decisions are made (Nolan *et al.* 1996b).

The second round of interviews (Sandberg *et al.* 2001) sought to under-stand better both the process of separation and spouses' efforts to maintain 'continuity' with their partner. The findings suggested that the process of 'separation' was not a discrete event but rather one that involved physical, emotional and psychological components. While the practical and physical demands of 'separation' were often addressed there was very limited dialogue and discussion between spouses about the placement itself, engendering a sense of betrayal among some spouses who were placing their partners in care. However, as carers often 'put on a brave face', the extent of their own emotional turmoil was hidden from their children and those professionals involved (Sandberg *et al.* 2001).

Following placement, 'keeping' emerged as a key activity explaining spouses' efforts both to maintain their relationship with their partner and to forge new caregiving roles in their interactions with care home staff. This 'keeping' took a variety of forms intended to keep their partner engaged with the world, and to keep their relationship special. Carers also 'kept an eye' on staff to monitor the quality of care that their spouse received. Although they were extensive, such 'keeping' activities were often kept hidden from staff (Sandberg *et al.* 2001).

Depending on the extent to which staff encouraged and facilitated carers' involvement with the home, and how much carers wanted to be involved, four types of staff/carer relationship emerged, termed: 'keeping your distance', characterized by limited interaction; 'keeping quiet', in which despite concerns about standards of care, families felt unable to discuss these openly with staff; 'keep on trying', whereby families worked hard to share their expertise with staff, and 'keeping things close', describing warm and cordial relationships between staff and families. Building on the theme of 'preparation for separation' that emerged from the initial interviews, the second set of interviews highlighted the importance of staff working actively with families to help them adjust. This was termed 'preparation for integration'.

Exploring the views and roles of adult children was the purpose of the third set of interviews (Sandberg *et al.* 2002a). From these data it emerged that adult children were often aware of the increasing difficulties that their parents faced and were concerned about the effects that caring was having on the main carer. They were also conscious that many spouses were reluctant to consider placement and therefore took a variety of actions to initiate the placement process, which varied by the degree to which adult children took a lead role.

- Allowing – involved creating an atmosphere in which placement could be discussed, but leaving the main decision to their parent.
- Initiating – involved children actively introducing the idea of placement.
- Pushing – involved children taking a lead role in the placement process.

However, following the decision to seek placement, adult children focused primarily on the practicalities rather than the emotional consequences of the move.

Following placement adult children generally had far fewer concerns than spouses about the instrumental care their parent received in the care home and were usually quite happy to delegate this to staff. Nevertheless, they still 'kept an eye' on the care delivered in ways similar to those described by the spouses in the earlier interviews. What was particularly interesting, however, was that following placement adult children no longer viewed their parents as a 'couple' and consequently developed quite separate relationships with their parents. For the community dwelling parent children often assumed increased responsibility for some roles previously undertaken by the parent now in a care home (for example, financial issues or gardening), while at the same time 'keeping an eye' on the parent in the community to see that they were coping adequately (Sandberg *et al.* 2002a). With regard to the parent now in care some adult children sought to improve their relationship while they still had time. This was termed 'making it special' (Sandberg *et al.* 2002a).

The fourth stage of the study elicited the perceived roles of community staff in the placement process (Sandberg *et al.* 2002b). As with children, many of the staff interviewed had been in contact with the family over a period of time and had noticed a deterioration in the caring circumstances. When this happened staff played an important but often subtle role in the placement process, comprising four components:

- Seeing the need            – recognizing carers' failing abilities, and that placement might be needed.
- Sowing the seed            – introducing the idea of placement to the carer.
- Nurturing the seed         – working to progress the idea of placement.
- Supporting the decision – helping carers to realize that they had made the 'right decision'.

These findings suggest that community staff play a significant and evolving role in helping family carers, particularly spouses, to make placement decisions. However, once the decision had been made relatively little attention was given to the carers' feelings about the move, and efforts were focused largely on instrumental aspects. Moreover, both the timing of the placement and the selection of a home were largely outside the carers' control, providing relatively few opportunities to initiate contact with the care home (Sandberg *et al.* 2002b).

The final set of interviews (Sandberg *et al.* 2002c) elicited the views of care home staff and explored their relationships with families, and their role in helping carers and older people to adjust to the move. Staff demonstrated varying levels of awareness about the needs of carers, termed:

- empathic awareness;
- guarded awareness;
- little awareness.

(Sandberg *et al.* 2002c)

The majority of staff demonstrated empathic awareness and recognized how hard the placement was for carers. Such staff were not only aware of the difficulties carers faced, but also actively sought to help the carer engage with the home. Other staff, while being aware of carers' difficulties, became defensive if carers raised their concerns, and tended to distance themselves from the families. Yet other staff showed little awareness of spouses' problems and emotional needs after the move to care and instead focused primarily on practical issues (Sandberg *et al.* 2002c).

## Improving the placement process

These diverse data revealed the complex, subtle, and often implicit or hidden processes that lie behind the placement experience, and clearly suggest that a far more coordinated and explicit approach to placement is needed if the needs of differing parties are to be more fully addressed. We would suggest that taking a temporal approach provides a useful framework, and that it is essential that the roles of all the key players are understood and integrated in order to provide a more complete understanding. Based on the data from the present study, Table 11.1 provides such an integration. This is followed by a discussion of the various roles involved.

### Making the decision

Unlike many previous studies, making the placement decision was not usually precipitated by an acute health crisis, but was rather the result of a growing awareness of the carer's inability to carry on in the caring role. In several cases care had been provided over a long period and carers described themselves as being exhausted (Sandberg *et al.* 2001). This gradual realization should in theory have provided sufficient time for a proactive and planned response. However, it was often not the carer who raised the possibility of alternative caring arrangements, and the matter was usually broached either by home helpers (Sandberg *et al.* 2002b), district nurses (Sandberg *et al.* 2002b), or adult children (Sandberg *et al.* 2002a). In many instances therefore the decision was primarily, if not exclusively, 'expert'-driven (Lundh *et al.* 2000; Sandberg *et al.* 2001; Sandberg *et al.* 2002a, b). Here the focus was primarily on practical issues with relatively little recognition of, or attention to, the severe emotions, described by some as a form of 'treachery', that carers experienced (Lundh *et al.* 2000). In cases where there had been fuller discussion with adult children and/or health and social care professionals, emotional reactions were less extreme and a more balanced perspective emerged (Lundh *et al.* 2000; Sandberg *et al.* 2001).

However, such discussions were usually limited, due both to the rather 'taken-for-granted' nature of placement in Sweden, and the fact that carers

**Table 11.1** The role of key players in the placement process: a temporal perspective

| Temporal phases | Carers' experiences | Key roles | |
|---|---|---|---|
| | | Adult children | Staff |
| 1 Making the decision | Pretending | Allowing | Seeing the need |
| | Dawning | Initiating | Sowing the seed |
| | Putting on a brave face | Pushing | Nurturing the seed |
| | Seeking solace | | Supporting the decision |
| 2 Making the move | In the hands of others | Advocating | Practical emphasis |
| 3 Adjusting to the move | Outsider | Advocating | Empathic awareness |
| | Keeping | Keeping an eye | Guarded awareness |
| | Changed relationships | Making it special | |
| | | | No awareness |
| 4 Reorientation | Establish new patterns of interaction with staff and spouse | Advocating | Importance of trust |
| | | Keeping an eye | |
| | | Making it special | |

often 'put on a brave face' for the sake of their partner and consequently did not reveal the true extent and depth of their emotions (Sandberg *et al.* 2001). Some carers did actively 'seek solace' from adult children, friends or professionals and when this was handled sensitively it was considered to be of great benefit (Lundh *et al.* 2000; Sandberg *et al.* 2001), but this was not the norm, and most of the help that spouses received was of a practical or instrumental nature (Sandberg *et al.* 2002b). Notwithstanding this, the data suggested that both children and professionals played a key role in the decision-making process and that they therefore have the potential to engage more fully with carers' emotional concerns and to provide a better 'preparation for separation'.

For example, in the majority of cases children either 'initiated' the decision-making process by raising their concerns, or took a far more active role and 'pushed' the process in order that events unfolded as quickly as possible. Such actions were invariably motivated by a concern for both parents' health, but paradoxically there was little exploration of the emotional sequelae of placement and the effects of separation from a lifelong partner.

Similarly, based on their personal knowledge of each carer's unique circumstances, and building on their experience of several similar situations, community staff also played an important role in decision-making. Conscious that carers would often not raise concerns themselves, staff were on the alert for 'signals' such as increased tiredness or irritability that suggested that the caring situation could not be sustained indefinitely. In this way they were often able to 'see the need' for a care home placement before carers themselves realized, or at least admitted, that it was necessary (Sandberg *et al.* 2002b).

Staff were usually reluctant to suggest placement and hoped that the family would realize the need themselves. But this was often not the case and, as they became increasingly concerned, staff would raise the issue and thereby 'sow the seed' of the need for placement. However, some carers were still resistant to the idea and in such circumstances staff would try increasingly hard to convince carers that this was the only logical step. Their role therefore became more proactive as it was necessary to nurture the idea of placement and to help it grow in the carers' minds (Sandberg *et al.* 2002b).

For the majority of carers who eventually made the decision that moving into a care home was the only option, there was still a need to feel that they had done the 'right thing', and staff played an important role in supporting and legitimizing the decision. Despite this, and the recognition of carers' conflicting feelings by some staff, emotional reactions to placement remained largely invisible (Sandberg *et al.* 2002b).

Clearly, therefore, although both adult children and staff demonstrated awareness and sensitivity, and took an active role in placement decisions, subsequently there was very little recognition of the emotional consequences and the focus was largely on the practical elements (Sandberg *et al.* 2002a, b).

*Making the move*

Carers described the move itself in almost invariably negative terms, reflecting their feelings of powerlessness over both the timing of the move and the location of the home (Lundh *et al.* 2000; Sandberg *et al.* 2001). In Sweden such factors are the responsibility of the case manager and are determined largely by local availability (Sandberg *et al.* 2002b). Consequently carers saw the move itself as being 'in the hands of others' (Lundh *et al.* 2000; Sandberg *et al.* 2001), and it took an assertive and persistent spouse to influence the selection process. The move itself was therefore made more difficult than it need have been by its uncertain nature and the indeterminate wait for a vacancy. Moreover, because the location of the home was often not known until shortly before the move there was little time for carers to establish prior contact with staff. Clearly, therefore, the way in which the system operates needs to be altered if maximum choice is to be offered. The move itself could also be eased if greater attention were given to carers' emotional concerns. For example, once the decision had been made, adult children played a largely instrumental role in helping with the logistics of the move and/or advocating on their parents' behalf to ensure that the move went as smoothly as possible. There was relatively little recognition of the feelings of separation and isolation felt by the family carer (Sandberg *et al.* 2002a).

The involvement of community staff at this critical time was further limited by the system as, once a care home place was accepted, community staff handed over all the relevant documents to the care home staff and played little further part (Sandberg *et al.* 2002b). Although some of these staff saw the need for emotional support at this time they mostly focused on the practical elements. This was in part due to their concerns that if they encouraged carers to discuss their emotional difficulties then they themselves might not be skilled enough to deal with these (Sandberg *et al.* 2002b). Conversely, other staff did not recognize any emotional difficulties and saw the move as being a relief for carers. Therefore, partly as a consequence of the system, partly due to a perceived lack of skill or a failure to recognize the emotional impact of placement, community staff did not maximize the opportunities available to support carers (Sandberg *et al.* 2002b).

### Adjusting to the move

Adjusting to the move was particularly difficult for most of the carers (Lundh *et al.* 2000; Sandberg *et al.* 2001) and many described feeling like an 'outsider', a feeling compounded by the powerlessness they had experienced during the move and the limited prior contact with the home, which was often limited to decisions about the furnishing of the room (Lundh *et al.* 2000; Sandberg *et al.* 2001, 2002a, c). The way in which the move itself was organized meant that most carers had not discussed their involvement in the care home, despite the fact that they all wanted to influence the care their partner received (Lundh *et al.* 2000; Sandberg *et al.* 2001). This was reflected in the various forms of keeping activity described earlier.

Despite the prevalence of carers' 'keeping', both staff and children were largely unaware of the importance they attached to maintaining a special relationship with their partner. Indeed, following the move adult children no longer seemed to view their parents as a couple but rather interacted with the parent in the community and the parent in the care home in quite distinct ways. This often posed a number of dilemmas. For example, children wished to provide extra support for their parent in the community, but at the same time did not want to reduce their independence, nor to compromise their relationships with their own family (Sandberg *et al.* 2002a).

With regard to the parent in care, adult children 'kept an eye' on the care they received both by direct observation during visits and through frequent contact with staff over the telephone. In cases where the adult children were unhappy with the care they would sometimes get involved in direct care delivery, but not to the extent described by their parents. Importantly, however, some adult children also wanted to enjoy their relationship with the parent in the care home, and went to considerable efforts to try and 'make' their relationship special. On rare occasions this could conflict with the desire of the community dwelling spouse to do the same.

Despite the limited prior contact between family and care home staff the data suggested that many staff were aware of the importance of the spouses' knowledge to achieving individualized care (Sandberg *et al.* 2002c), especially in the early days when staff had yet to get to know the older person. In order to help carers maintain their role staff often encouraged spouses to take the initiative after placement, even if this sometimes ran contrary to their own desire to be more fully involved. As noted earlier, many staff showed 'empathic awareness' (Sandberg *et al.* 2002c) and recognized that the carers' adjustment to the move was an ongoing process requiring continued discussion and negotiation between themselves and the family. By letting spouses adjust gradually to their new situation and role in this way the possibility of conflict and disagreement was reduced, and as spouses and staff got to know each other trust was established and spouses were encouraged to relinquish some of the care to staff. Establishing trust made it possible for the spouses to start to 'let go' and to accept more fully that the placement had been a good decision. Such a realization enabled carers to begin to reorientate to their new roles and relationships.

*Reorientation*

Following the move carers tried to reorientate themselves and to establish new patterns of interaction with their partner and the care home, while also trying to renew contacts in the community (Lundh *et al.* 2000). While all the spouses maintained some form of continued involvement with their partner, for many the placement also resulted in new possibilities to resume a more 'normal' life after years of caring (Lundh *et al.* 2000). For others adjustment was more difficult and they turned to their family as a source of meaning and purpose in their life, searching to rediscover their self-esteem and worth. However, even these efforts were unsuccessful for some informants who felt that their lives were effectively over and who could see no future beyond living life one day at a time (Lundh *et al.* 2000). Notwithstanding these differing reactions, the data suggest that more explicit attention to the adjustment process could enable more spouses to have a positive experience, thereby aiding the process of (re)-constructing roles and relationships.

## (Re)-construction of roles and relationships

The study on which this chapter is based has served to illustrate further the complex, subtle and often implicit interactions that lie behind, and influence, the placement process (Sandberg 2001). We would suggest that one of the key processes involved is that of '(re)-constructing roles and relationships', which operates at a number of levels and is experienced to a greater or lesser extent by all the major actors involved. The concept elaborates further the notion of (re)-constructive care, first suggested by Nolan *et al.* (1996a). The emphasis on (re)-constructing roles and relationships rather than 'reconstructing roles and relationships' is deliberate and is intended to capture the multifaceted nature of the placement process, particularly for spouses. Given that the experience of spouses was the point of departure for the study and that they remain its central focus, a brief explanation of the notion of (re)-constructing roles and relationships begins with a consideration of its relevance to the placement process as experienced by spouses (Sandberg 2001).

The duality implicit within (re)-constructing roles and relationships reflects the twin challenges facing spouses following placement in that they simultaneously have to 'reconstruct' existing roles and relationships in a variety of ways while needing to 'construct' both new roles and new relationships. As highlighted in the preliminary rounds of data collection (Lundh *et al.* 2000; Sandberg *et al.* 2001), spouses focus the greater part of their efforts on trying to ensure continuity and to maintain their relationship with their partner by 'keeping it going' and 'keeping it special' (Sandberg *et al.* 2001). At the same time they want to ensure that their partner's needs are well catered for by staff and therefore 'keep an eye' on their caring efforts. However, despite their best efforts to sustain their relationship by, for example, maintaining cherished routines and care practices, some reconstruction of relationships with their partner is inevitably needed. The extent to which such efforts were successful depended in no small measure on the roles carers adopted relative to care staff, and the relationships they constructed with personnel in the care home (Sandberg 2001).

Spouses tended to adopt a variety of roles and relationships with staff, which varied depending upon the extent to which they interacted with staff and were happy with the quality of care given to their partner. These interactions were described as 'keeping your distance', 'keeping quiet', 'keep on trying' and 'keeping it close' (Sandberg *et al.* 2001), with the latter being the closest and most cordial set of roles and relationships.

Moreover, although spouses devoted much of their time to (re)-constructing roles and relationships within the context of the care home, for a number of those interviewed the fact that they were now relieved of the 24-hour day-to-day care opened up new opportunities to re-engage with the community and this also required (re)-constructing roles and relationships, either with existing or prior contacts, or by constructing new contacts (Sandberg 2001).

However, while (re)-constructing roles and relationships are central to an understanding of the placement experience of spouses, adult children also engaged in such activity, albeit to a lesser extent. What was also notable, however, was that adult children often tended to 'deconstruct' the relationship between their parents. That is, they invested very little effort in, nor did they seem fully to appreciate the importance of, maintaining their parents as a 'couple'. Consequently, they adopted quite differing patterns of interaction with the parent in the community and the parent in the care home.

In terms of the parent in the community and the care home they 'kept an eye' on both but with differing purposes. For the parent in the community they attempted to strike a balance between providing necessary support, often by adopting roles previously undertaken by the parent in care, and also facilitating independence (Sandberg 2001).

For the parent in the care home they would 'keep an eye' on the quality of care provided and 'construct' relationships with care staff, whereby they would maintain regular contact, often 'at a distance', by using the telephone. Some adult children also appreciated that entry to care marked a major turning point in their relationship with their parent and had a desire to 'reconstruct' the relationship with their father or mother by 'making it special' before it was too late (Sandberg *et al.* 2002a).

The extent to which community staff (re)-constructed roles and relationships are less clear. Notwithstanding this, their ability to 'see the need' and 'sow the seed' was often rooted in an established relationship with the older couple that 'alerted' them to signs of fragility in the caring situation (Sandberg *et al.* 2002b). Consequently, there was a subtle shift in the nature of their relationship and the goals of care. This 'reconstruction' saw their role alter from being one of supporting and sustaining the couple in the community to one in which the aim was to initiate and move forward the placement process (Sandberg 2001).

For staff in care homes there was less emphasis on (re)-constructing roles and relationships and more need to 'construct' roles and relationships both with the older person entering care and especially with their family carers, both spouses and often adult children (Sandberg *et al.* 2002c). In contrast to previous studies in this area many of the staff interviewed demonstrated a carefully considered understanding of the feelings of spouses and in constructing their relationships used the skills of 'empathic awareness' (Sandberg *et al.* 2002c) whereby they facilitated the spouses' efforts to (re)-construct their own roles and relationships. In so doing, staff used a variety of tactics which acknowledged spouses' needs to share their expertise and knowledge while also continuing to provide care until such time as they felt ready to 'let go' of some of the more direct caring and focus their efforts on 'keeping it special'. Staff showing genuine 'empathic awareness' were also conscious that the process of (re)-constructing roles and relationships was an ongoing one, which would change as the caring trajectory unfolded post placement (Sandberg 2001).

## Discussion

The study, one of the few of its kind to be conducted in Sweden, suggests that potential difficulties arise at all phases of the placement process, and that such problems often go unacknowledged, or may even be unintentionally exacerbated by key persons. In exploring the roles and relationships between staff and relatives during the placement process (including spouses and adult children), the study has indicated that at times there are disagreements and apparent conflicts of interest between these key persons. However, disagreement is neither inevitable nor universal, and it is apparent that attention to important issues at key times could do much to improve the placement process (Sandberg 2001).

A lack of planning for entry to care featured prominently in the study, as did the largely ambivalent emotional responses to the move and the difficulties experienced in initiating and sustaining roles and relationships with staff after the move (Sandberg 2001). To date there has been little research evidence to suggest which type of support for carers would be most effective in reducing these potential difficulties. This is in part due to the way placement is viewed, with Schulz and Williamson (1997) suggesting that one of the most important directions for the future of caregiving research will be to focus on transitions, particularly those relating to the placement process.

The role of adequate preparation for separation is a central issue, and it is important to enhance practice to meet the carers' needs at this difficult time. It is necessary to help staff to appreciate and have the skills to address the ambivalent feelings that spouses experience following the decision to place. Carers need to be better prepared, not only for the separation, but also in (re)-constructing new roles and relationships in order to integrate with the care home (Sandberg 2001). Several factors have been associated with helping relatives come to terms with care home entry, including a perception of control over the situation and the acceptability of the care home (Naleppa 1996). These factors point to the importance of adequate information to allow relatives to make informed choices. Importantly, in a Swedish context, the study also highlights a need to reconsider the way in which the 'system' dominates placement and to give carers greater control over the timing of the move and the situation of the home.

This is essential if relatives are to be encouraged and enabled to make repeated informal visits to prospective care homes, and to be put in touch with the families of other residents before deciding which home is most suitable. The greater their knowledge and experience of different homes the more likely it is that the chosen home will meet the needs of the cared-for person and his or her relatives. In the present study the cared-for person was occasionally visited by the manager of the home prior to the admission thereby beginning the process of information exchange and 'getting to know' the spouses before the move. Such home visits also helped home staff to understand the caring context. Another important area that requires attention is the degree to which the older person being placed in a care home can be encouraged to be a more active participant. Although such participation is often limited due to physical or cognitive frailty, avenues need to be explored whereby more direct involvement in this important decision is facilitated (Sandberg 2001). Indeed, the absence of the voice of the cared-for person must be acknowledged as a major limitation of the present study and reduces its claims to be able to provide a more complete understanding of the decision-making process.

## Integrating into the care home

Kellett (1996) argues that creating a context in which carers feel empowered to exert influence in care homes is a key component of good care. However, following placement relatives often feel uncertain about how to find a role in their loved one's care. Moreover, having provided care for their spouse over several years, many carers are also left unsure of how to manage their time after the move. Relatives find themselves having to adjust to new and unfamiliar environments when they visit, but most expect staff actively to seek their 'expert' information and feel invalidated if this does not happen (Krause *et al.* 1999).

Helping carers to prepare for the separation from their spouses, as well as to develop new roles and relationships with their partner and staff, should be an integral and important part of the entire process of admission to care homes and subsequent adjustment (Nolan and Dellasega 1999). It is essential that staff not only recognize the importance of their interactions with relatives, but also have the time, skills and inclination to foster positive relationships. The notion of a more planned and systematic approach to 'preparation for integration' suggests the need for greater effort on the part of staff, both in the community and in care homes, to respond more fully to carers' needs at the time of the placement.

Part of the anxiety felt by relatives at the time of admission may be due to their unfamiliarity with the home and its policies. Showing relatives around and introducing them to staff and residents is likely to help them adjust to this new environment. Gaining knowledge about the sometimes ambivalent feelings they experience is also a step towards a better understanding of their situation. Often the admission process focuses mainly upon the needs of the resident with the difficulties that relatives experience being overlooked by care home staff (Tickle and Hull 1995), and there is some evidence to suggest that relatives' involvement is not always welcomed by staff (Hasselkus 1988; Tilse 1994; Tickle and Hull 1995).

Spouses in the present study sometimes described staff as a barrier or hurdle, highlighting the staff's reluctance to see them as partners in care and to recognize their expertise (Lundh *et al.* 2000; Sandberg *et al.* 2001). In marked contrast the interviews with care home staff suggested that the majority were actively aware of the difficulties families experienced and demonstrated what has been termed 'empathic awareness' (Sandberg *et al.* 2002c) in helping carers to (re)-construct roles and relationships (Sandberg 2001). This may in part be explained by the fact that it was not possible to interview spouses, children and staff who had been involved in the same placement process. Nevertheless, it is suggested here that the placement experience would be greatly enhanced if more staff demonstrated 'empathic awareness' in their interactions with families (Sandberg *et al.* 2002c).

Osis (2001) argues that practice in care homes has moved from a 'task-centred' to a 'person-centred' approach, but that there is a need to move towards a 'family-focused' model. This will mean changing current practice so that staff in both the community and care homes are aware of the needs of relatives and of their own role in addressing carers' needs. This will require closer collaboration between care providers, family carers and cared-for persons as summarized in Table 11.2.

The present study makes clear that one of the most important emotional consequences for carers following placement is the separation from their spouse and the feelings of loneliness this engenders, a conclusion recently reinforced in other studies (Osis 2001). None of the carers in the present study anticipated or were prepared for such feelings and their emotions were not sufficiently acknowledged by professionals or adult children. This suggests a need for more proactive 'anticipation' of placement (Nolan *et al.* 1996b) to ensure better 'preparation for separation'. This would be facilitated by greater recognition of carers' emotional needs and their status as 'experts' in providing care and support to their spouse throughout the placement process. While staff have an important role to play here, the present study also suggests that adult children often do not see their parents as a couple following placement and further research in this area is needed (Sandberg 2001).

Basically there is also a pressing need to develop service models that involve older people and family members as equal partners in care at all stages of the transition to a care home, from assessment to placement and beyond. In identifying and describing the skills of 'empathic awareness'

**Table 11.2** Enhancing the placement process

| Current situation | | Enhanced placement experience | Enhancing staff roles |
|---|---|---|---|
| 1 Decision making | Pretending | Preparation for separation and integration | Sensitive to the difficult nature of the placement decision |
| | Dawning | | |
| | Putting on a brave face | Opportunities to visit and select the home of choice | Efficient and timely support |
| | | | Attention to both practical and emotional needs of family and older person |
| | Seeking solace | More involvement of the older person | |
| 2 The move | In the hands of others | Prior contact and discussion with the home | Recognize and clarify roles and responsibilities |
| | Little active involvement | Orderly and planned move | |
| 3 (Re)-construction of roles and relationships | Outsider | Enhanced (re)-construction of roles and relationships | Awareness of carers' knowledge and expertise |
| | Keeping | Maintenance of 'couple-hood' if desired | Show 'empathic awareness' |
| | Changed relationships | | |

this study (Sandberg 2001) has elaborated upon the essential foundations of such partnerships, which require all those involved to:

- be sensitive to the difficult nature of the placement decision and the conflicting emotions that carers may experience;
- encourage carers to discuss these feelings if they wish;
- be aware of the limited preparation carers have for the move and their limited understanding of the nature, routine and philosophy of care homes;
- help carers to gain a better understanding of their role in the care home before and after the move;
- be aware that most carers wish to remain involved in care and to share their expertise with staff;

- be open and responsive to carers' knowledge;
- be proactive in initiating dialogue and in creating a first impression that makes carers feel welcome and invites participation;
- encourage carers to remain involved in care if they desire as a way of 'easing' the transition to their new role and of helping carers to 'let go' of certain aspects of care;
- recognize the potential for conflict between themselves and families and be sensitive to the fact that early complaints can be a manifestation of carers' own mixed emotions;
- actively facilitate compromise and negotiation in order to prevent or resolve conflict;
- recognize that adjustment and the development of trust takes time, and be sensitive to the ongoing need to (re)-construct roles and relationships.

However, it is not only staff who must demonstrate empathic awareness, but also families. Pillemar *et al.* (1998) argue that staff in care homes often feel that relatives do not always understand the constraints and difficulties under which they operate and recent Swedish work would suggest that while carers may be aware of such factors they rarely communicate this awareness, nor their appreciation, to staff (Hertzberg *et al.* 2001). It must therefore be remembered that (re)-constructing roles and relationships is very much a 'two-way street'.

This study has demonstrated that there are no easy solutions to the difficulties experienced in the placement process. However, increased knowledge about the complexities of the move and clear channels of communication between the key persons involved are likely to result in a more positive experience of care home placement. Hopefully, this study has provided some new insights into placing a spouse in a care home that will influence the way future partnerships are forged between family and professional carers.

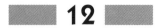 

# 12

# Creating community: the basis for caring partnerships in nursing homes

## Sue Davies

This chapter describes a typology of caring communities that can develop within care home settings. Drawing upon the findings of a study to explore family caregivers' experiences of nursing home entry, it outlines the factors that contribute to the development of a particular type of culture within nursing homes and suggests how this culture impacts upon older people, their families and staff working within such environments. The aim is to highlight ways in which the residents of care homes, their family caregivers and staff might work together creatively to forge cultures of care that enhance quality of life for frail older people and their carers, and also improve the job satisfaction and morale of staff.

The research underpinning this chapter was motivated in part by the limited existing literature on the experiences of relatives during and after nursing home placement, particularly within the UK. This represents an important gap in our understanding as temporal models of caregiving indicate that when carers assist an older person to move into a care home, they enter a new but still involved phase and require support to achieve a smooth transition (Aneshensel *et al.* 1995; Nolan *et al.* 1996b). However, there is little research evidence to suggest the type of support that is most effective during this often difficult period. The image of nursing homes as alienating places and the sense of failure carers experience following admission generate several tensions (Levine 1995; Nay 1995), and consequently studies of the effects of admission on relatives have shown that caregiver stress is not always alleviated to the extent that might be envisaged (Naleppa 1996; Nolan and Dellasega 1999). While there is as yet little research on this phenomenon, a small but growing literature suggests that the interactions between staff and carers are particularly influential (McDerment *et al.* 1997; Ryan and Scullion 2000). The desire to understand the nature of such interactions better was one of the primary aims of the study upon which this chapter is based.

The study began with a review of the existing literature (see Davies 2001), which initially focused primarily on the experiences of relatives around the time of admission and subsequently attempted to explain those experiences with reference to the context of nursing home life. However, as the study unfolded it became apparent that the care homes involved exhibited differing cultures of care and that these cultures significantly influenced the experiences of relatives, residents and staff. The empirical component involved two overlapping phases using the methodology of constructivist grounded theory (Rodwell 1998; Charmaz 2000). The primary purpose of a constructivist inquiry is to produce new insights that enhance the ability of individuals, in this case the residents of nursing homes, their relatives and staff members, to make informed choices that can lead to effective change. Methods included semi-structured interviews with 37 family caregivers who had placed a close family member in a care home, and ethnographic observational case studies within three nursing homes. This chapter draws mainly on the data generated from the case studies, although both phases of the study informed the other.

## Methods

In conducting the case studies I assumed the role of participant as observer. While the staff and residents of each home were informed of the nature and purpose of the research, it was felt it would be less intrusive and generate more insights if I actively participated in the day-to-day life of each setting. I therefore negotiated to spend time at each home in the role of a care assistant. Key features of the observation are shown in Box 12.1.

**Box 12.1** Key features of observational case studies

| |
|---|
| Accessing views of all stakeholders |
| Extended periods of time in the setting |
| Multiple methods of data collection |
| Checking out perceptions with participants |
| Feeding back case report |
| Offer of practice development |

I worked normal shifts, covering both differing times of the day and days of the week, including weekends. In total, an average of 15 shifts were spent at each home over a period of five to six months. During field-work brief notes were recorded and these acted as reminders for a more detailed written account which was prepared following each period of observation. Informal interviews were also conducted with staff, residents and their relatives as opportunities arose. Some of these interviews were tape-recorded with the participants' permission, while others were recorded as field notes. Access was negotiated to relevant documentation, including care plans, progress notes, written policies and procedures. These documents were examined and read during quiet periods and brief notes were made and then written up in full following each period of fieldwork. However, it was the direct observation of interactions, together with discussions with staff, residents and relatives within each home, that provided the most telling insights into the experiences of life and care within each setting. A reflective diary was also maintained throughout the period of observation, providing an audit trail of key decisions, both methodological and conceptual.

The case study homes were purposively selected to represent a range in terms of tenure, size and location (Table 12.1). However, in spite of sharing a similar day-to-day routine and providing care to residents with a similar range of needs, it quickly became apparent that the three homes differed from each other in a number of subtle ways. As data collection progressed ideas began to emerge about the factors that were influencing living and working within the home, the ways in which relatives experienced the

**Table 12.1** Key features of case study sites

| Characteristic | Ashtead Grange | Brookland Heights | Cross Glen |
|---|---|---|---|
| Number/type of places | 88 beds | 60 beds | 24 beds |
| | Dual registered 20 residential beds | Elderly frail | Recently registered as EMI but many residents remain from time of previous registration |
| Ownership | Owner manages two homes | Part of a large national chain of 90 homes | One of nine homes in small local chain |
| Location | Poor suburb of large city | Affluent suburb on outskirts of city | Reasonably affluent area two miles from city centre |
| Buildings | Part conversion/ new build | Purpose-built | Part conversion/ part new build |

admission process, and how subsequent roles and relationships developed.

In order to provide a context for the results a brief description of each home is presented, followed by a discussion of the key factors which influenced the experiences of residents, relatives and staff members. Based on these factors a typology of caring communities is outlined and the implications for developing partnerships considered.

## Ashtead Grange

The first case study was conducted in a large privately owned facility of 88 places. Part of the home was located within a converted eighteenth-century mansion, with the remaining rooms in a purpose-built attachment. In spite of the rather palatial impression afforded by the home's exterior, it was situated in one of the poorer areas of the city, although the social mix of residents was quite varied with a number of self-funding residents. The home had dual registration (i.e. it was registered for residential as well as nursing home beds), with approximately twenty places at any one time offering residential, rather than nursing care.

Throughout the period of observation, the home was run as two separate units divided between the ground and upper floors of the facility, although staff moved regularly between the two units. Observations focused largely on the 44-bed upper unit which provided exclusively nursing care. The home owner delegated day-to-day responsibility for running the home to an administrator and nurse manager. During the six-month period of observation, there were several changes among senior nursing personnel. Occupancy hovered around 70 per cent during this period and a significant amount of the nurse manager's time was spent trying to fill vacant places.

The layout of Ashtead Grange was potentially confusing, as it was arranged over three floors with long interconnecting corridors and several concealed staircases. There were four sitting rooms, two each on the first and second floors. These were light and spacious but chairs were generally arranged around the walls, which had the effect of limiting interaction between residents. Dining rooms (two on the ground floor and one on the first floor) were used only for meals, when they were quite crowded.

Rooms in the extension were all single rooms but were quite small with barely sufficient space for a single bed, a chair and a television. None were en-suite and toilet and bathroom facilities were shared by men and women. Residents' rooms in the older part of the home varied in size and some were very large; most had en-suite facilities. These larger en-suite rooms were more expensive and were occupied mainly by residents who were self-funding. Two double rooms in the old part of the house were occupied by married couples.

## Brookland Heights

This was a purpose-built nursing home for up to 60 residents situated in an affluent suburb of the city. The home was part of a large national chain, which owns and operates 160 care homes throughout the UK. The corporate influence was apparent in many of the features of the home, such as design and décor, and managerial staff reported that some management decisions were outside their control. Regional managers visited the home approximately monthly and a programme of staff training was in operation. Managerial functions were divided between a full-time clinical nurse manager and a full-time business manager. Relationships at this level were mutually supportive and the collaboration appeared to work well. A deputy nurse manager worked closely with the clinical nurse manager on practice development issues and staff recruitment.

The clientele were mostly self-funding and many were from affluent backgrounds. However, resident dependency was similar to Ashtead Grange and some residents were heavily dependent. The décor of the home was luxurious and first impressions were of a hotel-like environment. Occupancy here was about 90 per cent.

This home was particularly easy to navigate, with communal areas and offices located centrally, with residents' rooms either side of two corridors extending from two sides. Rooms were large and spacious and all were en-suite. Décor was similar for each room but most residents had personalized their private space with ornaments, soft furnishings and some larger items of furniture. The reception area located in the lobby opened into the administrator's office so there was usually someone to welcome visitors. A comfortable sofa situated in the lobby also provided a popular spot for residents to sit and 'watch the world go by'.

A large lounge on each floor was furnished with comfortable armchairs, one or two sofas, a large TV, music centre and video. However, most residents chose to remain in their rooms for the majority of the day and the sitting areas were rarely used. The dining room on each floor was also large and spacious with a servery at one end. Again, this room was not used between meals.

Staff accommodation was situated in the basement and included two rest rooms and separate changing rooms and toilets for men and women. The domestic supervisor and catering manager had offices here and a large laundry and hairdressing salon completed the 'service' areas. The home had pleasant grounds with outside seating and a sunny patio area adjacent to the dining room which was furnished with a barbecue, chairs and tables.

## Cross Glen

Cross Glen was the smallest of the three homes in the study with 24 places, and was part of a small chain of nine homes owned by two local general practitioners. The son of one of the owners acted as general manager and visited each home most days to deliver fresh fruit and vegetables and discuss any issues with staff. The home was situated within a culturally mixed, leafy residential area, two miles from the city centre.

Opened two years previously, Cross Glen had recently re-registered to provide care predominantly for elderly residents with a mental illness (EMI), but many residents remained from the previous registration, having made an active decision to stay. When the period of observation began the nurse manager had been in post for three months. The home was full, with a waiting list of eight.

A converted Victorian house provided the main communal accommodation, including two lounges and a large dining room, with the kitchen located off the dining room. Most of the bedroom accommodation was laid out on two floors of an additional wing completed two years previously. Residents' rooms had all been recently decorated in an individual style and residents had been involved in choosing the decorations wherever their cognitive ability allowed. Although individual rooms were not large, all had en-suite facilities.

Outside, an enclosed, secure courtyard allowed residents with dementia to walk around safely. The courtyard also housed a washing line and washing blowing on the line created a strong impression of domesticity. The home was very homely and comfortable with net curtains at the windows and ornaments adorning surfaces – very typical of many family homes.

## Comparing experiences

The cross-case analysis of data emerging from the observations suggested that, notwithstanding differences in size, location and client group, a number of factors influenced the experiences of residents, relatives and staff. These factors will be considered from the perspectives of the key stakeholders; however, first key features of the design and layout of each home will be compared.

## Design and layout of the home

The case studies indicated that the nature of the built environment and the use made of different areas within the home had an important impact on patterns of communication and on the way in which relationships developed. In particular the use to which communal areas were put acted either to encourage or to inhibit social interaction. The rather confusing layout of Ashtead Grange and the distance of communal areas from staff offices served to discourage communication between staff and visitors. Moreover, lack of seating in communal areas prompted visitors to take their relatives to their rooms for the duration of their visit, further limiting opportunities for interacting with staff. The limited communication between staff and families was compounded by the fact, that while staff rooms were located alongside residents' rooms on each floor, breaks tended to be taken in the nursing office, as staff were discouraged from having hot drinks in resident areas.

As already noted, Brookland Heights had a much more straightforward layout, identical on both floors. Communal areas, including a large sitting room and spacious dining room, were located centrally and close to the nurses' station, but these were used only infrequently, with most residents preferring to stay in their rooms during the day. Reasons for this were unclear but staff were rarely available in such areas. Alternatively, as suggested by staff, the limited use of communal areas might have been due to the desire for privacy among residents. The exception was the small smoking lounge where a few residents and regular visitors congregated from time to time. However, even here contact between staff and relatives was usually limited to a welcome on arrival, unless the relative specifically sought contact.

Cross Glen also had a central area with a large dining room and sitting area off to one side and two separate lounges, all leading off a central corridor. The main difference here was that the majority of residents chose to spend most of their day in this central area, only returning to their own room at night. As a result, visitors also congregated here, and this facilitated interaction between visitors and staff, as well as between visitors and other residents and their relatives. In particular the large dining area was used for sitting and conversing between meal times and most staff chose to take their breaks here. A staff room on the upper floor was used mainly for storage.

These data suggested that while the physical layout may have an influence on staff/resident/relative interactions, it was the customs and routines of staff that played the central role.

### The influence of routine on the relationship between staff and residents

The case studies revealed subtle differences in staff/resident relationships within the three homes, particularly relating to the exercise of power and control during interactions and caring activities. At Ashtead Grange, many residents voiced the feeling that they had no choice but to fit in with the routine of the home, a contention which was certainly supported by observations of practices such as weekly bathing. On occasion, and despite loudly voicing their disapproval, residents were taken to the shower room and continued to protest throughout the procedure, with little response from members of staff. For some residents it appeared that the 'routine' operated to suit the needs of the staff, rather than themselves:

I've been in [N] hospital a while since, but if you happened to say, 'Oh I can't go to sleep', they go round in the night and she'd say, 'Wait a minute.' And she'd bring you a lovely mug of tea. But they won't do that here. I only asked once and she said, 'I've my work to do, get to sleep.' Oh she was nasty. 'I've my work to do. I can't be getting you cups of tea.'

At Brookland Heights, the daily routine was certainly more flexible, but many residents felt that staff spent little time just 'chatting' with them:

I don't get no company, that's the point; I'm on my own. I might as well be at home in my own bedroom. People don't take the time to talk. That's the trouble, I've nobody to talk to. I'm on my own so much and I like a bit of company. I've nobody at home. Nobody comes now to see me. Still, I suppose they have other things to do.

The high turnover among carers, who provided the majority of day-to-day care, meant that residents found it difficult to build relationships with individual members of staff, or risked being upset when they left the home.

In contrast, staff at Cross Glen seemed much more aware of the individual likes and dislikes of different residents and care was more orientated to meeting their personal preferences. Even though residents here were more cognitively impaired than at either of the other homes, staff went to great lengths to ensure that, whenever possible, they were able to exercise choice in relation to their day-to-day routine.

Despite these obvious differences, a good deal of affection between certain staff and residents was evident in all these homes:

Martin, he cheers me up. He comes in and he always gives me a cuddle and a kiss. He's special.

However, at Ashtead Grange, such affection between staff and residents was rather selective, with certain residents being singled out for attention, while others seemed to be actively disliked by some members of staff. Cross Glen was the only home where there did not appear to be 'unpopular' residents and all residents were treated with equal respect and affection. Therefore, while a 'family' feeling was apparent to some extent in all the homes, it was only at Cross Glen that everybody was treated this way.

## Relationships between staff and relatives

Observation and interviews with relatives at each of the three homes revealed considerable variation in experiences. For example, at Ashtead Grange visitors often had no contact with staff unless they deliberately sought them out. Even then most of the observed interactions occurred around the nurse's office, most frequently with staff sitting in the office and the visitor or relative speaking from the doorway. This did not encourage lengthy communication or the consideration of private or sensitive information. There were indications that staff remained largely unaware of the needs of relatives, both at the time of admission to the home and subsequently. Relatives who actively sought greater involvement could be labelled as troublemakers, and were seen as a threat to the authority of staff. The limited contact relatives had was confined largely to qualified staff, and care assistants were rarely observed interacting with visitors to the home.

In marked contrast, at Brookland Heights, the majority of relatives were treated like respected guests and staff were always welcoming. Visitors had to pass by, or close to, the nurses' station in order to make their way to a resident's room or to the lounge areas and so qualified staff were usually aware that they were in the building. This enabled visitors to request information about their relative's condition and sometimes such information was volunteered spontaneously by staff. Subsequently, however, most visits took place in residents' rooms, and this had the effect of limiting further interaction between staff and visitors, with staff apparently being reluctant to enter individual rooms during visits for fear of invading privacy. A small minority of relatives who were regular visitors sought out the staff more frequently and made a deliberate effort to get to know them. Once again, however, the onus was on visitors to take the initiative.

Because most visitors to Cross Glen spent their time in the communal areas of the home, interactions with staff and with other residents and visitors were much more frequent and prolonged. While residents were able to take visitors to their room for added privacy, this was rarely observed. More commonly visitors would choose to sit with their relative at one of the tables in the spacious dining room, which became an all-purpose room outside mealtimes. This allowed relationships to flourish:

> I liked that it was small and homely and it felt very welcoming. Now it feels like they are family. All the residents get a bit of love – there are no favourites. I look forward to coming here – it gives a bit of structure to my day. I catch the bus about eleven and I'm here to help Will with his lunch. They always offer me a meal, although I usually just have a cup of tea. They're like my family.
>
> (Spouse Carer, Cross Glen)

The lack of opportunity to share time with staff in communal areas at Ashtead Grange and Brookland Heights seemed to contribute to a sense of isolation for visitors, and while the privacy of being left alone during visiting may be welcomed, relatives who find visiting difficult may miss the opportunity to engage in conversation with others.

The daily routine within each home also impacted upon relatives' experiences. To some extent a fixed routine can facilitate the process of visiting and supporting a family member living in a care home, as relatives know what to expect. However, if routines are so rigidly adhered to that individual preferences cannot be accommodated, this is likely to inhibit relatives' spontaneity. The extent to which routines dominated day-to-day life varied between the homes. While some routine was evident in all three homes, and was valued by residents and relatives, there was far greater flexibility and choice, such as when to get up or go to bed and whether or not to have a bath, at Cross Glen. There was also a greater willingness to negotiate a relative's level and type of involvement, so that they were not under pressure to participate if they did not wish to.

When staff and relatives were able to work in partnership, then this usually resulted in mutual support and regard. For example, at Cross Glen relatives were fully involved in discussions about care and retained a sense of shared ownership over key decisions. This was the only case study home with an active relatives' committee. The regular contact between staff and relatives evident at Cross Glen enabled relationships to develop, which in turn meant that staff were more 'in tune' with relatives' needs and better able to respond quickly to signs of anxiety or distress. However, this was reciprocal, with relatives also being sensitive to situations where staff were obviously under pressure and prepared to offer practical support. At Ashtead Grange on the other hand, where there was little contact between relatives and staff, relatives' needs for support often went unnoticed. Similarly, relatives frequently seemed unaware of the various pressures on staff and consequently were less likely to be sympathetic and more likely to complain.

## Relationships between staff

The extent to which staff members work effectively together has obvious implications for the experiences of residents and their relatives, and the job satisfaction and morale of staff. At Ashtead Grange relationships between staff were acknowledged to be hierarchical and, at times, adversarial, and the nurse manager spoke of the difficulties she experienced in motivating care assistants to meet the standards which she felt were appropriate. There were also 'cliques' among the carers and some hostility between individual members of staff. An arrangement whereby selected carers who had achieved NVQ Level 3 were appointed as senior carers was unpopular with many of the junior staff and surfaced as a repeated 'bone of contention'. Compounding matters, a number of care assistants were of the opinion that qualified staff did not fully appreciate their contribution:

Since I've been here I've had a run-in with one of the qualifieds because they talked down to me and I didn't like it. If they want respect they've got to respect us as well. We know these residents better than they do. We're with them seven hours a day and if they're ill we can tell. We're not qualified but you know when they're not right, don't you?

(Care Assistant, Ashtead Grange)

While still hierarchical, relationships between staff members at Brookland Heights were generally friendly and mutually supportive. At Cross Glen relationships between staff were acknowledged to be good and there was a strong sense of teamwork. The nurse manager repeatedly praised her staff and gave them the credit for standards of care within the home. The qualified staff felt well supported by the owners and manager.

The degree of staff autonomy also varied between the three homes. Senior staff at Ashtead Grange, for example, were constrained by a lack of resources, even for some essential items of equipment, and there was effectively no budget for staff training and education. The proprietor was something of a distant figure who visited the home occasionally but delegated routine management to an administrator. Neither of these individuals played much part in the day-to-day life of the home but they nonetheless seemed to control access to resources quite fiercely. Perhaps as a consequence, junior nursing staff and care assistants at this home often felt powerless to make any changes to the daily regime:

There should be more activities available, something they can do. Perhaps some of them would like to knit. There should be something they can do like ask for it or just get up and get it. Because they're that bored, some of them, it must finish them off. They're just looking at the walls.

(Care Assistant, Ashtead Grange)

At Brookland Heights, the clinical nurse manager and business manager enjoyed a degree of autonomy in relation to some practices within the home, particularly clinical matters. The home was well equipped and a rolling programme of in-service education could be accessed by any member of staff. However, these sessions focused largely on health and safety issues and on policies within the home rather than the development of practice. There were obviously some areas where the managers felt constrained by the 'corporate culture' of the parent company. For example, targets for bed occupancy, incentive schemes and budgets were all determined externally. Nonetheless there was some evidence here of staff acting on their own initiative to improve experiences within the home. In marked contrast, staff at Cross Glen were in daily contact with the son of the proprietor, who acted as general manager, and they were consequently able to make a case for additional resources, which were rarely denied. The proprietor trusted his staff and obviously perceived that they were the experts in relation to residents' needs:

They can have anything they want – we don't give them a fixed budget. They may have to wait for it but they can usually have it in the end. I don't mind what they buy as long as it's used.

(Owner/Manager, Cross Glen)

Because of the close relationships that had developed at Cross Glen between members of staff of all grades and relatives, everyone felt that their opinion mattered and that they could influence what went on in the home. This was apparent in the often lively discussions during hand-over reports and during breaks. Because staff felt valued, they also felt that their opinions would be taken into account. Similarly, senior staff were careful to keep junior staff informed of decisions in relation to the care of individual residents and check their understanding and viewpoint.

Not surprisingly, pressures on staff at all three homes arose from staff shortages and the complexity of residents' needs. Staffing levels varied between the three homes and were difficult to compare due to the different numbers of places within the homes and variations in occupancy during the observation period. Shift patterns also varied, with staff at Brookland Heights and Cross Glen working twelve-hour shifts. At Ashtead Grange there was usually one qualified member of staff and seven or eight care assistants providing care for the 44 residents on the upper two floors during the morning shift. The nursing home manager was supernumerary to these figures for two out of five shifts per week. At Brookland Heights, the figures were: one qualified nurse and five care assistants for 30 residents. Once again, the nurse manager was super-numerary for three of five shifts, and the business manager worked on a full-time basis. At Cross Glen, one qualified nurse and three care assistants provided care for 24 residents with the nurse manager being super-numerary. The input of activity coordinators at each home was additional to these staffing levels. Overall, Cross Glen had a slightly better qualified nurse to resident ratio than the other two homes. There certainly appeared to be a reduced sense of 'being under pressure' at Cross Glen but all staff at all homes felt that the thing that would most improve the experience of residents and relatives was having more staff.

Within the case studies, the contribution of qualified nursing staff to direct patient care emerged as an important influence on the care practices of unqualified staff. At Ashtead Grange and Brookland Heights, for example, the role of the qualified nursing staff appeared to be largely managerial: during each shift, a fair amount of the qualified nurse's time was taken up with completing paperwork and liaising with people outside the home. The main clinical tasks involved wound dressings and the administration of medication. Care assistants met most of the direct care needs of residents and worked largely without direct supervision. Also at Ashtead Grange and Brookland Heights, qualified staff encouraged care assistants to undertake the National Vocational Qualification (NVQ) level two and three programmes, but at Ashtead Grange, the fact that staff had to pay the fee for this themselves acted as a disincentive. The NVQ programmes involved supervision and assessment with some theoretical sessions; however, these were structured largely around activities of daily living and there appeared to be little emphasis on psychosocial aspects of care.

Brookland Heights had an operational manager (who was not a nurse) and a clinical nurse manager. The clinical nurse manager worked on the floor for some of her shifts but others were spent largely in the office completing paperwork and recruiting staff. The qualified nurse on each floor spent most of the shift at the nurses' station, ostensibly coordinating the shift, although little direction and communication with carers was observed. At both Ashtead Grange and Brookland Heights the qualified staff appeared to give very little direction to carers. Handover reports were brief to the point of being perfunctory and carers were rarely fully involved in the process. This had important consequences for their awareness of the needs of individual residents:

> You have to find out about the residents as you go. I think it would be good if the qualified staff would sit you down and run through the care plans with you on a daily basis, to get to know what their needs are. But that's not being done.
>
> (Care Assistant, Ashtead Grange)

The nurse manager at Brookland Heights suggested that it would be inappropriate for care assistants to have access to detailed information about residents' nursing needs and social circumstances and revealed that some relatives had actually complained that such information had been shared with care assistants. To some extent, relationships followed a corporate model, with grades of staff being aware of their responsibilities but with little interaction or discussion about working practices taking place. Directives were awaited 'from above' and employees at the level of the home felt they could only operate within corporately defined limits.

At Cross Glen the qualified nurse on a shift and the nurse manager both appeared to have much more direct contact with residents and visitors to the home. Again, this was partly due to the layout of the home, which meant that all activities took place in reasonably close proximity. However, it was the only home where qualified staff were observed to be regularly involved in helping residents to get up in the morning and bathing residents, providing opportunities for role-modelling care to more junior members of staff. Handover reports were detailed and all staff actively engaged, with carers contributing their knowledge of individual residents and making suggestions. Furthermore, unofficial breaks were often spent discussing the needs of individual residents and relatives. These breaks also provided opportunities for informal teaching sessions.

## Creating community

In comparing the experiences of residents, relatives and staff across the three case study sites, patterns began to emerge which highlighted structural characteristics and care practices, which in turn suggested the values and beliefs underpinning care. Importantly, the nature and quality of relationships between residents, staff and family caregivers emerged as a central factor. Collectively, these influences shaped the type of culture or 'community' that was dominant within each home. Three types of 'community' could be discerned and the most significant dimensions of each type are included as Table 12.2.

**Table 12.2** A typology of communities of care within care homes

| Characteristics | Model | | |
| --- | --- | --- | --- |
| | Controlled community | Cosmetic community | Complete community |
| Practice as | Control | Service | Enablement Nurture |
| Objectives | Maintenance | Customer satisfaction Profit | Growth and development Partnership |
| Important values | Minimizing risk Maintaining the status quo | Quality Privacy | Well-being Interdependence |
| Organization of work | Task-centred Routine | Customer-centred Individual | Person-centred Relational |
| Relationships between staff and residents | Authoritarian Favouritism | Attendance | Reciprocal |
| Relationships between residents | Fellow captives Competitive | Fellow guests Reserved Critical | Family Intimate |
| Relationships between staff | Hierarchical Segregation of roles Occasionally hostile | Hierarchical Corporate | Collegial Blurring of roles |
| Relationships between staff and relatives | Distant Sometimes combative | Stage-managed Cordial but superficial | Natural Spontaneous Equal Affectionate |
| Quality as | 'Good geriatric care' | 'The satisfied customer' | 'Community of equals' |

Similar to Stanley and Reed (1999), Table 12.2 represents an attempt to disentangle the community types in terms of their key characteristics. However, this form of presentation runs the risk of under-representing the subtlety of these models and the way in which they coexist, intertwine and provide counterpoints to each other within a single organization (Stanley and Reed 1999). It is important to reiterate that all of these models can operate to some extent within a single care home. They are presented here as 'ideal' types and as an aid to thinking about care in order that:

> ... we can make some more open and reflective choices about the way we want practice to go, rather than be caught up in the momentum of a set of ideas that no one has articulated or challenged.
> (Stanley and Reed 1999: 73)

Elements of the community types have been described previously (see for example Townsend 1962; Miller and Gwynne 1972; McDerment *et al.* 1997; Stanley and Reed 1999), however, these earlier accounts tended to focus primarily upon the experiences of residents rather than consider the ways in which the values, expectations and perceptions of all the main stakeholders inter-relate to create a 'culture of care'. By considering the nature of these inter-relationships, previous analyses can be elaborated upon and used to suggest the most appropriate model for supporting frail older people and their families. The key characteristics of each type of community are now briefly described.

### Controlled community

The 'controlled community' reflects many of the characteristics of the 'warehouse' model described so vividly by Miller and Gwynne (1972). Safety and containment are prime objectives within this model, often at the expense of personal autonomy. Care is characterized by the operation of a standardized series of task-centred activities with some evidence of personalized care, but within an overarching and pervasive routine. Work scheduling is orientated to 'getting through' a series of tasks, most of which have to do with meeting the basic physical necessities of life rather than residents' social and emotional needs. Minimizing physical risks to residents is an important goal and is prioritized above autonomy and personal growth. Relationships between staff and residents are characterized by power and authority, with staff having strong likes and dislikes for individual residents. This in turn promotes competition between residents for staff approval. However, it can also result in strong positive relationships between residents as they realize that they are 'in this together'. Staff lack the necessary skills to maintain a positive culture and have lost confidence in the capacity of the institution to change (Stanley and Reed 1999). Staff relationships are hierarchical, critical and sometimes punitive. Relatives are perceived as visitors and outsiders, and seen as interfering as they constitute a threat to the objectives of the institution. Such a model is legitimized by the perception that residents lack the ability for self-control, which needs to be provided by an external agency (Stanley and Reed 1999). The views and preferences of service users are secondary to the institutional view of how life and care are best ordered. This model often reflects an isolated community with only tenuous links with the outside world.

*Cosmetic community*

The 'cosmetic community' resembles the tariff model derived from contemporary service industries such as hotel and travel services (McDerment *et al.* 1997). Its focus is individual rather than communal and it seeks to satisfy individual needs according to means. Privacy for service users is highly valued, but this may be at the expense of facilitating meaningful relationships, which tend to be reserved. Residents are generally less tolerant of each other, and of what they perceive to be inadequacies on the part of staff. Consequently, complaints are an accepted feature. Staff relationships with relatives can be influenced by expressed expectations and are largely cordial but superficial. The cosmetic model reflects the business culture that has developed in the care industry, which emphasizes service specifications and the need to demonstrate concrete, measurable services and outcomes. However, the model may be divisive since some residents may be excluded on the basis of cost. The language of 'customer care' has implications for the 'homely and welcoming' atmosphere so valued by residents and relatives alike. Nonetheless, the cosmetic community is likely to appeal to some older people and their families, particularly since it is predicated on the illusion of the 'customer' retaining control.

*Complete community*

The 'complete community' is relationship-based and community-focused. Relationships are affectionate and mutually reinforcing. Care is orientated towards enabling and nurturing residents to achieve their optimal quality of life and is person-centred. Relationships between residents and staff aim to empower residents and afford them as much control as possible, but also result in benefits for staff. Relationships with relatives and other community dwellers are fostered and encouraged to promote the mutual benefit that such relationships afford. Roles within the home are relatively interchangeable and everyone feels that they have a voice. Relationships between staff are mutually supportive and reciprocal. Effective leadership is a key element to the achievement of the complete community and this involves ensuring that staff are valued and supported. The result is a community of equals in which every member – resident, relative or staff – makes an important and recognized contribution.

It is important to recognize that these core values and objectives, being more abstract than the practices and interactions which were observed in each of the homes, can only be inferred from those events and have not been confirmed by the participants in the case studies. Furthermore, some features of each model were observed at each home, but the predominant model in evidence at any particular home most closely matched one of the three model types. Moreover, it is possible that there are alternative types of community which were not apparent within the data gathered for this research. Nonetheless, observations and interviews during the second phase of the study suggested that it is the 'complete community' which is likely to result in the most positive experiences for older people, their relatives and staff working with them.

The typology of communities within care homes described here is at an early stage of development and requires further empirical testing and elaboration. Nevertheless, there is sufficient evidence within the case study data to suggest that the dominant model of care within a nursing home, whether implicit or explicit, has important consequences for residents and their close relatives, as well as for the experiences of staff.

## Discussion

An important finding of the current research is that relatives' experiences of nursing home entry cannot be considered in isolation from the experiences of the older residents and staff of care homes. Furthermore, the results suggest that these experiences are largely a consequence of the dominant model of care in operation within a given home.

The importance of an explicit common philosophy and shared goals for residents, their relatives and staff finds support within the literature. For example, relatives have highlighted their desire for residents and families to be the agency's top priority rather than making money and profits (Rantz *et al.* 1999). Rantz compared staff and relative perceptions of what constituted a quality service and found that relatives recounted anxieties about negative experiences such as accidents and loss of belongings, whereas these issues were not highlighted by staff. In a similar study comparing the views of relatives and staff, Ryan and Scullion (2000) found that while the resident was the focus of care for both family and nursing staff, delivery of that care was guided by different considerations:

> Nursing staff followed and were inhibited by policies and pro-
> cedures within a professional relationship. In contrast, families
> derive their caregiving role from existing family structures, values
> and established relationships. Staff perceptions of care reflected
> the culture of the institution, whereas family care reflected a more
> complete human concern.
>
> (Ryan and Scullion 2000: 632)

More than a decade previously, Minichiello (1987) argued that such discrepancies arise from managers' attempts to standardize and routinize services, resulting in the creation of unintended rules. Such rules rarely serve the goals of both the institution and the interests of individual clients. Rigid policies and inflexible rules have repercussions for both residents and relatives. Nelson (2000) suggests that residents often try to enlist family members to help them to win concessions: however, these family allies are often frustrated because they are, relatively speaking, without resources themselves. The result is often an 'impotent retreat' or 'angry retaliation' with the complaint carried higher and higher in the chain of command. This parallels the experiences of relatives within the current study who were forced either to 'put up with it' or 'battle it out' (Davies 2001). Nelson, after Litwak (1985) attributes this situation to the bureaucratization of care and a clash of value systems:

> It is apparent that most nursing home complaints stem from the institution's poor translation of an essentially intimate family care-giving function into the impersonal mechanisms of a bureaucracy (Litwak 1985). The impersonal and incomplete care that results creates frustration surrounding issues of autonomy, better service, and individualized care – the core rewards in the consumer's value system. Conflict arises from clashes between this value system and the facility's value system that embraces efficiency, profit, risk management and proper care as well as other medical, managerial and professional prerogatives. Although these goal sets are not always in conflict, the provider's concern for the individual patient's interest is inherently limited by facility priorities and the need to sustain managerial power and control.
>
> (Nelson 2000: 48)

Nelson argues that patient (resident) advocates are essential in order to achieve an appropriate balance which meets the needs of the older person, the person's family and the organization.

Taken together, the findings of the current study and the existing literature suggest that the potential to create appropriate cultures of care for older people and their relatives is unlikely to be realized unless the needs of all stakeholders, including staff members, are taken into account. Significantly, a recurrent theme within recent literature is the need to acknowledge the emotional component of work with older people and family caregivers if true partnerships are to be created (Brechin 1998; Gattuso and Bevin 2000). Gattuso and Bevin (2000), for example, suggest that the kinds of phenomena which must be accounted for in a theory of emotional labour include the blurring of 'public' and 'private' in women's experiences and maternal models of care. They argue that the welfare of the recipients of 'gerontic' nursing is linked to the well-being of the nurse carer but that a cultural change is needed so as to recognize and value emotion work. These arguments resonate with Brechin's assertion (1998) that any analysis of care must address the experiences of all those involved so as to tease out the tensions and pressures which mitigate against good care in order to help identify and build appropriate support. Other studies have also identified a need to expand the current conceptualization of caregiving to place a greater emphasis on emotional support (Oldman *et al.* 1998; Keefe and Fancey 2000):

> There is still too much emphasis in quality standards, on the quality of physical care and not enough on the need for good social relationships, having enough to do, going out of the home. These issues are not easily addressed.
>
> (Oldman *et al.* 1998: 64)

The difficulties for practitioners of reconciling the realities of practice with traditional care models has also been highlighted (Hasselkus *et al.* 1996). More than a decade ago Safford (1989) recommended practice models to overcome such tensions by coordinating and joining the shared functions of formal and informal support. The important thing is to ensure that the selected model reflects the concerns of all the main stakeholders.

## Implications

As with much existing research in this field, the findings of the present study reinforce the need to prepare older people and their relatives for what to expect from nursing home care, including educating the general public about what goes on in care homes. Stanley and Reed (1999) argue persuasively that what goes on in care homes is a societal responsibility.

The importance of creating partnerships is also clear. In particular, developing partnership between residents, relatives and staff members is crucial. However, we must also think creatively about ways in which care homes can link with local communities, perhaps involving volunteers or local schools. Many care institutions are largely self-contained and some have limited interactions with the outside world. In such a context it is easy for the language and customs of the institution to become entrenched. Links with local communities can ensure that inappropriate practices are challenged and also inject new ideas.

Finally, there is a need to consider how we might change the culture of care within a care home to create the most appropriate type of community. In some cases this will involve education and support to ensure that staff are prepared to work in fundamentally different ways. Models which might provide the basis for developing practice in this field are beginning to emerge and require evaluation (McDerment *et al.* 1997; Stanley and Reed 1999; Nolan *et al.* 2002b). Stanley and Reed (1999), for example, identify a number of themes essential to an understanding of how to change the nature of care institutions. These include the need for redistribution of power, the need to trace the relationship between individual and institutional values, the importance of creating an ethos or culture of care which is open and supportive and the need to recognize ways in which implicit and explicit models of care impact upon practice.

Whatever model is chosen, creating community within the context of a care home has the potential to enrich relationships and to enhance quality of life for frail older people and their carers, as well as improving job satisfaction and morale of staff. We must strive to ensure that this potential is fully realized.

# 13

## Forging partnerships in care homes: the impact of an educational intervention

## Ulla Lundh, Åsa Påulsson and Ingrid Hellström

It is now widely recognized that placing an elderly relative into a care home does not mark the end of family caregiving, but rather signals a new but still involved stage (Aneshensel *et al.* 1995; Dellasega and Nolan 1997; Sandberg 2001). However, the degree of involvement varies and while most family carers visit regularly (MacDonald *et al.* 1996; Naleppa 1996; Ross *et al.* 1997; Wright 1998; Sandberg 2001), many feel uncertain about their role within the care home, and unsure of how to relate to professional carers (Aneshensel *et al.* 1995; Hertzberg and Ekman 1996; Naleppa 1996; Dellasega and Nolan 1997; Sandberg *et al.* 2001). Consequently family carers may experience problems in establishing mean-ingful relationships with professional caregivers (Hertzberg and Ekman 1996), and interactions are often of a superficial nature, focusing primarily on practical issues. As a result, carers can feel that their efforts to provide detailed information about the preferred lifestyle, personal circumstances, needs and wishes of their relative are met with indifference or even dis-missed by professional carers (Hertzberg and Ekman 1996; Lundh *et al.* 2000), and that their expertise and experience as caregivers is not fully acknowledged or utilized by staff (Ross *et al.* 1997; Pillemar *et al.* 1998; Lundh *et al.* 2000).

This situation arises in part because most carers have only limited con-tact with the care home before placement and they feel uncertain about what to expect from the staff, as well as what is expected of them. There-fore misunderstandings can occur between family and professional carers (Ehrenfeld *et al.* 1997; McDerment *et al.* 1997; Pillemar *et al.* 1998). A number of studies have suggested that if this situation is to improve then family carers need support and encouragement when visiting care homes, and help to understand the nature of their future relationship with the cared-for person (Naleppa 1996; Wright 1998; Sandberg 2001).

For most family carers it is very important that they maintain their relationship with their relative (Sandberg *et al.* 2001; Sandberg 2001), but professional carers may not appreciate the significance of this and often assume overall responsibility. All too frequently, therefore, family carers are not given any support or advice about how best to maintain their relationship with the cared-for person (McDerment *et al.* 1997; Wright 1998; Sandberg 2001).

This chapter considers the impact of an educational intervention designed to create closer working relationships between family and professional carers in care homes for people with dementia in Sweden. The study was supported by the Swedish National Board of Health and Welfare and was conducted in seven care homes. The intervention itself was based on a study package, *Partners in Care* (Woods *et al.* 1999), developed as part of an EU-funded project involving the UK, Eire, Spain and Sweden. The package explores how partnerships can be created between family and professional carers in care homes for people with dementia, and was based on national consensus conferences held in each country and involving practitioners, policy makers and family carers. These conferences identified a number of key issues that informed the design of the final study package.

The aims of the package were:

- to raise awareness of issues concerning family involvement in dementia care among relatives, staff and cared-for persons within care homes;
- to highlight examples of good practice when involving families in long-term care, and to encourage and support greater family involvement;
- to stimulate discussion about current practice regarding family involvement within participating homes;
- to identify and highlight areas for improvement, and to develop new partnerships between staff and family carers resulting in planned action to initiate change.

The material within the package comprised both text and video-based learning resources addressing several issues, and suggesting ways of increasing cooperation between family and professional carers which would result in closer working relationships and enhanced care for the person with dementia. The material was designed for use in study groups involving both staff and relatives, and was intended to be used in a flexible way to facilitate the exchange of views and experiences within particular contexts. While the study pack contains suggestions for its use, it could therefore be adapted to suit local circumstances and the needs and preferences of individual groups. However, underpinning the package are four main themes, and it is recommended that each group completes at least four sessions of about 1½ hours which focus on one of the four themes each session. The four themes are as follows:

*Theme 1 – Sharing information*

This theme highlights the need for staff to provide relatives with information about the care home at the time of placement in order to help families and the cared-for person understand their new environment. The importance of sharing information with staff is also stressed in order to help staff provide personalized, individual care. The session includes topics for discussion about the best ways of sharing information.

*Theme 2 – Sharing the care*

This theme emphasizes the value of families and staff sharing the care and highlights differing ways in which this might be achieved. The concluding section suggests ways of encouraging relatives to participate in caregiving, identifying potential barriers to shared care, and suggests how these might be overcome and current practice improved.

*Theme 3 – Developing supportive relationships*

This session provides further insights into how to develop partnerships between staff and relatives, stressing the importance of helping relatives to adapt to their new caring role, as well as suggesting ways in which staff can cope with the demands of their work. Both emotional and practical problems are addressed, and the changing nature of staff/family relationships over time considered.

*Theme 4 – Making it work*

The focus in this theme is on practical ways of sustaining partnerships, and it highlights the need for good channels of communication and a shared understanding of the needs and wishes of all parties. This final theme reinforces the fundamental principles upon which successful partnerships between relatives and staff are based, such as 'flexibility and understanding' and 'dealing with concerns, complaints and conflicts'.

Following a consideration of the above themes, each group is asked to identify an action plan for implementation within their care environment.

Within this study the intervention was implemented using a 'study circle' methodology, developed in Sweden by Jansson *et al.* (1998), as a means of facilitating communication between family carers and community volunteers working in the field of dementia care. Each 'circle' was led by a Deacon from the Church of Sweden, who had received additional training in the care of people with dementia. The circles met for three hours each week over a period of five weeks and provided a forum in which family carers could share their experiences with each other and also with interested volunteers. The hope was that by developing trust and understanding the volunteers would be able to provide appropriate and sensitive services for family carers, such as in-house respite care. Evaluation suggested that the study circles were seen as being very success-ful by both parties. The volunteers considered that they had gained important new theoretical and practical knowledge, while relatives were pleased at being able to share experiences and perspectives. As a result they had greater confidence in the quality and appropriateness of the respite care provided.

Similar methodologies have also been used in care home settings. For example, Pillemar *et al.* (1998) organized two parallel, but initially separate, study circles, one for staff and one for family carers in which each group considered the advantages of closer working, and identified barriers and facilitators. Following this separate consideration of the issues involved the groups met to decide on the action needed to improve cooperation and partnerships. The content of the intervention used by Pillemar *et al.* (1998) in many ways reflects that in the current package, for it comprised the following elements:

- introduction to the intervention;
- sharing successful family and staff communication techniques;
- advanced listening skills;
- saying what you mean clearly and respectfully;
- cultural and ethnic differences;
- handling blame, criticism and conflict;
- understanding differences in values;
- planning a joint session;
- holding the joint session.

The sessions were led by a social worker facilitator employed in the six homes within which the intervention was field-tested. The intervention was evaluated using questionnaires at the end of the sessions and two months later, together with in-depth interviews with 31 (of 41) family members and 24 (out of 66) staff using telephone interviews. The satis-faction of both groups was high, with virtually all participants feeling confident and comfortable with the intervention and claiming to have gained new insights into the world of the other, which gave them a changed perspective and a differing approach to staff/family interactions. These sometimes resulted in concrete changes such as regular meetings, development of a family handbook, a bulletin board with staff names and pictures, the formation of a family council and monthly support groups.

In addition to these positive benefits the evaluation also highlighted the importance of institutional commitment to the programme and to the cost of the training (especially the social worker's time). It was particularly important to involve the administrators at an early stage and to gain their complete cooperation. Last but by no means least was the need to consider the sustainability of the intervention and the need to repeat it regularly, especially in the light of staff and relative turnover.

Both of the above studies highlighted the potential benefits of working to create better understanding and enhanced relationships between family carers and either volunteer workers or paid staff, and a similar model underpinned the intervention in the present study.

## The present study

In the present study, study circles were formed in seven homes for people with dementia, with each circle comprising eight participants; there was equal representation from staff and families. In contrast to the work of Pillemar *et al.* (1998), where a social worker was employed as the facilitator of the group, in our case one member of each circle was nominated as a facilitator by the group. While previous experience of such a role was an advantage, this was not considered to be essential. Rather, it was more important that the group itself determined the most appropriate way for the sessions to be organized and run. So, for example, it was possible for each session to be facilitated by a different individual, who could either be a staff or relative member of the group, or indeed someone external to the group. This provided a rather less prescriptive model than that of Pillemar *et al.* (1998). However, it was stressed that in order for maximum benefit to be gained the facilitator should familiarize him/herself with the material for the next session in advance. In the event each group nominated one of its members to act as facilitator, in one instance this was a relative and in the other six groups it was a member of staff. Subsequently, each facilitator attended a briefing day in which he or she was introduced to the learning material and the four main themes upon which the intervention was based. The study circles themselves were introduced into the homes in Autumn 2000 and were completed by the end of the year. Subsequently, a six-month period was allowed in order for the action phase to be introduced.

In order to evaluate the impact of the study circles two focus groups and reflection days were organized by the research team. These brought together three groups of people: group facilitators, staff members and family members. During the early part of the day each group, led by a member of the research team, considered the benefits and disadvantages of the intervention separately. Later in the day the groups were brought together to share their thoughts and move towards a consensus. These days were held in January 2001, following the end of the sessions, and in August 2001, following the six-month action phase. The data collected during the focus group meetings with members of the study circles suggested that the intervention had a number of positive effects, particularly on the communication patterns between staff and relatives. These are now described below.

## Benefits of the intervention

*Enhanced communication between relatives and staff*

As noted earlier, the study guide and the video placed considerable emphasis on the importance of good communication between relatives and staff, and the benefits each group could gain from the other's experience in ensuring that the cared-for person received the best possible care. However, such sharing of knowledge and information is not always easy, as staff may work differing shifts and relatives may not know who to contact. The study circles reinforced the need to share information and also provided a forum within which both groups could begin to understand the needs of the other. Staff, for example, became more aware of the families' desire to share their knowledge of the person with dementia (PWD):

> I can see that relatives have lots they want to talk about when they meet like this.

Relatives also stressed the benefits of being able to enlighten staff about their caregiving practices, and in so doing they were able to have greater confidence in the quality of care given:

> My experience is that all the practical things, like diet and sleeping and all that, were sorted out right at the start. Then of course this is added to as you get to know each other. Gain confidence. Perhaps you don't tell everything in the beginning. It's just how it is.

The study circles therefore became a forum for information exchange. However, not all staff groups were represented and this was seen as a limitation. For example, no nurses participated in the groups, as homes often did not have a dedicated nurse practitioner but rather received help and advice on a peripatetic basis. All the participants thought that this was an oversight:

> I would say they should include everyone, including the nurses. They cooperate in the work, don't they, staff and nurses? It's a mistake, I think.

The study guide stressed the importance of families being given detailed information on a range of fronts including the nature of dementia, the philosophy of the care home and also other sources of information, such as relevant literature, family support groups and other contacts. The rationale was that this would better prepare families for likely future changes in their relative's condition. The participants valued this and considered that this should become part of the routine practice within the care homes:

> Personally, I feel that this should spread like rings on the water.

It was suggested that one way of facilitating and enhancing the sharing of information was to create a sponsored support scheme, which would involve nominating a named staff contact person for every resident, and asking experienced family carers to provide support to relatives of newly admitted residents:

> We had suggestions from relatives that they'd like to have a support system among themselves. So when someone new is admitted, you would choose a contact among those who already have a loved one with dementia living here, and with whom you'd think that the new family would perhaps have something in common. So that this relative would take care of the new family as a sort of introduction . . .

In addition to providing more information for the relatives, staff also wanted to gain insights into the life of the PWD. For example, it was suggested that it would be a good idea for relatives to attach notes to various objects belonging to the resident, including information about the origin of these objects, pictures and so on. In another home relatives began writing a simple diary following their visits, and staff did the same by providing details of forthcoming events and activities in the home, such as outings and the like. Both families and staff used these notes as a source of conversation with the PWD, as well as a way of communicating between themselves. Staff in this home felt that the notes were very useful and could also potentially save time:

> I can write down if anything happens, and then any of her siblings can read my notes and write back to me, when they're visiting their sister. It's a good channel of information, isn't it, and it saves time as well.

Both staff and relatives felt that the improved channels of communication helped to clarify mutual roles and formulate agreed goals for care, thereby avoiding misunderstandings and allowing relatives the opportunity to influence the care given. For example, in one study circle relatives were able to convey to staff their perceptions that the staff were occasionally over-protective and did not allow the PWD to take risks:

> We were told in our circle, weren't we, that we're obviously over-protective.

Because of the more open relationships between staff and families within the study circles this revelation was not seen as a threat or criticism, as the following quotes illustrate:

> . . . how easy it is just to keep going on in the same old rut. It's not always about what you do, but how you do it.

> We can also learn. I mean, if we're not criticized, we'll keep on thinking that we're ever so good, won't we?

The data therefore provided clear examples of better partnership working and it was apparent that the aim of the first major theme, that of sharing information, had been achieved. The second and third themes were intended to promote a 'sharing of care' and the development of supportive relationships between staff and relatives. The data also suggested that progress had been made in these areas.

## Creating partnerships and sharing the care

As a result of the intervention relatives felt that staff were more interested in their experiences and views on both the content and delivery of care. The need to forge working partnerships and to 'share the care' was highlighted in the video, as was the importance of creating an environment of trust:

> I think it's a question of mutual give-and-take. I felt positive about it [the study circles], because you get new ideas, both how they [staff] feel about the situation, and also how they regard relatives; one does tend to get a little blind in both respects, after a while.

In addition to sharing information and experiences with staff, relatives also valued the opportunities the study circles provided to talk to other relatives. Realizing that others experienced similar difficulties and problems was perceived as very supportive:

> To me, this has meant that I don't feel that I'm alone. Just to hear others talk about how they manage . . . I feel it's most important for me as an individual.

However, it was the staff that relatives really wanted to get to know in order that they could build up trust and confidence in them to provide good care for the PWD. The study circle proved very effective in this regard:

> So, I know, obviously, that Mum's incredibly well taken care of. I often say that she couldn't be taken better care of. In fact, if I were afflicted, I'd really consider living there . . .

However, in some cases relatives still worried about their loved ones' care, particularly during the night shift when they felt that there were not enough staff, and that the staff could not watch all the residents. This resulted in some relatives finding it difficult to sleep themselves:

> What worries me a lot is nights. Because then there are only two nurses on four wards, and I often think about that when I go to bed at night – what could happen.

Generally, though, the study circles allayed many concerns and also enabled relatives to feel that staff had their welfare at heart, as staff encouraged relatives to think more about themselves, and not focus their life solely around their loved ones. Staff would suggest that they should relax and be more proactive in looking after their own health. For instance, staff would encourage relatives to take a break from their visiting routine, and to use the day to do something completely different, such as meeting friends, which they might not have been able to do on a regular basis:

> Yes, this she tells me, do think about yourself for a while. You come here every day so you risk becoming burnt-out doing too much . . .

It was also apparent that interactions within the study circles helped to forge a greater sense of community within the participating homes.

## Creating a sense of community

The evaluation suggested that the study circles contributed to an increased sense of community and partnership between families and staff. Families in particular had a much clearer sense that staff and relatives were working towards the same goals, and that they could now have much more open and frank discussions:

> Yes, you feel, don't you, that you can bring it up and talk about it. You think about, and you discover that you're perhaps not alone thinking about some specific question or problem, and you actually find other ways of bringing it up. And this is felt even more when the staff also are really dedicated to make changes to make things better. Because what you don't know, you can't change, obviously. You have to talk about it, don't you?

Staff described increased feelings of partnership with families both during the time of the study circles and afterwards:

> This has certainly made us feel closer to each other. Even if we thought that we had a good cooperation before this, we have become even closer now, I think, both the staff and the relatives.

Furthermore, while staff now demonstrated their concern for the families' welfare, families in turn began to appreciate the problems faced by staff. Consequently, staff felt more appreciated and supported, particularly in difficult times such as the death of a resident:

> One thing that was brought up by the relatives was this question of who really cares about how we feel – they said so then, didn't they, how they'd never thought of that before, about our feelings – they never even mentioned that before.

This again is consistent with the work of Pillemar *et al.* (1998) who found that an unanticipated benefit of their intervention was the opportunity it provided for relatives to let staff know how much they valued their support. It has recently been noted in Sweden that many of the problems that arise between families and staff in care homes are attributable to the lack of overt appreciation that is shared between the two groups (Hertzberg *et al.* 2001). These researchers found that although families may have some awareness of the difficulties staff face, and genuinely appreciate their efforts to provide good care for their relative, they often do not convey this to staff. It was apparent that the study circles provided a mechanism for doing this.

Another important way in which the study material helped to create better mutual understanding was in helping staff to appreciate why some relatives only visited the home rarely. Staff felt that it was very important to find out why some people did not visit regularly, without at the same time making them feel guilty. One possible explanation was that some relatives lived far away, and thus found it difficult to visit frequently, or to participate in family meetings or study groups:

> Then there is the question of where they live. If you live far away it's not so easy. Otherwise we would have wished for those who live far away to visit, as well.

Staff also began to appreciate more fully the importance of previous relationships:

> Of course you can't judge everyone alike; they may not have had any relationship at all before they moved in, and then we can't expect them to have one afterwards. You can't force too much on them, can you?

In addition the study material suggested that some relatives found it very painful to see the changes that dementia causes, and that seeing a loved one with problems in communicating with a parent or spouse can create severe strains. Furthermore, the PWD may have profound changes in his/her personality, and behave in ways which the families find difficult to accept. Consequently, the psychological strain caused in such circumstances may inhibit families from visiting, as is highlighted below:

> One relative told me that 'There is this knot in my stomach; it'll never go away, but [that] after many, many conversations and perhaps thanks to this study circle, things have begun to ease up a bit.' But he still doesn't come very often; he can't take it, because his mum is acting very aggressively and he clearly can't cope.

## Finding new roles

The text and video material stressed the importance of family carers and relatives being able to find 'new roles' when their loved ones move into a care home, and sought to raise staff awareness of how they could assist in this process, particularly by enabling relatives to make a direct contribution to care if they so desired. This involves agreeing on ways in which staff and families can work together and, if necessary, giving 'permission' to the family:

> . . . it's just that they didn't really know what they were allowed to do, so that they just didn't do anything for fear of stepping on our toes.

This often involved a delicate balance so that staff felt that they could relinquish some of their traditional roles, without feeling threatened, while at the same time not making families feel obligated:

> They can help, but you have to be careful about asking them. It's not a question of them taking over our duties; they are most welcome to help at any time, or when we're planning a party or something. They are happy to assist if only they know how.

Relatives also need to understand why it appears that staff do not act in certain circumstances, and this is essential to consolidating trusting relationships:

> There's this woman who screams and shouts. We know that she has been fed and washed, but then there are her shouts and her other sounds and noises. Someone coming from the outside would perhaps think, 'Oh dear! The staff aren't doing anything to help her . . .'

Conversely, while many family members wanted to make a direct contribution to care, others were happy for staff to take the responsibility for the physical aspects of care:

> Then when her mother gets worse she hands over all responsibilities but she still visits. So she says to me, as I'm her contact person, 'You know exactly what my mum needs. You make her feel good. You know you do.' So, that part of the care she has handed over completely to me, but she still visits her mother.

The initial evaluation of the study circles themselves therefore provided a clear indication of the progress made towards addressing three of the four main themes underpinning the intervention (sharing information, sharing care, developing supportive relationships). However, the fourth element, 'making it work', involved the creation of action plans and their implementation after the study circles had been completed.

## Evaluating the action plans

Following the discussions of the fourth of the study themes ('making it work'), the groups were assigned the task of creating an action plan with a view to maintaining future collaboration within the care home. The idea was for each group to formulate a number of specific goals that would promote ongoing cooperation between relatives and staff. Six of seven groups submitted their action plans, which contained a number of ideas, including:

- mechanisms for ensuring verbal and written information was given to relatives;
- providing a checklist of actions when moving into a care home;
- having a noticeboard displaying staff names;
- conducting assessments and follow-up reviews with relatives on a regular basis;
- scheduling and organizing home visits and a 'host' scheme when moving into a care home;
- displaying the names of the personal contact for each resident;
- highlighting family information, by the use of photos, pictures on the walls, and awareness of personal histories;
- organizing a forum for conversations and information exchange.

The implementation of the above plans varied across the homes, and in some instances little happened, as staff considered that the current situation was satisfactory. However, in others, several activities were introduced. For instance, noticeboards were put up displaying the names of staff and their duties on various units, staff schedules and/or information about their shift patterns. In some instances staff names and photographs were displayed, but in others staff did not think this was required:

> No, I don't know, I think you get to know them so very quickly – I don't feel the need for it . . .

On the other hand this was seen as essential within some of the groups:

> This was a priority among the relatives in our group.

Building on some of the ideas from the study circles in three of the care homes, each resident had an individual diary or guest book, where family and staff noted important facts and information, for example visitors, or family and staff attending activities together with the resident. One relative commented:

> Yes, I keep a diary. How others do I don't know, but I do, because it was brought up and discussed in our group.

Keeping a diary was one way to facilitate communication between the PWD, his/her family, and staff. The staff emphasized that this activity was an individual decision and that relatives should not feel obliged to do this. However, it was seen to be very useful:

> Only yesterday I read one and then I understood. There was a plate of cakes and biscuits in her room, and I thought, 'Where does this come from?' and I looked in her guest book and it said she'd had two

visitors. They'd written that they'd visited and brought these cakes and it gives you something new to talk about, doesn't it?

Other action plans were also intended to improve interaction and co-operation between families and staff. For example, some care homes now provided an information file for relatives when a new resident moved in, together with scheduled follow-up meetings between families and their contact person. In one home staff designed an information brochure giving a general background about life in the home and facts that may be important for relatives to know. For example, the nature of the work in the home, and the relevant care routines and practices.

Overall both relatives and staff felt that these actions plans had helped to sustain the momentum generated by the study circles. Several examples of this were cited. For example, two of the care homes now provided information about staff contacts in the residents' rooms, which made it easier for relatives to liaise with the right person:

> . . . now there's a contact for each person. It's one staff member who's assigned responsibility for this particular person, and who you should turn to from now on.

Similarly staff considered that the study circles had contributed to improving their contacts with relatives, and had now started to invite relatives to participate in information groups about the care home before a new resident moved in. As a result relatives felt that they were able to have a greater say in the way the home was run. For instance, one relative had been asked to become a member of the board of users, which discusses the implementation of care guidelines and consists of representatives from the local authorities, the staff and relatives of residents. This individual eagerly awaited the first meeting:

> I wait, wait and wait, because I want to become involved, be able to have an influence.

Relatives were also able to influence other aspects of care such as diets within the homes, and the level and type of activity that was available. For example, one relative was highly critical about the way religious services were organized, especially the lengthy sermons, considering that they excluded PWD. This was brought to the attention of the churches involved:

> . . . just from short verses of poetry or something and not these long services. I've made this clear so now they'll bring it up and inform the various churches.

Some of the homes had established more formal mechanisms whereby staff and families meet to plan care jointly for the PWD:

> I had a chance to tell them how I felt and the staff told me how they saw my mother. It was a great opportunity to talk to each other.

It was noted that these meetings did not always result in changes to the care given, but that they at least helped to facilitate full and frank discussion.

## Sustaining improvements

One of the key messages contained in the study material was the need for ongoing and regular meetings between relatives and staff after the completion of the study circles. This has not as yet been achieved by any of the groups, even though several relatives recognized that it was important:

> At least once every three months or something like that would be a good idea, I think.

Staff considered that establishing good channels of communication between relatives and staff could solve existing problems and difficulties, and they also wanted the study circles to continue, as they provided dedicated time for discussion, that was often missing within the homes:

> You felt more secure in the study group, all being together. I definitely think that this was the case.

> Sometimes you don't have enough time and perhaps you say the wrong things – that's how it is. Then you need some more inspiration – or how should I put it – by listening to how others manage.

Of necessity membership of the study circles had been confined to a small number of staff and relatives but there was widespread acknowledgement that all staff should at least view the video. However, despite enthusiasm within the circles themselves it did not prove easy for staff to motivate their colleagues. The need for further training, for both staff and relatives, was highlighted during the evaluation, and relatives felt that some of the skills staff had learned, for example the use of therapeutic massage with the PWD, would also be valuable to relatives.

It was also interesting to note that the focus group evaluations, which brought together staff from the participating homes, were themselves seen as providing a valuable opportunity to share good practice. Staff working in care homes can often feel isolated from peers and there are few chances for them to exchange their views with colleagues. This is an area which merits further development.

In addition to considering the effects of the study circles and the action plans, the evaluation also identified areas in which the material itself, and the organization of the study circles, could have been improved.

## The study material and organization of the study circles

As noted earlier, the study pack was the result of an international collaborative study but the video footage itself had been filmed mainly in the UK. Consequently, not all the material was seen as relevant to a Swedish context. For example, the interiors of the homes differed, as did the ways in which care was delivered. Some staff therefore found it difficult to relate to the scenarios used, and considered that they were not always as realistic as they could have been:

> I felt that it was extremely selective. I did not recognize myself in it. Obviously, it only shows the 'nuggets of truth'.

> The films didn't show daily work as it is, did they? No washes, or such things. It was as if everything was touched up, made to look better than it really was.

Generally, however, the video was used primarily as a trigger for discussion, and it seemed to work well in this context:

> I think it was very good, introducing the video from the start. You watched in silence together, and then it opened up what to say and what to talk about at the meeting.

Some of the scenes evoked powerful responses, which had obviously left a lasting impression on staff:

> That lady at the end of the film who was devastated because the staff had to help her husband in the bathroom . . . showed a lot of different feelings. I think this reflected the reality of the situation; that they must 'hand over', imagine handing over your husband . . . In this way the material was good to use afterwards when we were discussing this.

Relatives had also clearly found some of the video footage useful in thinking about how care could be improved:

> The ideas of, for example, writing what the pictures show. It could even be a piece of furniture that has a special meaning and family history, anything . . . we focused on this in our group and agreed that this was positive.

Staff realized the importance of all their colleagues being given the opportunity to join a study circle and also suggested that this would be a useful way of initiating good staff/family relationships in new care homes.

> It's so very important to be able to include new ones. This mustn't end here, you must keep it running all the time.

> It would be good if this could be developed, especially for those residents who have relatives visiting every day.

The evaluation data therefore provided several insights into the value of study circles and the study materials as a way of creating closer working relationships between staff and families in care homes. However, they also suggested that sustaining momentum requires continued commitment and an investment of time and energy from all those involved.

## Discussion

This study demonstrates that there are numerous ways in which families can take an active part in the life of a care home and that when a family member with dementia moves into a care home there are several possibilities to develop mutual and constructive partnerships and interactions between the staff, relatives and residents. This is likely to result in the best possible care and thereby optimize the quality of life for an older person with dementia. At the same time, should they wish, families can assume a more active role in the care process, providing staff with important personal information about their relative which should also enable staff to experience enhanced job satisfaction and find greater meaning in their work.

While cooperation between staff, families and residents is central to the provision of high-quality care, there may be several barriers to achieving this. Staff and families may have quite different expectations about what constitutes good care and of the roles they see each other playing. Both parties have differing forms of knowledge and expertise, acquired in differing ways: staff through training and professional experience, and families by personal knowledge of the particular life of their family member, as well as, in many cases, by their own experience as caregivers (Liaschenko and Fisher 1999). When placing a relative into a care home, family carers leave their personal domains of competence and security (Lundh 2001) and enter the arena of the care home staff (Sandberg *et al.* 2001). Ensuring that both parties appreciate and value the expertise of the other is unlikely to happen by chance and relies on entering a climate of mutual trust and recognition. As families often have little experience of life in a care home, the initial onus is on staff to provide information to show that the families' experience is respected and valued. If the opinions and care practices of family carers are acknowledged in this way relatives will feel a greater sense of security, and see that a relationship of mutual trust can be created between themselves and staff. Unfortunately daily care is often based on staff routines, with little or no consideration of individual wishes and an expectation that new residents and their families will adapt to the prevailing rules and routines. However, the study circles demonstrate that with effort on both sides this need not be the case.

It is clear that a basic prerequisite for increased cooperation is the provision of information for residents and their families, so that they can become familiar with the way life is organized and identify ways in which they can contribute. This often does not happen and some of the biggest sources of complaint about care homes in Sweden is the lack of adequate information (SOU 1997: 51). It is therefore important that care homes gear themselves up to provide information and that there are staff assigned to do this, ideally those who are identified as the named 'contact person', for each resident. However, there is little standardization in the way such a role is defined and operates, and, as the study circles demonstrated, many families do not know who their contact person is. The fact that information of this kind is not made available suggests that staff do not always understand and empathize with the perspective of relatives, a situation which existed in several homes in the study prior to the introduction of the study circles. Staff often have their own culture, with little or no tradition of family involvement, and this suggests that staff are unaccustomed to involving families rather than unwilling to do so. Staff in this study showed great consideration to residents and their families, but in a rather paternalistic fashion, and needed help to promote a more egalitarian way of working. To initiate and sustain a new culture of care requires training and freedom to innovate. This study demonstrates that the use of study circles is one way of achieving this.

Using study circles as a working method has the advantage of developing both formal and informal channels of communication and information exchange but was limited in its present form by the number of participants. Other mechanisms need to be developed that promote the inclusion of all those who might want to be involved. The role of facilitator is also a crucial one and it has yet to be determined whether this role is best fulfilled by a staff member, a relative, or someone external to the home. In the present study the facilitators, with one exception, were staff, and this might not be an easy role for a relative to fulfil. However, there is always the risk that facilitators who are also staff may have a restraining effect on family representatives. On the other hand, if family representatives are encouraged to accept the role as facilitators they may feel empowered by this, as well as acquiring a new role in the care home.

In the present study we did not try to influence the composition of the study groups, apart from the fact that there should be an equal number of staff and family representatives. As information exchange had been very limited in the care homes studied the meetings raised several questions, and not all the answers could be provided. For example, questions were asked in the circles about the responsibilities of nurses and other professionals, and why they were not included in the group. However, there is a risk that the balance of power between staff and families may shift if senior staff such as doctors, counsellors and, to some extent, nurses and managers are included as regular members of study circles. We feel that separate forums for the exchange of specific information would probably be a better solution, but that the involvement of nurses and managers in study circles should be encouraged.

Our experience would also suggest that study circles are most effective, at least initially, when they have a clear focus. The learning material worked well in this regard as the participants could prepare by studying the text beforehand if they wished, and the four themes provided a direction for the meetings, enabling group members to raise often delicate issues that might otherwise have proved difficult. It appeared that the video often served to legitimate but not personalize sensitive questions and concerns in a way which was less threatening to both staff and relatives. This is important as studies in Sweden have shown that fear of personal disclosure can inhibit some families from joining support groups (National Board of Health and Welfare 2001).

One of the key objectives of the study circles was to provide suggestions for further development of activities in the care home, based on specific action plans. It was hoped that these plans, including the division of responsibilities and agreeing a time frame, would facilitate future work. Six of the seven study circles produced an action plan, but despite this these did not prove easy to implement, for several reasons. For example, one of the groups found it difficult to hold their meetings as the employer would not allow meetings during working hours. Consequently, staff had to participate in their own time, with the result that the group did not achieve its expected results. In other cases, while the meetings were sustained, subsequent action was not encouraged by senior staff within the home. Therefore ensuring the full support of management appears absolutely essential.

## Education and further training

Within the elderly care sector, as in all other professions, ongoing training is an absolute prerequisite if staff are to keep up to date with the latest knowledge and practice innovations, especially in dementia care, where there are often limited opportunities for ongoing education (Nolan and Keady 1996). Working with people with dementia can be very demanding and requires specific awareness and knowledge about the illness, its symptoms, and how patients are best treated. Staff require ongoing supervision and education to be able to communicate effectively with PWD, and to be able to solve problems arising within the care home and in their contacts with both families and residents. It is also essential that care homes do not operate in isolation.

The focus group evaluations allowed staff from different dementia homes to meet and they found this to be of great value, facilitating the exchange of experiences and knowledge, and stimulating ideas for change. Staff wanted such opportunities on a regular basis in order to develop a network of contacts with colleagues from different homes, to share mutual experiences and support each other, as well as providing inspiration for change and development. This has resource implications and it is therefore essential that the need for ongoing support becomes widely recognized and funded in the care home sector.

## Conclusions

Although relatively small-scale, the present study has provided several important insights into: the benefits of better partnerships between families and staff in care homes; the mechanisms whereby such partnerships might be created; and the potential barriers to both initiating and sustaining changes. Interestingly, despite their differing genesis, cultural contexts and modes of delivery, several of our conclusions and recommendations mirror those of Pillemar *et al.* (1998) from the USA. They clearly highlight the fact that much is to be gained from collaborative working, but that it will require commitment and ongoing investment if changes are to be sustained. Moreover, several important questions such as the role of the facilitators, or whether to form initially separate staff and family groups or create joint ones from the outset, remain to be addressed. Despite this we are encouraged by our results and are currently exploring avenues for the more widespread use of the package in care homes in Sweden. The search for better partnerships has only just begun.

## Acknowledgements

This study was supported by grants from the Swedish National Board of Health and Welfare.

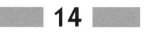

# 14

# New directions for partnerships: relationship-centred care

## Mike Nolan, Gordon Grant, John Keady and Ulla Lundh

Because the future of family caregiving is likely to become more complicated and multifaceted than it has been, practitioners and researchers can best serve caregivers and care-recipients by developing strategies that will optimally enhance the quality of life for the care-recipient and caregiver.

(Berg-Weger *et al.* 2001: 271)

Thus the caregivers not only had to deal with the demands and stresses related to the care of the ill person, they also had to battle the healthcare system and the professionals who worked within it. Rather than becoming allies and partners, the health professionals were seen as a barrier to what the caregivers considered to be necessary care and the best interventions for the cared-for person.

(Jeon and Madjar 1998: 703)

Optimal care depends on family and professional caregivers communicating well. If they are to communicate well they must operate with the same concepts and use a common vocabulary.

(Zgola 1999: x)

As we noted in the Introduction, our motivation in producing this book was to explore, and if possible to begin to explain, a number of 'unresolved' issues (Pearlin *et al.* 2001) in relation to family care. Our hope was to provide insights that might shed light on the currently paradoxical situation where, despite several decades of intensive investigation, there is still remarkably little 'evidence' for the type of help and support that is most useful to family carers and those for whom they provide care. We argued that answers were likely to be forthcoming if caring was understood as a temporal experience, where needs and demands change over time, as do the dyadic and triadic relationships between those in need of care and support and those family and paid carers who provide it.

In Chapter 13, Lundh *et al.* suggested that 'the search for better partnerships has only just begun'. This is a view with which we concur. However, we believe that the various contributors to this book have done much to advance debate. Our task in this concluding chapter is not simply to summarize what has gone before but rather to distil some 'threads of continuity' and to suggest how a further understanding might emerge if we apply a 'relationship-centred' approach to family care (Tresolini and the Pew-Fetzer Task Force 1994). In so doing we will draw upon recent conceptual and empirical work which resulted in the elaboration of the 'Senses Framework' (Nolan *et al.* 2001, 2002b), and its application to caregiving.

Promoting a relationship-centred approach recognizes that the ways in which the various parties involved 'interface' (Clarke 1999c) is a crucial determinant of successful partnerships. As the quote above by Jeon and Madjar (1998) suggests, relationships between family and formal carers are not always as positive as they might be. Indeed, the interactions between family carers and what Wuest (2000a, b) terms 'helping systems' are often fraught with difficulties. The resultant 'system induced setbacks' (Hart 2001) frequently stem from the seeming inability of existing systems of support to acknowledge the proactive strategies that 'lay' people, both disabled individuals and family carers, use to manage their situation. Several examples of such 'active' strategies, for example 'working' (Keady and Nolan, Chapter 1), 'seeking' (Brereton and Nolan, Chapter 3) and 'keeping' (Sandberg *et al.*, Chapter 11), together with the wide variety of coping tactics carers employ (see, for example, Grant and Whittell, Chapter 5; Nolan *et al.*, Chapter 7), have been described in the preceding chapters. So have numerous accounts of how 'helping systems' fail fully to consider such activities when providing support to disabled people and family carers.

Wuest and Stern (2001) suggest that support, whether from formal or informal sources, will only be seen as helpful if carers perceive it to be 'connected' to their concerns and congruent with their expectations. Unfortunately, all too often the support offered is viewed by family carers as disconnected and distanced (Jeon and Madjar 1998; Wuest and Stern 2001). As Brereton and Nolan (Chapter 3) argue, family carers need to be convinced that paid carers are 'up to the job' of providing suitable care for their relative, and this requires that they have both confidence and trust in them. Confidence is largely a facet of the perceived skills and abilities of paid carers, that is, whether they have the training and competence to provide good care. Confidence is a necessary but not a sufficient condition for trust to develop. Trust can only be 'earned' when family carers are convinced that paid carers have the best interests of the cared-for person at heart, and respond in positive ways to carers' own expertise and knowledge. Both confidence and trust are fragile commodities and can easily be lost, particularly when there is a lack of continuity in relationships.

Such fragility was tellingly portrayed by Grant and Whittell (Chapter 5), who noted how insensitive or untimely professional support in the early stages of caring can colour interactions over the life course. Reinforcing the importance of the temporal dimensions of care, they argued that families and 'helping systems' often operate using different 'calendars' which are frequently out of 'synch' so that the most relevant type of help is not necessarily provided at the most appropriate time. They suggest the need for a longer term commitment to supporting families of both children and adults with learning disabilities.

The importance of such a longer term view to an understanding of how certain groups of carers negotiate and experience their involvement with formal services was further highlighted by Llewellyn (Chapter 8). She illustrated the 'caregiving biography' of older 'parent-carers' of people with learning disabilities and eloquently described how, despite the uniqueness of each caregiving situation, carers nevertheless shared certain common experiences. First, there was the way in which their child was cast as being 'less worthy' by formal services, thereby evoking a protective response among 'parent-carers'. Secondly, despite the growing expertise of parent-carers, they all considered that they remained outside the 'inner circle' of experts – the professionals, a situation which provoked hurt and deep frustration. Lastly, there was the changing face of the policy and practice rhetoric which, over a lifetime of caring, successively promoted very different, and often contradictory, values and goals.

Thus for most parent-carers their 'biographies' began at a time when the prevailing wisdom was to separate parent and child and place the disabled child in an institution. Currently, however, policy has turned full circle and promotes a philosophy of independence for the person with learning disabilities, such that parent-carers are now seen as being 'overly protective' if they resist these developments. The failure of professionals to appreciate the impact of such factors on 'caregiving biographies' was a major source of discontent for Llewellyn's informants, and resulted in many 'parent-carers' not planning proactively for the future.

The challenges carers face in future planning for people with learning disabilities were also considered by Bigby (Chapter 9), who noted the limited options available and stressed the importance of 'helping systems' fostering succession planning among informal caring networks. Difficulties in future planning of a differing sort formed the substance of the chapters by Pearson *et al.* (Chapter 10) and Sandberg *et al.* (Chapter 11), which focused on carers' experiences of helping a relative move into a care home. Once again, many of the problems they encountered could be attributed to 'system induced setbacks', ranging from the practice of individuals to a policy discourse that continues to portray institutional arrangements as 'the last resort', thereby rendering them all but unacceptable as viable alternatives to care at home.

However, 'system induced setbacks' and a lack of congruence between the needs and desires of disabled people, family carers and 'helping systems' are not inevitable, and several contributors to this book have described how better partnerships can be developed (see Clark *et al.*, Chapter 2; Lundh and Nolan, Chapter 6; Davies, Chapter 12; Lundh *et al.*, Chapter 13). Moreover, misunderstandings do not only arise between family and paid carers but also on occasion between carers and, for example, people with dementia, sometimes resulting in their working 'separately' or 'alone', rather than 'together' (see Keady and Nolan, Chapter 1).

In order to illuminate ways in which 'system induced setbacks' might be reduced and better partnerships forged, this final chapter will focus on the relational context of care. Temporal dimensions will not be forgotten but will form the backdrop for a consideration of a relationship-centred approach. The chapter begins with a brief consideration of some of the more recent literature on dyadic and triadic relationships in caregiving contexts, and highlights their implications for the development of more appropriate and sensitive forms of support based on partnerships between disabled people, family and paid carers. Subsequently a relationship-centred approach (Tresolini and the Pew-Fetzer Task Force 1994) based on the 'Senses Framework' (Nolan *et al.* 2001, 2002b) is described, and suggestions are made as to how it might be implemented.

## The importance of relationships

In the Introduction to this book we suggested the emergence of a 'paradigm' shift in the ways in which relationships between disabled people, family carers and 'helping systems' are conceptualized, noting that while there is still a need to recognize the important contribution of a 'stress/burden' model, more holistic and dynamic approaches are now being developed which challenge many taken-for-granted assumptions about the rationale for, and nature of, services to support disabled people and family carers. Despite this shift in emphasis, several authors still attribute the relative failure of the research endeavour to isolate the characteristics of 'effective' interventions to methodological flaws (see introductory chapter). Their proposed solution is to design better 'trials' using more 'robust' measures, and to apply ever more sophisticated statistical models to the analysis of the results.

However, several dissenting voices argue that limitations persist *because* most studies are still anchored in 'closed ended' methods (Reinhardy *et al.* 1999) that place too much reliance on the language of variables, frequencies and statistical significance (Russell *et al.* 1999), and attempt to explain the complexities of caring relationships in terms of composite (Berg-Weger *et al.* 2001) or summary (Croag *et al.* 2001) scores on standardized 'measures' which decontextualize caring (Ayres 2000a, b) and fail to account for the subtle and dynamic nature of caring relationships.

The importance of the 'relational context' (Allen and Walker 1992), or 'relationality' of care (Jeon and Madjar 1998), to a better understanding of individual reactions to the giving and receiving of help (Martini *et al.* 2001) and the nature and quality of interactions between disabled people and both family and paid carers (Efraimsson *et al.* 2001) has been increasingly recognized. But as Lawrence *et al.* (1998) argue, relationships remain the 'overlooked' variable in many studies, with very few having explored the dynamics between the main parties involved (Snyder 2000). An over-reliance on the measurement of burden and the continued dominance of a professional view as to which factors are important has perpetuated a narrow view of caring relationships (O'Neill-Conger and Marshall 1998).

There remains a particular dearth of work on the perspectives of disabled people (Nunley *et al.* 2000), as the continued discourse of dependency has effectively silenced their voices (Shakespeare 2000). More recently, however, several studies have highlighted the active part played by those who are typically seen as being rather passive recipients of care (Russell *et al.* 1999; Efraimsson *et al.* 2001). Indeed, such individuals often perceive themselves to be very much 'in charge' and work proactively to present themselves as competent, despite their disabilities (Lewinter 2001). As Shakespeare (2000) argues, it is important to recognize that we are all 'variously' dependent and therefore it is essential that we understand better the types of 'interdependencies' that result (Mintz and Marosy 2000). An appreciation of the complex, dynamic, interactive, contextual and temporal elements of such interdependencies is needed in order to develop better and more effective partnerships. It is just such interdependencies that are captured in the 'Senses Framework' (Nolan *et al.* 2001, 2002b). However, before considering the relevance of relationship-centred care and the Senses Framework, attention is turned to the more recent literature on the relationships between disabled people, family carers and helping systems, beginning with those between family carers and disabled people.

## Achieving a balance in caregiving relationships

Notwithstanding the overriding concern with the burdens of care and the difficulties carers face, the importance of potential satisfactions and rewards has been recognized for some time. For example, we have already highlighted the seminal contribution of Hirschfield (1983) (see Keady and Nolan, Chapter 1) who, in applying the concept of mutuality to family care, demonstrated that carers who are able to find 'gratification and meaning' in what they do find caring less stressful and are more likely to continue to provide help and support. Since then several other authors have reached similar conclusions, and our own studies using the Carers' Assessment of Satisfactions Index (Nolan and Grant 1992a; Nolan *et al.* 1996a; Grant *et al.* 1998; Nolan and Lundh 1999; Lundh and Nolan, Chapter 6 this volume) have demonstrated the diverse and pervasive nature of caregiving satisfactions.

Such findings are of more than theoretical interest for, as already noted, carers who experience satisfaction are often less stressed and others have argued that efforts actively to 'enrich' caregiving relationships can be therapeutic (see, for example, Cartwright *et al.* 1994).

Over the last decade several studies have sought to shed further light on the dynamics of the relationships between family carers and those they help and support, often explaining variation in relationships using concepts such as reciprocity or mutuality.

For example, Allen and Walker (1992) explored the relationship between mothers and their caregiving daughters, suggesting that three broad types of relationship could be identified, which were determined largely by the degree of mutuality and reciprocity that existed and the perceived costs and conflicts within relationships. 'Intrinsic' relationships existed where daughters perceived their interactions to be mutually rewarding and reciprocal with few associated costs and limited conflict. 'Ambivalent' relationships were characterized by limited mutuality and relatively high costs/conflicts, whereas in 'conflicted' relationships rewards were few, costs were perceived as high, and conflicts were frequent.

In an interesting variant on the above study Martini *et al.* (2001) considered the relationships between daughters and their relatively independent older mothers and examined the reactions of both the giving and receiving of help. They identified two key factors which they termed 'perspective taking' and 'attribution'. 'Perspective taking' refers to the ability of an individual to recognize and respond to the feelings of the 'other party' about giving or receiving help, while 'attribution' is concerned with the perceived motives behind the actions of others. Martini *et al.* (2001) argue that both mothers and daughters want to maintain an element of personal control in their relationships and that if the giving or receiving of 'help' is seen to threaten this perception then feelings of competence and independence are undermined. It is here that perspective taking and attribution are important.

The authors suggest that mothers are often better able to take the perspective of their daughters, as they are likely to have been in a similar situation themselves, whereas daughters have relatively more difficulty in taking the perspective of their mothers. They found that where mothers were able to appreciate the 'costs' to their daughters of providing help and could understand their motives then daughters were more satisfied with their relationships, but mothers reported no differences. Conversely, in situations where daughters could appreciate the potential difficulties that their mothers had in accepting help and were sensitive to the manner and form of the support they provided, then mothers were more satisfied with their relationships. If difficulties existed in relationships and behaviours were seen as being 'dispositional', that is they were attributed to a deliberate act, then more negative helping relationships emerged.

On the basis of their results the authors promote the need for more open discussion between mothers and daughters about their feelings regarding the giving and receiving of help. Martini *et al.* (2001) suggest that there is a need for further studies which explore in greater detail the ways in which help is given and received in relatively independent relationships as this may have important implications when more sustained help is required. They also argue that it should be possible to provide 'attributional training' in order to avoid the development of negative (dispositional) attributions among mothers and daughters, and to develop methods that would help enhance each group to take the perspective of the other. We will return to this suggestion later.

Adopting a not dissimilar stance, Lee *et al.* (2001) suggest that although the notion of 'empathy' has been extensively studied in formal caregiving contexts it has received little explicit attention within family (informal) caring relationships. They go on to suggest that helping carers to empathize better with the cared-for person is likely to enhance their positive appraisal of their situation. In particular they promote the idea of 'cognitive empathy' whereby carers take a balanced, rather than a purely emotional, view of their situation and thereby set more appropriate expectations of themselves and the cared-for person.

In a study exploring a number of differing caregiving situations, such as Alzheimer's disease, stroke, spinal injury, diabetes and cancer, Ayres (2000a) sought to identify the 'meanings' that carers ascribe to their roles and identified three 'types' of relationships, each shaped by the expectations that carers hold and the types of interaction that they experienced.

In the 'ideal life' carers had few expectations of the cared-for person and were motivated largely by feelings of love and affection. Negative aspects of care were played down, rewards enhanced, and difficult behaviours understood primarily in terms of the illness itself. Such carers often saw their lives as being better now than previously. Interestingly, although the total sample size was small ($n = 36$), the 'ideal life' was only found among sons ($n = 2$) caring for their mothers, providing a counterpart to other studies which have considered the reactions of daughters providing care for their mothers (see Allen and Walker 1992; Martini *et al.* 2001).

The largest number of relationships were categorized as 'normal/ ordinary', where carers had flexible expectations of the cared-for person and saw their relationship as reciprocal, with the disabled person making an active contribution. While they recognized that caring had both positive and negative effects they rejected the notion that it was burdensome.

In 'compromised' relationships carers held unrealistically high expectations of the cared-for person, and if these were not met then a sense of failure prevailed. Consequently, carers were dogmatic and actively 'policed' the behaviours of the cared-for person. These carers tended to dwell on the difficulties they experienced, and saw life as providing few satisfactions. Importantly, Ayres (2000a) suggests that they were also likely to reject offers of help either because they believed that no one else could understand their situation or because they felt that they were not 'worthy' of receiving support.

A fourth group of 'ambiguous' relationships were also identified where there was a lack of fit between the expectations of carers and the 'explanations' they sought for the behaviour of the cared-for person. In many cases carers were often 'new' to their role and Ayres (2000a) believes that intervention at this point could help to shape future relationships proactively so that they were more likely to be seen as 'normal' as opposed to 'compromised'.

In a related paper, Ayres (2000b) further elaborated upon the expectations carers bring to their role, the explanations they draw upon to understand their changing relationships, and the strategies they adopt when providing care. She concluded that carers' expectations provide an essential context which frames both the explanations they accept and the caring strategies they adopt. If their expectations are not met then the willingness of carers to seek a flexible explanation is critical to ongoing positive relationships. On this basis Ayres (2000b) suggested that interventions could be targeted at helping carers to reframe their expectations and also to pursue differing forms of explanation where no blame was attributed to the cared-for person.

While the terminology used in the above studies may differ, the similarities between notions such as 'perspective taking', 'attribution', 'cognitive empathy', 'expectations' and 'explanations' are readily apparent, as is their potential not only to provide a better understanding of the dynamics of caring relationships, but also to offer differing forms of intervention and support. This is an area to which we will return later.

All of the above studies, either implicitly or explicitly, were underpinned by the idea of 'balance' within relationships, often described in terms of reciprocity and mutuality, and manifest in the congruence between expectations and behaviours. It therefore seems important to understand how such 'balance' is achieved.

This was the goal of a study by O'Neill-Conger and Marshall (1998) which focused on the impact of sudden and unexpected severe illness on the lives of both the 'new' carer and the newly disabled person. They noted the limitations of existing research with its focus on the caregiver, its emphasis on burden/stress, and the dominance of a professional view as to what counts as 'quality' in care. Based on their data they described how both carer and care receiver actively engaged in a process of 'recreating life' whereby they sought to regain integrity in their relationship and, if necessary, to re-pattern their 'biographical trajectory'. This often required a redefinition of self (for both parties) and relationships. This was an iterative and ongoing process.

Redefining self involved two activities. First, dependent on the severity of the condition, there was a need to 'let go' of old lifestyles and roles. The focus at this point was mainly on the disabled person. People who needed to 'let go' were more likely to construct differing biographical horizons and move on to the second stage of 'becoming', in which a new biographical trajectory was shaped. At this stage 'new' caregivers focused mainly on the skills they perceived themselves to need, and the data suggested that it was only when carers felt confident and competent to care that they could focus on higher order activities and look to their own future needs. Interestingly, these findings mirror closely carers' need to feel 'up to the job', as described by Brereton and Nolan (Chapter 3). The first stage of 'recreating life' therefore required both carer and care recipient to acknowledge existing changes and to begin to create a new and positive biographical trajectory.

The second phase of 'redefining relationships' began before redefining self was fully complete and comprised two major elements, 'collaborating' and 'evaluating'. Collaborating was associated with supportive interactions between carer and care recipient in which both demonstrated that they still cared for and valued the other, and were 'vigilant' in protecting the interests of their partner. This required that they were able to share and communicate their thoughts and to renegotiate the basis for their relationship. Couples successful in this were subsequently able to 'evolve' and create shared meanings which, in the best situations, brought them closer together and allowed a new perspective on life to emerge. Thus, as the authors note, 'through identifying values and creating shared meanings, couples engaged in redefining their relationship' (O'Neill-Conger and Marshall 1998: 540). The similarities between this and the '(re)-constructive' care described some time ago (Nolan *et al.* 1996a), and the idea of (re)-constructing roles and relationships outlined by Sandberg *et al.* (Chapter 11), are readily apparent.

O'Neill-Conger and Marshall (1998) argue that, while their findings mirror the notion of 'protective' care described by Bowers (1987), the activity they describe is more overtly reciprocal than the protective care Bowers portrayed. They concluded that there is a need for further studies that explore positive adaptation and the strengths and resilience that families draw upon.

The above studies attest to the dynamic and reciprocal nature of many caring relationships, especially when both the carer and the disabled person are able to reciprocate, not only tangibly but also emotionally and cognitively. However, as studies in the areas of dementia and learning disability have shown (see, for example, Hirschfield 1983; Motenko 1989; Scorgie and Sobsey 2000), such attributes are not essential to the perception of reciprocal relationships.

In an interesting study of carers of premature infants with cognitive impairments, Neufeld and Harrison (1995) explored reciprocity in two caregiving situations where opportunities for overt reciprocity were limited. They also considered the extent to which reciprocity existed between carers and their informal networks of family and friends.

With regard to family and friends, carers considered it very important to maintain some form of 'balance' and 'give and take' in their relationships, even if this took the form of some future return. If a mental 'balance' sheet could be maintained it enhanced carers' self-esteem and made it easier for them to ask for, and accept, help. If, however, they identified an 'imbalance' in their perceived reciprocity then help was less likely to be requested and relationships often deteriorated. However, with respect to carers' interactions with the care recipient, quite differing forms of reciprocity emerged. In some instances reciprocity was 'waived' as there was little expectation of return due to the nature of the illness, and in such cases 'difficult' behaviours were understood largely in terms of the condition. In other cases a purely 'altruistic' form of reciprocity existed.

But in the most positive caregiving situations carers were able to 'construct' reciprocity based on the 'supportive actions' of the care recipient, which carers took as indicators of the benefits of their care. Such 'supportive actions' could be as simple as a smile or outward sign of pleasure from the cared-for person. Parents of premature children also constructed reciprocity based on the future development of their child, whereas carers of people with dementia often constructed reciprocity on the basis of their past relationship. The authors suggested that constructed reciprocity was associated with higher caregiver satisfaction and enhanced relationships. Constructed reciprocity therefore involved others observing for subtle clues which could be interpreted as 'supportive actions'; waiting for future opportunities for reciprocity; or remembering past examples of positive relationships.

Once again these conclusions highlight the importance of the temporal dimensions (past, present and future) of caring relationships, and also resonate with ideas of active (re)-construction as a major but essentially invisible element of caring (Nolan *et al.* 1996a).

Neufeld and Harrison (1995) contend that the presence of reciprocity within carers' social networks, and the existence of constructed reciprocity in their relationship with the cared-for person, was associated with higher caregiver satisfaction, a higher perceived ability to care, better self-esteem, and with the caregiver being more likely to ask for and accept help. Although this was an exploratory study the authors conclude that it should be possible to help carers to build constructed reciprocity and to perceive reciprocity with members of their social networks, thereby providing another potentially useful form of support.

Lavoie *et al.* (2001), concerned that most published work on caregiving portrayed relationships as largely non-reciprocal, explored reciprocity in caring and identified several forms of reciprocity: 'immediate reciprocity' involved simultaneous exchange, such as sharing pleasurable activities; 'deferred reciprocity' was seen as being in lieu of previous help given by the care-recipient; whereas 'generalized reciprocity' related to the return carers gained from helping others. The authors also describe two forms of hypothetical reciprocity, one in which carers believed that if the situation were to be reversed then the care recipient would do the same for the carer, the other in which carers believed that providing help now would reap some future return of a more metaphysical nature. The study concluded that although reciprocity is in part a function of social and family mores, it is primarily determined by the nature and quality of relationships between carer and care recipient.

As will be apparent by now, there is still considerable conceptual ambiguity concerning the various 'types' of reciprocity or mutuality that exist, with terms often being used in interchangeable ways. Nevertheless, there are distinct 'threads of continuity' in all the above studies, as well as in studies cited in other chapters in this volume. All of these attest to the centrality of the relationship between the carer and disabled person, not only to a better understanding of the dynamics of caring interactions, but also to the development of differing and innovative forms of help and support. Small wonder then that there are increasing calls for consideration of such relationships to be a core component of any assessment of the need for help and support (Nunley *et al.* 2000; Snyder 2000). For situations where good relationships are 'lost' then carers are more likely to feel trapped and to experience a diminished sense of self-esteem (Narayan *et al.* 2001). A fuller consideration of these issues will conclude this chapter.

However, Uehara's (1995) review of reciprocity is of relevance here. Adopting a deontological perspective, she asserts that moral beliefs held by people enable, constrain or otherwise influence their interactions. She criticizes Gouldner's (1960) classic statement on reciprocity for assuming that moral reciprocity obligations must be met by providing return directly to those who have provided benefit. She illustrates how the timing, form and focus of reciprocity can vary between individuals, and that indirect and delayed reciprocity are quite common. From the collective evidence she suggests that people tend to become more distressed by ties from which they 'over-benefit' rather than by those from which they 'under-benefit'. This suggests that it would be useful to pose questions about the range of moral norms or beliefs that inhibit people from accepting moral support, or about what makes support 'morally available' to people even when it is physically and socially available.

Having considered recent work on the nature and quality of relationships between carers and disabled people attention is now turned to the relationships between carers/disabled people and the 'helping system'.

## Resolving tensions

The paradoxical situation whereby carers, despite often being in need of help and support, frequently do not make use of available services was highlighted in the Introduction to this book. It was suggested that, while there are explanations for this situation, the two most compelling are that carers either did not see the available services as relevant to their needs (Pickard 1999; Braithwaite 2000), or that they did not consider services to provide care of sufficient quality (Moriarty 1999; Pickard 1999; Qureshi *et al.* 2000). Throughout this book we have reiterated the idea, suggested by Hart (2001), that 'system induced setbacks' are often the result of tensions between the values and expectations of family carers and those of 'helping systems', which serve to reduce the confidence and trust that carers have in the support available. Difficulties are compounded when the support provided is not sufficiently flexible and responsive to meet carers' needs.

Lay participation in health and social care has been actively promoted in recent years (Allen 2000b), a prime example in the UK being the notion of the 'expert' patient (DoH 2001d). However, barriers to successful participation remain, especially the resistance of formal care providers to other forms of 'expertise' (Wilson 2002). In part the problem arises from a lack of conceptual clarity as to what participation means, for while 'expert' patients and carers are expected to work with 'helping systems', they are usually not treated as 'knowledgeable partners' (Allen 2000a), and existing relationships are often implicitly exploitative, and underpinned primarily by economic concerns (Ward-Griffin and McKeever 2000). For example, families are viewed as either a help or a hindrance, depending largely upon the extent to which their efforts assist professional carers to achieve their self-defined goals (Tamm 1999).

However, it is also important to look at the way in which services and support are delivered (Raynes *et al.* 2001; Newbronner and Hare 2002). Qureshi *et al.* (2000) describe these 'service process outcomes' as critical determinants of whether carers see services as acceptable or not. Unfortunately the way in which services are delivered often leaves much to be desired. Coyle (1999), for example, argues that the contact that disabled or ill people have with the healthcare system can leave them feeling dehumanized, disempowered and devalued.

For family carers in particular many difficulties arise from the general failure to recognize their own expertise, and from the discrepancies between their goals and values and those of professional carers (Jeon and Madjar 1998; Ward-Griffin 2001). Even when both groups aspire to similar goals there are often differences of opinion as to how such goals are best achieved (see, for example, Lundh *et al.*, Chapter 4). As a result, relationships may be characterized by uncertainty, tensions and power struggles (Ward-Griffin 2001).

Of course this is not always the case and relationships between family and paid carers can range from fragmented and non-existent to close and supportive (Efraimsson *et al.* 2001), as indeed can relationships between family carers and their informal support networks (Wuest and Stern 2001). Others too have suggested that relationships between family and formal carers can be either 'integrated' or 'disintegrated' (Gilmour 2002), or 'connected' or 'disconnected' (Wuest and Stern 2001). Important determinants of such relationships appear to be the extent to which there is agreement between parties as to the goals of care (Wuest and Stern 2001), and whether or not professionals value and accord status to the knowledge that family carers possess (Ducharme *et al.* 2001; Ward-Griffin 2001; Gilmour 2002; Kirk and Glendinning 2002). Relationships appear to work best when professionals actively promote equality, and where family carers feel that paid carers are familiar with the preferences of the disabled person and genuinely appear to have their welfare at heart (Efraimsson *et al.* 2001), as has been noted at several points in this book. Conversely, tensions can arise when professionals are perceived as being critical or judgemental of family carers (Rose 1998; Farvis 2001).

In the context of hospital or institutionally based interactions between disabled/ill people, family carers and professionals, it is suggested that there is a need to create an environment promoting 'empathetic understanding' that recognizes the anxieties and frustrations of both disabled people/families and professionals who are often struggling in the face of competing demands and scarce resources (Coyle 1999). Elsewhere Grant *et al.* (1994) have shown in the case of family carers of people with learning disabilities that the 'perceived empathy' of their key workers was the overriding link in explaining how service quality was judged across a range of service quality indicators. This resonates closely with the notion of 'empathic awareness', highlighted by Sandberg *et al.* in Chapter 11. Similarly Allen (2000b) promotes the need for a 'participatory' caring context in which staff demonstrate respect for the patients' perspective and knowledge, and work with patients in an open, flexible and approachable manner.

In a community setting Nicholas (2003) has highlighted the benefits that can accrue from genuine partnership working, which she believes can unlock the 'innate creativity' of both family and professional carers, resulting in much more inventive and innovative forms of help and support. However, she argues that achieving this requires a subtle change in practice orientation, with professional carers adopting a more facilitative role.

One way of moving towards such a facilitative role is to adopt a 'strengths-based' approach to work with family carers (Berg-Weger *et al.* 2001). Consistent with many of the arguments advanced in this book, a 'strengths-based' model acknowledges both the difficulties and rewards of caring, but seeks to build primarily on the latter. It recognizes the wide range of coping strategies that carers use and helps carers reflect upon these in order to reframe and find 'balance' in their situation. It also helps carers to consider the many and varied forms of competence they possess (Berg-Weger *et al.* 2001). In promoting such a philosophy Berg-Weger *et al.* stress the need to develop a more extensive range of strengths-based assessment tools to help introduce such a way of working to routine practice. As we will argue later, we believe that instruments such as the Carers' Assessment of Satisfactions Index (CASI) and the Carers' Assessment of Managing Index (CAMI) (Nolan *et al.* 1996a, 1998) have potential in this regard.

In a similar vein, Wuest (2000a, b) believes that much could be done to improve the relationship between family carers and 'helping systems' (both formal and informal) if there was a better understanding of the various forms of 'negotiation' that carers employ, and the 'expert' strategies they use in order to 're-pattern' their relationships with 'helping systems' (Wuest 2000a). Such 're-patterning' involves several activities such as anticipating future caring demands, establishing 'ground rules' for relating with helping systems, and being able to 'juggle' time to achieve best results. Carers need to be able to recognize their need for help and trust others to provide certain types of care (relinquishing), while also acknowledging the importance of time for themselves and the benefits of reflecting on the rewards of caring (replenishing) (Wuest 2000a). Wuest contends that re-patterning is an important form of 'expert' caring of which professionals should be more aware in order that they can work creatively with family carers and help them to 're-pattern' more effectively.

Elaborating upon the above arguments Wuest (2000b) provides a more detailed account of the various forms of 'negotiation' that family carers employ in order to reduce their 'fraying connections' with helping systems, and to facilitate support that they find acceptable. According to Wuest (2000b), such negotiations largely determine the quality of relationships and comprise four strategies:

- 'Reframing responsibility' – whereby carers 'weigh up' their expectations of themselves and of the 'helping system'. The need for such 'reframing' often arises out of the disillusionment and frustrations carers experience during their early contact with formal services (or informal support networks). Successful reframing does not result in carers rejecting all forms of help but rather enables them to become a more 'active player' in shaping the nature and type of help that is provided.
- 'Becoming expert' describes the ways in which carers learn more about their situation and involves three processes:
  - 'Learning the rules': both formal, such as eligibility criteria and the availability of support, and informal, such as the attitudes of professionals. Carers learn the rules by actively gathering information, consulting others, and also by 'observing' how informal rules are enacted. There are distinct similarities between such activity and

the various forms of 'seeking' behaviour described by Brereton and Nolan in Chapter 3.
- 'Networking' in order to 'tap' into various forms of information, assistance and support.
- 'Experimenting' to determine what works or does not work.
- Harnessing resources comprises the next stage in which carers actively draw upon their developing expertise in order to interact most effectively with 'helping systems'. This may involve rejecting an unacceptable service or engaging in a variety of differing approaches such as being assertive or confrontational, or bargaining with the formal or informal support systems.
- Eventually if the above strategies fail then carers may 'take on more' and either work actively within existing systems to try and change them or go outside the system and seek alternative forms of help and support.

Wuest's (2000a, b) studies portray carers as being increasingly proactive and she suggests that negotiation is a process that is relevant in differing caring contexts and at several points in time.

Recently a more complete understanding of the delicate interplay between family carers and both formal and informal 'helping systems' is beginning to emerge, and it is clear that much depends on a more flexible interpretation of the rationale for, and delivery of, support services. This will require a change in current practice orientation. However, changing practice is not of itself sufficient as there also needs to be time and continuity (Piercey and Woolley 1999; Russell *et al.* 1999; Nicholas 2003), two increasingly scarce resources. Critically there has to be recognition of the delicate interpersonal skills required, not only from professionals, but also from paid care workers who require training and support in fulfilling an often difficult role (Piercey and Woolley 1999). Before considering how the 'Senses Framework' can help to promote positive relationships, attention is turned to the more limited work on triadic relationships between disabled people, family carers and 'helping systems'.

## Towards an understanding of triadic relationships

In summary, during the past 40 years, research has only scratched the surface regarding our understanding of the caregiving experience. Caregiving touches a wide variety of social and psychological areas and has the potential to teach us much about the 'human experience'.
(Pruchno 2000: 207)

In presenting a case for this book we suggested, notwithstanding the extensive research on family care, that there remained much to learn about the nature and form of caregiving, and the interactions between those providing and those receiving help and support. In seeking a better understanding we have adopted an explicitly temporal and relational approach and in so doing acknowledged the influence of several authors. In the introduction we noted the contribution of Kahana and Young (1990) who, in drawing attention to the often static and uni-dimensional models of family care that existed at the time, argued for a more holistic approach. Their vision was of a more dynamic, interactive and contextual exploration of dyadic, and eventually triadic relationships, and recently this is a position that other authors have supported (Brandon and Jack 1997; McKee 1999; Fortinsky 2001).

As the preceding sections have illustrated, there is now a better appreciation of several forms of dyadic relationships, although there is still a dearth of research focusing on the experiences of receiving care (Litvin 2000; Nunley *et al.* 2000; Lyons *et al.* 2002). All too often those in receipt of care have been cast in a passive role and few studies have considered the effect on their self-identity of accepting the help and support that they need to remain within their own homes. As we pointed out earlier, frail older or disabled people are often active strategists in balancing their need for help with their desire to remain independent, and while some studies suggest that it is important for those in need of help to maintain a view of themselves as independent (for example Seale 1996), others argue that this does not necessarily result in an altogether positive psychological state, and that people who are able to accept the need for help while engaging in a series of negotiations and compromises to sustain the quality of their relationships often feel more satisfied with their life (Litvin 2000). Roe *et al.* (2001) describe a number of reactions to the need for help among older people, including positive acceptance, resigned acceptance, and passive acceptance. They stress the complex interplay between notions of independence, dependence and interdependence in older age.

Recent work has also suggested that those in need of help and support actively manage their relationships with both family and formal carers. For example, Lewinter (2001) provides an eloquent account of how frail older people act as both givers and receivers of care in their interactions with family carers and home helpers in Denmark, and in so doing she describes direct and reciprocal relationships between older people and both types of carer. For Lewinter (2001), 'reciprocity is what oils social relationships, that is keeping them functioning. In order to be able to participate in social relationships one has to be able to reciprocate' (p. 7). Moreover, she argues that personal dignity is inherently anchored in social relationships and that dignity therefore hinges on the ability to reciprocate.

She goes on to describe how, during their interactions with older people, home helpers perceive several types of reward which include feeling needed and appreciated by the older people, and a self-perception that they are doing something of value for society. Furthermore, home helpers often described how they enjoyed and learned from the company of the older people and looked on them as role models for 'ageing gracefully'. In return home helpers 'gave of themselves' by listening to and valuing the contribution of the older people, thereby promoting their dignity and self-esteem. Conversely, if home helpers considered that the older people treated them primarily as 'servants' then less positive relationships developed.

Family carers, mostly children in this study, talked primarily in terms of returning help that they had previously received, and consequently it was the nature and quality of prior relationships that were the major influence on the quality of current relationships.

In their interactions with both home helpers and their children, older people worked hard to present themselves as competent, well-orientated individuals in charge of their lives, and spoke in terms of their active role in both the giving and receiving of support. In particular they stressed the importance of maintaining the 'small reciprocities' of everyday social life, which could often be as simple as offering coffee and biscuits to the home helper. Lewinter (2001) contends that being able to engage in everyday reciprocities forms the perceived basis of independence in frail older people who, although they may need extensive help, are nevertheless able to conceive of themselves as making an active contribution. In order to be able to maintain such reciprocities older people need two fundamental forms of security (Lewinter 2001). They need 'economic security', which provides them with sufficient financial wherewithal to be able to provide for the small reciprocities of daily life, and they need 'care security', based on established relationships which have an element of continuity, which enables them to feel secure in the knowledge that help will be provided in a way that maintains and promotes their dignity and personal worth.

## Is person-centred care enough?

The recent policy and practice rhetoric has actively promoted a vision of services underpinned by a 'person-centred' or a 'patient-centred' approach (Easterbrook 1999; DoH 2001b) which seeks to individualize care by focusing on individuals and their needs (DoH 2001b), giving rise to a range of ways of conceptualizing the nature of interpersonal ties required (Mead and Bower 2000; Coyle and Williams 2001; Martin and Younger 2001). However, we would suggest that this approach may fail to account for the sorts of negotiations, interdependencies and reciprocities that characterize the best dyadic and triadic relationships. Interestingly, in espousing 'person-centredness' as a cornerstone for the support of people with learning disabilities, the thinking behind *Valuing People* (DoH 2001c) and the guidance on person-centred approaches (DoH 2001e) appears to embrace a more socially embedded perspective that recognizes the importance of people's support networks and how these can shape a person's support, opportunities, inclusion and quality of life. As Brechin (1998) contends, 'good' care has to be considered at both an inter- and intra-personal level, for as she notes:

It will be apparent that in some circumstances care is mutually rewarding, coterminous with personal and social expectations and not overwhelming to the personal identity or needs of the carer or the person cared for. In some other circumstances the reverse may be true.

(Brechin 1998: 171)

On this basis she believes that 'good' care can best be understood in terms of the inter-relationship between those giving and those receiving care, particularly in longer term caring relationships when, consistent with the arguments presented by Qureshi *et al.* (2000), Brechin concludes that there is a need to consider both the processes and outcomes of care for all those involved. While Brechin (1998) frames her arguments primarily in terms of dyadic relationships we would suggest that, although they are inevitably more complex, similar considerations would apply to triadic relationships. This requires an understanding both of the outcomes of care and of the interpersonal and intra-personal experiences and processes of care and their impact on self-esteem and identity. Brechin (1998) argues that it is important to acknowledge that 'differences' exist in caring inter-actions while at the same time promoting a 'working alliance' that focuses attention on the 'fundamental similarities' that underpin the best caring relationships. It is just such 'fundamental similarities' that are reflected in the 'Senses Framework' (Nolan *et al.* 2001, 2002b).

## The emergence of the 'Senses Framework'

It is clear from the above that the notion of 'person-centred care', while intended to represent a positive approach to the provision of help and support, fails fully to account for and capture the dynamics of caring relationships. It was recognition of this that prompted the emergence of 'relationship-centred care' (Tresolini and the Pew-Fetzer Task Force 1994), which seeks to redefine the provision of health and social care in a way that values and attests to the relationships that form the context in which care is provided. According to the authors, relationship-centred care addresses the interdependencies between the psychological, social and biological aspects of health and 'captures the importance of the inter-actions amongst people as the foundations of any therapeutic or healing activity' (Tresolini and the Pew-Fetzer Task Force 1994: 11). They believe that models of practice and education should equip practitioners with the skills, attitudes and beliefs necessary to promote positive relationships that have as their basis 'a shared understanding of the meaning of illness' (p. 22).

The quotation by Zgola (1999) with which this chapter began suggested that the essence of positive relationships is good communication and that this relies on people operating with the 'same concepts'. The 'working alliances', advocated by Brechin (1998) require, as she notes, the 'identification of some fundamental similarities in caregiving work and experiences', and it is here that we believe that the 'Senses Framework' has a contribution to make.

The 'Senses Framework' (Davies *et al.* 1999; Nolan *et al.* 2001, 2002b) is intended to capture the subjective and perceptual dimensions of caring relationships and reflects both the interpersonal processes involved and the intra-personal experiences of care. The 'Framework' is underpinned by the belief that all parties involved in caring (the ill or disabled person, family carers, and paid or voluntary carers) should experience relationships that promote:

- a sense of security – to feel safe within relationships;
- a sense of belonging – to feel 'part' of things;
- a sense of continuity – to experience links and consistency;
- a sense of purpose – to have a personally valuable goal or goals;
- a sense of achievement – to make progress towards a desired goal or goals;
- a sense of significance – to feel that 'you' matter.

Although initially developed as a means of promoting a rationale for the provision of care within longer term institutional settings (Nolan 1997), the Framework has since been the subject of extensive empirical testing which has highlighted its value in understanding good quality caring relationships in acute hospital settings for older people (see Davies *et al.* 1999). Basically it is now apparent that although what creates a sense of security, belonging, continuity, purpose, achievement and significance will vary across differing groups and caring contexts, such 'senses' are nevertheless prerequisites for relationships that are satisfying for all parties involved.

Following an extensive consideration of the relevant literatures in relation to older people which involved an initial overview of some 22,000 references and a more detailed reading of approximately 2000, Nolan *et al.* (2001) summarized the 'senses' as in Table 14.1.

Subsequently the 'Senses Framework' was subjected to detailed empirical study involving interactive focus groups and workshops to determine if the dimensions of the Framework captured those elements of relationships that participants considered important. In addition participants were asked to consider whether the 'senses' resonated with their experiences and 'spoke' to them in a language that they understood and related to. In total 196 people took part in these various activities, comprising older people, family carers, a diverse multidisciplinary set of professionals, and paid but unqualified care assistants in both institutional and community settings (see Nolan *et al.* 2002b for a detailed account).

While there was very strong endorsement for the senses, participants thought that the language used was a bit 'heavy going' in places, especially for older people and their carers. Some 'fine tuning' was therefore suggested, as were subtle changes in emphasis, with some additions to

**Table 14.1** The six senses in the context of caring relationships

*A sense of security*

- For older people:    Attention to essential physiological and psychological needs, to feel safe and free from threat, harm, pain and discomfort. To receive competent and sensitive care.
- For staff:    To feel free from physical threat, rebuke or censure. To have secure conditions of employment. To have the emotional demands of work recognized and to work within a supportive but challenging culture.
- For family carers:    To feel confident in knowledge and ability to provide good care ('To do caring well' – Schumacher *et al.* 1998) without detriment to personal well-being. To have adequate support networks and timely help when required. To be able to relinquish care when appropriate.

*A sense of continuity*

- For older people:    Recognition and value of personal biography. Skilful use of knowledge of the past to help contextualize present and future. Seamless, consistent care delivered within an established relationship by known people.
- For staff:    Positive experience of work with older people from an early stage of career, exposure to good role models and environments of care. Expectations and standards of care communicated clearly and consistently.
- For family carers:    To maintain shared pleasures/pursuits with the care recipient. To be able to provide competent standards of care, whether delivered by self or others. To ensure that personal standards of care are maintained by others. To maintain involvement in care across care environments as desired/ appropriate.

*A sense of belonging*

- For older people:    Opportunities to maintain and/or form meaningful and reciprocal relationships. To feel part of a community or group as desired.
- For staff:    To feel part of a team with a recognized and valued contribution. To belong to a peer group, a community of gerontological practitioners.
- For family carers:    To be able to maintain/improve valued relationships, to be able to confide in trusted individuals to feel that you're not 'in this alone'.

*A sense of purpose*

- For older people:    Opportunities to engage in purposeful activity facilitating the constructive passage of time. To be able to identify and pursue goals and challenges. To exercise discretionary choice.

**Table 14.1** Continued

| | |
|---|---|
| • For staff: | To have a sense of therapeutic direction, a clear set of goals to which to aspire. |
| • For family carers: | To maintain the dignity and integrity, well-being and 'personhood' of the care recipient. To pursue (re)constructive/reciprocal care (Nolan *et al.* 1996a). |

*A sense of achievement*

| | |
|---|---|
| • For older people: | Opportunities to meet meaningful and valued goals. To feel satisfied with one's efforts. To make a recognized and valued contribution. To make progress towards therapeutic goals as appropriate. |
| • For staff: | To be able to provide good care. To feel satisfied with one's efforts. To contribute towards therapeutic goals as appropriate. To use skills and ability to the full. |
| • For family carers: | To feel that you have provided the best possible care. To know you've 'done your best'. To meet challenges successfully. To develop new skills and abilities. |

*A sense of significance*

| | |
|---|---|
| • For older people: | To feel recognized and valued as a person of worth; that one's actions and existence are of importance; that you 'matter'. |
| • For staff: | To feel that gerontological practice is valued and important; that your work and efforts 'matter'. |
| • For family carers: | To feel that one's caring efforts are valued and appreciated. To experience an enhanced sense of self. |

(From Nolan *et al.* 2001: 175)

the definitions being made. For example, it was generally agreed that some of the longer definitions would be more useful if they were presented in 'bullet point' form and that they would be more user friendly if they were personalized, so that the definitions were presented in the first person rather than the third person.

The senses were seen as highly relevant to the care of older people, and comments from the workshops mirrored the feelings of participants that the senses provided a means of highlighting important, but often taken-for-granted, aspects of care that participants felt were often lost in debates about evidence-based care. For example:

'the senses could help us to celebrate success';
'they can help us to define best care';
'they make the seemingly insignificant significant';
'I feel a connectedness to these';
'I can identify with this [Senses Framework] as it relates closely to my practice';
'they highlight what gets lost in evidence-based care'.

Participants believed that the senses were implicit within their existing philosophy of care but that the Framework helped to make their contributions more explicit.

Significantly, in those workshops involving professionals, much of the discussion focused around the value of the senses for staff themselves, with participants believing that they could provide a means of overcoming the prevalent 'NHS blame culture' by helping staff to 'feel good about what we do'.

Overall participants at all the workshops saw the need for a new vision and direction for work with older people, which provided a greater sense of therapeutic potential and more subtle and appropriate indicators of 'success'. While it was recognized that this would require a change of culture among staff, several participants felt that if staff were valued and supported themselves they would be better able to value and support older people. There was much talk of the need for strong and visionary leadership and of a supportive culture which celebrated success rather than concentrating on failure, and which recognized mistakes as learning opportunities rather than seeking to apportion blame. Several ways in which such a culture could be achieved were suggested during the workshops. However, the key was seen to be vision and leadership, and the 'senses' were acknowledged as providing a way of realizing a 'vision' of care in which 'fundamental' elements were valued and accorded status. Furthermore, their relevance for several stakeholder groups was endorsed, as was their potential to promote a better shared understanding. For example, having applied the senses to their own situation, participants, especially staff, felt better able to relate the senses to older people and their carers. It is with the perceptions of this latter group that we conclude this section.

Although carers who participated in the workshops represented a range of caring relationships, they had all, at one time or another, experienced the relative insensitivity of services to their needs, and those of the person that they cared for. Although examples of good practice were provided, each carer had his or her own account of how services often failed fully to recognize and appreciate the complexities of caring, and described help which lacked flexibility and cohesion. It was in better attuning paid carers, whether professional or not, to the needs of carers and of cared-for persons that the senses were seen to have the greatest potential. Based on detailed analyses of the carers' experiences, as recounted at the focus groups, together with the written comments subsequently posted by a number of attendees, the senses were therefore revised further. These revised senses are presented better in Table 14.2, as these reflect both the processes and outcomes that carers considered the 'bedrock' of good services and support.

**Table 14.2** Revised senses

| For the person you care for | For carers |
|---|---|
| *A sense of security – feeling safe* | |
| To ensure that the person you care for is safe and free from threat, harm, pain or discomfort | To have your own needs recognized and acknowledged |
| To ensure that the person you care for receives competent, sensitive and consistent care | To feel confident that you have the information, knowledge and skills to provide good care, when you need them |
| To reduce unnecessary risk but ensure that the person you care for is able to make choices about what they do | To have appropriate, sensitive and timely support |
| To ensure that the person you care for is clean, comfortable and well turned out | To feel able to say 'no' to caring if you want |
| For paid carers to respect the wishes of the person you care for | For others to recognize that your needs, and the needs of the person you care for, may not always be the same |
| To be confident that paid carers have the skills to provide good care for the person you care for | To be able to maintain your own physical and emotional health |
| | To have time for yourself without feeling guilty |
| | To have rapid access to support in an emergency |
| | To know that good support will be available if you are no longer able to care |
| | To feel safe to criticize services without fear that they will be discontinued, or that it will be 'taken out on' the person you care for |
| | To know that services will arrive on time, and as promised |
| | To be given an honest account of what services and options are available |
| *A sense of belonging – to feel part of something, to have a place* | |
| For the person you care for to have opportunities to socialize and mix with others | To be able to maintain meaningful and valued relationships with the person you care for, family and friends |
| For the person you care for to be able to keep in contact with their friends | To have someone to turn to if you need to talk things over |
| To maintain contact with family, especially grandchildren if appropriate | To feel that you are not 'in this alone' |
| To maintain valued relationships with non-human companions, such as pets | To feel an active and equal partner in caregiving |

**Table 14.2** Continued

| For the person you care for | For carers |
| --- | --- |

*A sense of continuity – linking the past, present and future*

| For paid carers to know the person you care for as an individual, with personal likes and dislikes | To be able to maintain shared pleasures and interests with the person you care for |
| For one paid carer (or a limited number) to provide support for the person you care for | To be able to ensure consistent standards of care, whether given by yourself or others |
| For paid carers to have time to care properly, and not 'clock watch' | To be actively involved in their care if the person you care for is in hospital or a nursing home. To have your views listened to and acknowledged |
| | To receive help and support in a way which fits in with your routines and needs |

*A sense of purpose – a goal to aim for*

| For the person you care for to be able to do the things they enjoy | To ensure the dignity and individuality of the person you care for |
| For the person you care for to feel stimulated and challenged | To ensure that the person you are caring for receives the best possible care |
| For the person you care for to feel that they have something to offer | To be able to achieve a balance between caregiving and other important parts of your life |
| For the person you care for to be able to 'have a say', that their opinions are listened to | To be able to work or pursue interests outside of caring |
| For paid carers to take full account of the wishes of the person you care when planning services | To be able to plan for the future, with general knowledge of the possible options |

*A sense of achievement – to feel you're getting somewhere*

| For the person you care for to be able to make a valued contribution, due to how they are acknowledged by others | To know that you are providing/have provided the best possible care |
| For the person you care for to maintain their independence, and sense of self | To develop new skills and abilities |
| | To be able to meet competing demands successfully |
| For the person you care for to feel that they are able to grow and develop | To have your caregiving abilities and expertise acknowledged and valued, and to pass this on to other carers where appropriate |
| For the person you care for to experience pleasure and happiness | To feel satisfied with the care that you are giving |
| | To feel that caregiving is appreciated by the person you care for, family, friends and others |

**Table 14.2** Continued

| For the person you care for | For yourself |
| --- | --- |
| *A sense of significance – to feel that you matter* | |
| For the person you care for to be recognized and valued as a person, and their dignity maintained | To feel that you are recognized, valued and listened to as a person |
| For the person you care for to feel that they are important | To feel that your actions and existence are important |
| For the person you care for to feel that they 'matter', that their life has value and meaning | To feel that you 'matter' |

## Taking the 'senses' further: implications for partnerships between 'helping systems' and disabled people/family carers

> Caregiving does not emerge with a life of its own, but takes place within an historical context.
>
> (Horowitz and Shindehan 1983: 18)

> The interpersonal relationship among caregiver, care-receiver and health professionals can contribute significantly to the outcome of the informal caregiving situation.
>
> (Davis 1992: 8)

Our primary aims in producing this book were to highlight the benefits of viewing family care from a temporal and relational perspective, and also to suggest ways in which services for family carers and disabled people might be enhanced by the creation of better partnerships with 'helping systems'. As the two quotes above illustrate, our central messages are hardly new but we believe that the temporal model of care that we initially described (Nolan *et al.* 1996a) and have elaborated upon here, in conjunction with the notion of relationship-centred care (Tresolini and the Pew-Fetzer Task Force 1994) as operationalized via the 'Senses Framework' (Nolan *et al.* 2001, 2002b) have considerable potential to inform new and better ways of working to support family carers and disabled people.

In addition, several other subtexts have appeared throughout this book, including: the need to pay greater attention to the positive aspects of caring; the need to recognize and acknowledge the expert, proactive strategies adopted by both family carers and disabled people; and the need for more research into the experience of receiving care. All these form key elements of the 'paradigm shift' that we believe is gathering momentum.

However, as we also pointed out in the Introduction, we feel that another book on family care is necessary because, notwithstanding the emergence of a more holistic approach, we believe that 'it is still the voices of researchers and their search for ever more "sophisticated" methodologies, or policy makers/practitioners, who determine what counts as evidence, that hold sway' (p. 12 this volume). Two recent and potentially highly influential papers suggest that our concerns are well founded.

The first, by Sörensen *et al.* (2002), presents an updated 'meta-analysis' on the effectiveness of interventions to support family carers. Once again considerable attention is paid to the methodological limitations of existing studies such as the relative failure to address multiple outcomes, the limited attention given to the differences that might be expected between varying types of intervention, and the need to account for a number of 'moderating' factors such as the intensity of the intervention, adherence to treatment regimes and the reliability and validity of the outcome measures used. On this basis it seems that 'closed-ended methods' remain predominant (Reinhardy *et al.* 1999), with a continued reliance on the language of variables, frequencies and statistical significance (Russell *et al.* 1999), which reduce outcomes to composite or summary scores on standardized measures (Berg-Weger *et al.* 2001; Croag *et al.* 2001). The influence of the pathological model of care is also still apparent, with 57 of the 78 studies included in Sörensen *et al.*'s (2002) review incorporating measures of carer burden, while 40 included indicators of carer depression. Conversely, only three considered the 'uplifts' or satisfactions of care. Similar findings emerged in Helff and Glidden's (1998) review of published research on family care of people with learning disabilities. While the Sörensen *et al.* review makes some interesting points about the need for greater specificity in intervention work, and stresses the fact that virtually none of the studies included considered the timing of the intervention in relation to the stage of caring, the overriding emphasis is nevertheless methodological rather than conceptual.

The second of the two reviews focuses on 'intervention research' in relation to dementia care (Schulz *et al.* 2002), but most of its messages are relevant across caring contexts. Given that several recent systematic reviews have painted a rather bleak picture of the effectiveness of interventions in dementia care (see, for example, Charlesworth 2001; Cooke *et al.* 2001; Pusey and Richards 2001). Schulz *et al.* (2002) set out to 'take stock' of the field and to identify the strengths and weaknesses of current intervention studies. In so doing they suggest that perhaps too much reliance has been placed on 'statistical significance' and that in the future it will be important to pay greater attention to the 'clinical significance' of interventions.

In support of this potentially important and far-reaching suggestion they draw upon Kadzin's (1999) definition of clinical significance, which 'generally refers to the practical value of the effects of an intervention, or the extent to which an intervention makes a "real" difference in the everyday life of an individual' (Schulz *et al.* 2002: 590). Subsequently they outline four dimensions of clinical significance, which are:

- symptomatology – the extent to which individuals return to normal functioning or experience a change in symptoms;
- quality of life – the extent to which interventions broadly improve an individual's quality of life;
- social significance – the extent to which interventions are important to society, as evidenced by their impact on service utilization, for example, admission to care;
- social validity – the extent to which treatment goals, procedures and outcomes are acceptable, as assessed by the client or expert ratings of the interventions and their effects on participants' lives.

(Schulz *et al.* 2002: 590)

They acknowledge that research and service communities may have very different views about the relative importance of the above dimensions, but say very little about the views of carers themselves.

The other issue they raise is how large an effect has to be before it can be considered as 'clinically significant', and they suggest that judgements of effect size are best made in the context of the problem being studied. Great store is placed on the 'meaningfulness' of the outcome, and the authors acknowledge that 'it is possible to identify a clinically unimportant effect as statistically significant by having sufficiently large samples, or greatly restricting the variability in the sample' (Schulz *et al.* 2002: 590).

Paradoxically, although 'meaningfulness' provides the central tenet of their argument, Schulz *et al.* (2002) exclude case studies and qualitative studies from their review. However, perhaps the ultimate irony is that having illustrated how a reliance on statistical significance may result in the identification of 'clinically unimportant effects' they subsequently only include studies with statistically significant results in their review, noting: 'To be considered clinically significant an outcome had to have first achieved statistical significance according to the published report' (p. 590).

Moreover, judgements about the 'meaningfulness' of any effect were based upon 'a common metric of percentile change attributable to the intervention'. The marginal relevance of meaningfulness, as determined by the recipient of the intervention, i.e. carers themselves, was reinforced in the value the authors accorded to 'social validity':

Most studies met criteria for social validity. Study participants consistently rated the interventions as beneficial, helpful or valuable. Researchers and policy makers would likely agree that social validity is important but that it is probably not the most valued indicator of clinical significance.

(2002: 598)

It would seem that Post's (2001) call for an 'epistemology of humility' has fallen on deaf ears, at least in respect of intervention research. Further evidence of this is provided in the authors' main recommendation, which is to establish a consensus panel to define clinical significance in caregiver research. The hegemony of a professional view is reinforced in their conclusion that, most importantly of all, 'researchers should set as their goal the achievement of reliable and clinically significant outcomes, preferably in multiple domains' (Schultz *et al.* 2002: 599).

Despite the tensions and obvious contradictions inherent in the above arguments, we find the notions of 'meaningfulness' and 'social validity' useful. However, we would take a fundamentally different position to Schulz *et al.* (2002) and propose that meaningfulness be defined primarily by carers and disabled people themselves, together, where appropriate, with those paid carers with whom they are in 'partnership'. Therefore 'social validity' should be the main criterion upon which judgements of 'clinical significance' are made.[1]

Notwithstanding our concerns about the sentiments underpinning Schulz *et al.*'s (2002) position, their paper nevertheless provides a somewhat different spin, despite the fact that they focus primarily on the types of intervention that Snyder (2000) aptly terms 'the usual suspects'. However, despite Schulz *et al.*'s (2002) call for 'conceptual enlargements', it is the failure to expand conceptual horizons that represents the major flaw in their thesis. This particularly relates to the notion of 'social validity', which is more than a simple post-intervention polling of views, and should incorporate the processes and outcomes that carers and disabled people see as important. We would suggest that the adoption of something like the 'Senses Framework' provides a mechanism whereby a far more expansive approach to 'social validity' could be promoted.

## Designing meaningful support for family carers and disabled people

The problems created by 'system induced setbacks' (Hart 2001) have been raised at various points in this book, and we have suggested that the 'Senses Framework' provides one potential way of promoting better 'caring' partnerships predicated on the belief that if paid carers do not feel secure, that they belong, and that they have a sense of continuity, purpose and achievement in their work, then they are unlikely to create similar experiences for disabled people and/or family carers. Essentially the 'Senses Framework' proposes that in the best partnerships all parties perceive benefits and that if this does not happen then relationships are compromised.

Too often services fail to aspire to the types of outcomes suggested by the senses or other work such as that of Qureshi *et al.* (2000), and little attention is paid to the 'processes' of care and the manner in which services are delivered (Qureshi *et al.* 2000; Newbronner and Hare 2002).

---

[1] We would reject this term and instead prefer Kadzin's (1999) key dimensions of practical value, or making a 'real' difference to the lives of individuals.

Some time ago it was suggested that from a carer's perspective service effectiveness could be viewed along a continuum ranging from facilitative, through contributory and inhibitory, to obstructive (Nolan *et al.* 1996a). Facilitative services are those in which there are overt, planned and systematic attempts by service providers to complement carers' efforts and to provide support that is sensitive and responsive to the caregiving dynamic and the 'expert' knowledge held by carers. While some of these characteristics apply to contributory services, these arise largely by chance or good fortune rather than resulting from negotiation and agreement. Inhibitory services rarely achieve the attributes of facilitative support but are sometimes accepted out of necessity or desperation. Obstructive services are seen by carers to be at odds with their own goals and quality standards and are generally summarily rejected. It seems to us that the 'Senses Framework' begins to elaborate upon some of the essential dimensions of facilitative services. However, we would add two other important considerations that we term 'symmetry' and 'synchronicity'.

In many respects the 'senses' capture important elements of 'symmetry' within caring relationships, relating to the extent to which the parties involved are able to both give and receive help and support. This is more likely to be achieved when people feel secure, experience continuity, and perceive their interactions to have a valued purpose which promotes a sense of achievement and significance. These are not simply abstract ideas but are very 'meaningful' to older people, family carers and paid carers, as suggested by Nolan *et al.* (2002b). There is of course a need to explore further the ways in which the 'senses' might be achieved, and their relevance to caregiving relationships that do not involve older people. However, the wider literature would support the notion of 'symmetry' as important to caregiving relationships, both in terms of reciprocity and mutuality and with regard to the negotiation of shared expectations, values and beliefs, which underpin the best relationships.

Reflecting the importance of the temporal dimensions of care, which lie at the heart of this book, a second key characteristic of meaningful support for carers and disabled people is 'synchronicity', that is the extent to which service systems work to the same 'calendars' as family carers and disabled people (Grant and Whittell, Chapter 5). As Grant and Whittell point out, existing services are often 'out of synch' with the needs of carers, a contention reinforced by others. For example, in considering future directions for caregiving interventions Czaja *et al.* (2000) suggest that it is essential to take greater account of the changing nature of caring demands and to recognize that different approaches might be more appropriate at different phases of caring. They also contend that support should continue after placement or the death of the cared-for person. However, despite widespread acceptance of the benefits of early support for carers (Kuhn 1998; Brown and Stetz 1999; Ayers 2000a, b; Tebb and Jivanjee 2000), both in shaping their perceptions of caring and providing them with the necessary knowledge and skills, such help is rarely forthcoming, and services remain largely reactive rather than pro-active and preventive. It is of course possible to think of services as being 'out of synch' in several ways, some minor, some major. For instance, services often take little account of carers' daily routines and are not sufficiently flexible or responsive. At a differing level there can be major mismatches in 'calendars', as portrayed by Grant and Whittell (Chapter 5), or, on an even longer term basis, a failure to account for the influence of a caring biography that might span 50 years or more (see Llewellyn, Chapter 8).

Taking the dimensions of 'symmetry' and 'synchronicity' and pre-senting them as an axis is helpful in determining whether services are likely to be considered facilitative or not. This is represented in Figure 14.1.

As is suggested in Figure 14.1, we would argue that when there is agreement as to the intended goals and outcomes of services, and when timelines are in 'synch', then services are likely to be facilitative. Con-versely, when neither of these two characteristics are met, then services are likely to be seen as obstructive and therefore rejected. Further we would suggest that agreement as to the goals of care is probably more critical than timing, or at least that issues of timing are more readily resolved, so that services in which there is agreement as to goals and values, but which are

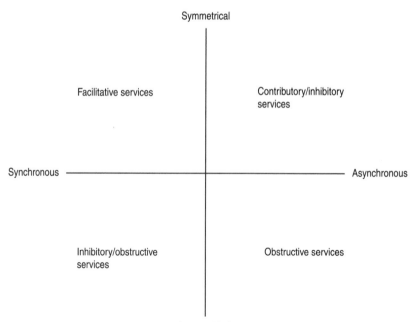

**Figure 14.1** The influence of symmetry (balance) and synchronicity (timing) on service delivery

potentially 'out of synch', are likely to be viewed more positively than when the reverse is true.

On this basis we would suggest that balance and timing in services are essential determinants of whether support is seen as meaningful by family carers and disabled people. However, while these may be necessary conditions, we would not see them as being sufficient, as the manner in which support is provided is another essential consideration.

Some time ago Smale *et al.* (1993) suggested that the assessment process, during which service decisions are made, follows one of three models: the questioning model; the procedural model, or the exchange model. In the questioning model the assessor is the 'expert' who asks a series of questions to which the carers or disabled person respond, with the appropriate service being determined largely on the basis of their answers. Here the power lies essentially with the individual assessor. The procedural approach is dominated by the expectations of the service agency which provides a relatively fixed set of eligibility criteria which determine the right to services. Once again the balance of power does not lie with the carer/disabled person. In contrast the exchange model assumes that all parties have important considerations which will influence the type of service that is needed, and that all of these should figure in the final determination.

Mirroring a questioning or procedural approach, current assessment processes seem to us to produce services that are either 'allocated' or 'imparted'. The 'allocation' of services is formulaic and based primarily on considerations such as the amount or intensity of help and support that the family carer provides. Here eligibility criteria relate mainly to the objective circumstances of care and the support provided is more likely to be instrumental in nature. This is typical of the currently dominant approach to the assessment of carers' needs in the UK, in which services are targeted primarily at carers providing 'regular and substantial' care, which is generally equated with more than 20 hours of care per week (Hirst 2001). We would see the above model as being inherently reductionist.

The 'imparting' model is underpinned by the belief that the service pro-vider is in possession of information or other expertise that the carer or disabled person needs. Such a model implicitly or explicitly underpins several psycho-educational interventions targeted at family carers. How-ever, for new carers and newly disabled people the 'imparting' model may be important, as there is general consensus that all carers (and we would add disabled people) are likely to benefit from knowledge of their disease condition, the caregiving role, the resources available, and some training on problem solving and related skills (Schulz *et al.* 2002). Of course the timing of such interventions is essential and existing research has paid little attention to this (Czaja *et al.* 2000; Sörensen *et al.* 2002). Several authors stress the benefits of early intervention (Kuhn 1998; Brown and Stetz 1999; Ayers 2000a, b; Tebb and Jivanjee 2000), although it must be acknowledged that finding carers at an early stage does provide challenges. It also has been suggested that carers are unlikely to focus on their own needs until they feel they have the skills they need to provide adequate care and support for their relatives (O'Neill-Conger and Marshall 1998; Brereton and Nolan, Chapter 3 this volume).

This sentiment was captured by Schumacher *et al.* (2000: 192) thus:

> Providing care well is important to caregivers and developing caregiving competency, knowledge and skill is a central concern for those in the process of becoming a caregiver.

Schumacher *et al.* (2000) present what is probably the most detailed and comprehensive analysis of caregiver skill, and as a result of their analysis they identify nine dimensions of caregiving skill as follows:

- monitoring – keeping an eye on things in order to know how well the care receiver is doing;
- interpreting – making sense of what is observed;
- making decisions – choosing a course of action;
- taking action – carrying out caring decisions and instructions;
- providing 'hands-on' care – giving care safely and with comfort;
- making adjustments – and progressively refining care until it is 'fine-tuned' to the care-receiver's needs;
- accessing resources – such as information, equipment and help;
- working together with the care receiver – and providing care appropriate to the needs of both parties;
- negotiating healthcare systems – working with the system and getting the most out of it.

Although this is a very useful taxonomy it is orientated primarily at the 'quasi-clinical' elements of caring, with effectiveness being defined in terms of 'optimal symptom management, prevention of injury, early detection of problems, and so forth' (p. 199). Schumacher *et al.*'s (2000) intention is to assist carers to 'do' caring well, and they envisage a crucial role for professionals (nurses) in providing not only a brief introduction to caring, but ongoing 'coaching' of family carers.

Clearly the above 'skills' are essential in many circumstances, especially when carers are supporting people who are increasingly 'technologically dependent' (Kirk and Glendinning 2002). Indeed, there is emerging evidence that even when family carers develop a higher level of technical competence than the professionals supporting them, they still value information and practical and emotional support from paid carers (Kirk and Glendinning 2002). Once again, however, the manner in which such support is delivered appears to be of crucial importance.

> First and foremost, it was of the utmost importance that professional nurses recognized and openly acknowledged parents' expertise, not

just their technical skills but their expertise in applying those to their child. It was this recognition of this individual expertise which was so important and which underpinned positive and supportive parent–professional relationships.

(Kirk and Glendinning 2002)

Although such 'skills' are clearly important we would argue that it is essential to look beyond the 'doing' of care and to consider the 'being' aspects. It is here that a relationship-centred approach offers considerable potential for, as several authors have noted, a greater focus on the intra- and interpersonal dynamics of caring relationships provides opportunities for new and potentially powerful forms of intervention and support (Ayres 2000a, b; Berg-Weger *et al.* 2001; Martini *et al.* 2001).

## Moving beyond the 'usual suspects'

Most family caring relationships, by definition, do not emerge from the ether but 'take place within an historical context' (Horowitz and Shindehan 1983). Indeed, this is clearly recognized in our temporal model of care which acknowledges the importance of 'building on the past' (Nolan *et al.* 1996a). However, the need for care usually heralds a change in roles and relationships which may develop suddenly or more gradually. The speed with which such changes occur significantly influences the ways in which carers 'recognize the need' (Nolan *et al.* 1996a), and also the point at which they have first contact with 'helping systems'. What is now quite clear is that the nature of these initial meetings between family carers, disabled people and various 'helping systems', is an important determinant of future relationships.

All too often there is a failure to create an 'empathetic understanding' of differing needs and expectations (Coyle 1999), or to foster a 'participatory caring context' (Allen 2000b), thereby sowing the seeds of 'system induced setbacks' (Hart 2001). The scope for creativity within triadic relationships is further limited by an over-reliance on a 'questioning' or 'procedural' model of initial assessment and the failure to engage in the negotiations upon which an exchange model is predicated. This is likely to perpetuate the 'allocation' or 'imparting' of services, and inhibit the development of what might be termed 'relational' support.

The literature suggests several forms that 'relational' support might take, such as enhancing carers' ability to 'construct' reciprocity (Neufeld and Harrison 1995), or helping both carers and cared-for persons to reconsider the 'attributions' they make and better enable them to take the 'perspective' of the other (Martini *et al.* 2001).

Similarly, helping both parties to shape their expectations and to seek more flexible explanations may have much to commend it, so that 'ambiguous' caring relationships are avoided and 'normalized' ones promoted (Ayres 2000a, b). Such approaches may well lay the foundations of an empathetic relationship (Kuhn 1998; Lee *et al.* 2001), which creates a more balanced view and results in more realistic expectations (Shyu 2002). Including a 'strengths-based' model of working (Berg-Weger *et al.* 2001) within a relational approach is likely to provide an even more holistic and empowering perspective.

However, for genuine progress to be made, 'helping systems' need to leave the security of the eligibility-based 'allocation' model and the professionally dominated 'imparting' model and fully recognize the importance of relationships to an understanding of family care and to the delivery of 'meaningful' forms of help and support. This will inevitably mean a reconsideration of the goals and outcomes of current services, in particular what constitutes 'success'. Greater recognition is required of the need for good quality services to be underpinned by the proper investment of time, energy and 'self' by paid carers. This has financial and emotional implications. We believe that the 'Senses Framework' provides a vehicle which will open up debate and focus it on the interdependencies on which good triadic relationships depend.

However, if practitioners are to assist carers and disabled people in 'perspective' taking, and in promoting a 'strengths-based' approach, they too need to be able to take the 'perspective' of the other and to have at their disposal mechanisms that will help carers and disabled people to explore their perspectives and to identify both their strengths and areas where help is needed. We believe that this cannot be achieved using 'standardized measures' that reduce the caring relationship to a 'summary score'.

Nevertheless, alternative ways of working with family carers do exist and the usefulness of instruments such as CADI, CASI and CAMI and related approaches in shaping the perspectives of both family carers and professionals has been clearly demonstrated in a number of studies (see Qureshi *et al.* 2000; Guberman *et al.* in press; Nicholas 2003; Lundh and Nolan, Chapter 6).

Of course there is a need for further work that pays greater attention to the experiences of giving and receiving care within both dyadic and triadic relationships. If 40 years of research has indeed 'only scratched the surface regarding our understanding of the caregiving experience' (Pruchno 2000: 207) and we desire further insights, we would be wise to show greater humility (Post 2001) and recognize that the questions that 'matter' are not determined by researchers or policy makers, and 'significance' is not confined to 'statistical' or 'clinical' concerns.

We would suggest the notion of 'social validity' (Schulz *et al.* 2002) has a great deal to commend it and should be developed as one of the key criteria for framing the relational aspects of the interactions between disabled people, family carers and 'helping systems'. However, there is a need for a far more expansive definition of what counts as important in this context that recognizes and is responsive to the temporal dimensions of care as they unfold over time, much as described in this book. We believe that further elaboration of the Senses Framework in order to establish its relevance and utility with respect to past, present and future triadic relationships provides an important direction for the ongoing exploration of the dynamics of care.

# References

AAMR (American Association on Mental Retardation) (1992) *Mental Retardation. Definition, classification, and system of supports*, 9th Edition. Washington, DC: AAMR.

Abel, E.K. (1995) Representation of caregiving by Margaret Foster, Mary Gordon, and Doris Lessing. Special Issue: Qualitative Methodology, *Research on Ageing*, 17(1): 42–64.

Adams, T. and Clarke, C.L. (1999) (eds) *Dementia Care: Developing Partnerships in Practice*. London: Balliere Tindall.

Allen, D. (2000a) Negotiating the role of expert carers on an adult hospital ward, *Sociology of Health and Illness*, 22(2): 149–71.

Allen, D. (2000b) 'I'll tell you what suits me best if you don't mind me saying': 'lay participation' in healthcare, *Nursing Inquiry*, 7: 182–90.

Allen, K.R. and Walker, A.S. (1992) An analysis of interviews with elderly mothers and their daughters, in J.F. Gilgun, K. Daly and G. Handel (eds) *Qualitative Methods in Family Research*. Thousand Oaks: Sage Publications.

Almberg, B., Grafström, M. and Winblad, B. (1997) Major strain and coping strategies as reported by family members who care for aged demented relatives, *Journal of Advanced Nursing*, 26: 683–91.

Alzheimer's Disease Society (1995) *Right from the Start: Primary Health Care and Dementia*. London: Alzheimer's Disease Society.

Alzheimer's Disease Society (1996) *Younger People with Dementia: Care Learning Programme*, Carer Resource Book. London: Alzheimer's Disease Society.

Anderson, R. (1992) *The Aftermath of Stroke. The Experience of Patients and their Families*. Cambridge: Cambridge University Press.

Aneshensel, C.S., Pearly, L.I., Mullan, J.T., Zarit, S.U. and Whitlach, C.J. (1995) *Profiles in Caregiving: The Unexpected Career*. San Diego, CA: Academic Press.

Anson, M. (1995) Nursing homes are for nursing people, *Elderly Care*, 7(3): 37.

Antonovsky, A. (1987) *Unravelling the Mystery of Health*. San Francisco, CA: Jossey-Bass.

Antonucci, T. and Akiyama, H. (1987) Social networks in adult life and a preliminary examination of the convoy model, *Journal of Gerontology*, 42: 519–27.

Archbold, P.G., Stewart, B.J., Greenlick, M.R. and Harvath, T.A. (1992) The clinical assessment of mutuality and preparedness in family caregivers of frail older people, in S.G. Funk, E.M.T. Tornquist, S.T. Champagne and R.A. Wiese (eds) *Key Aspects of Elder Care: Managing Falls, Incontinence and Cognitive Impairment*. New York, NY: Springer.

Arksey, H., Hepworth, D. and Qureshi, H. (1999) *Carers' Needs and the Carers (Recognition and Services) Act 1995: An Evaluation of the Processes and Outcomes of Assessment*. York: Social Policy Research Unit.

Ashman, A., Suttie, J. and Bramley, J. (1993) *Older Australians with a Learning Disability. A Report to the Department of Health, Housing and Community Services, Research and Development Grants Committee*. Brisbane: Fred and Eleanor Schonnell Special Education Research Centre, University of Queensland.

Askham, J. (1998) Supporting caregivers of older people: an overview of problems and priorities. *Australian Journal of Ageing*, 17(1): 5–7.

Audit Commission (2000) *Forget Me Not: Mental Health Services for Older People*. London: Audit Commission.

Australian Law Reform Commission (1995) *The Coming of Age: New Age Care Legislation for the Commonwealth*, Report No. 72. Canberra: ALRC.

Ayres, L. (2000a) Narratives of family caregiving: four story types, *Research in Nursing and Health*, 23: 359–71.

Ayres, L. (2000b) Narratives of family caregiving: the process of making meaning, *Research in Nursing and Health*, 23: 424–34.

Baker, B.L., Blacher, J., Kopp, C.B. and Kraamer, B. (1997) Parenting children with mental retardation, in N.W. Bray (ed.) *International Review of Research in Mental Retardation*, Volume 20. San Diego, CA: Academic Press.

Baker, C., Wuest, J. and Stern, P.N. (1992) Method slurring: the grounded theory/phenomenology example, *Journal of Advanced Nursing*, 17(11): 1355–60.

Banks, P. (1999) *Carer Support: Time for a Change of Direction*. London: King's Fund.

Banks, P. and Roberts, E. (2001) *A Break for Carers: An Analysis of the Local Authority Plans to Use the Carer's Special Grant*. London: King's Fund.

Barber, C.E. (1993) Spousal care of Alzheimer's disease patients in nursing home versus in-home settings: patient impairment and caregiver impacts, *Clinical Gerontologist*, 12(4): 3–30.

Barnes, C.L., Given, B.A. and Given, C.W. (1995) Parent caregivers: a comparison of employed and not employed daughters, *Social Work*, 40(3): 375–81.

Barnes, M. (1999) *Public Expectations: From Paternalism to Partnership, Changing Relationships in Health and Health Services*. Policy Futures for UK Health, No. 10. London: Nuffield Trust.

Bartlett, M.C. (1994) Married widows: the wives of men in long-term care, *Journal of Women and Ageing*, 6(1/2): 91–106.

Bartlett, M.C. and Font, M.E. (1994) Hispanic men and long-term care: the wives' perspective, *Journal of Multicultural Social Work*, 3(4): 77–88.

Barusch, A.S. (1995) Programming for family care of elderly dependants: mandates, incentives, and service rationing, *Social Work: Journal of the National Association of Social Workers*, 40(3): 315–22.

Bayley, M. (1997) Empowering and relationships, in P. Ramcharan, G. Roberts, G. Grant and J. Borland (eds) *Empowerment in Everyday Life*. London: Jessica Kingsley.

Beange, H. and Taplin, J. (1996) Prevalence of learning disability in northern Sydney adults, *Journal of Learning Disability Research*, 40(3): 191–7.

Beck, C. (2001) Identification and assessment of effective services and interventions: the nursing home perspective, *Aging and Mental Health*, 5(Supplement 1): S99–S111.

Benner, P. (1984) *From Novice to Expert: Excellence and Power in Clinical Nursing Practice*. Menlo Park, CA: Addison-Wesley.

Berg, S. and Sundström, G. (1999) Sweden, in J. Schroots, R. Fernandez Ballesteros and G. Rudinger (eds) *Aging in Europe*. Amsterdam: European Commission Directorate-General XII, Science, Research and Development, IOS Press.

Bergmark, Å., Parker, M.G. and Thorslund, M. (2000) Priorities in care and services for elderly people: a path without guidelines? *Journal of Medical Ethics*, 26(3): 312–18.

Berg-Weger, M., Rubio, D.M. and Tebb, S.S. (2001) Strengths-based practice with family caregivers of the chronically ill: qualitative insights, family in society, *Journal of Contemporary Human Services*, 82(3): 263–72.

Bernard, M. and Phillips, J. (2000) The challenge of ageing in tomorrow's Britain, *Ageing and Society*, 20(1): 33–54.

Best, D.G. (1994) The development of a guide for stroke survivors and their families, *Canadian Journal of Cardiovascular Nursing*, 5: 35–8.

Bigby, C. (1996) Transferring responsibility: the nature and effectiveness of parental planning for the future of adults with learning disability who have remained at home until midlife, *Journal of Intellectual and Developmental Disability*, 21: 295–312.

Bigby, C. (1997a) When parents relinquish care. The informal support networks of older people with learning disability, *Journal of Applied Learning Disability Research*, 10(4): 333–44.

Bigby, C. (1997b) In place of parents? The sibling relationships of older people with learning disability, *Journal of Gerontological Social Work*, 29(1): 3–22.

Bigby, C. (2000) *Moving On without Parents. Planning, Transitions and Sources of Support for Middle-aged and Older Adults with Intellectual Disability*. Sydney: Maclennan and Petty.

Blumer, H. (1969) *Symbolic Interactionism. Perspective and Method*. Englewood Cliffs, NJ: Prentice-Hall.

Bond, J. (2000) The impact of staff factors in nursing home residents, *Aging and Mental Health*, 4(1): 5–8.

Borgermans, L., Nolan, M.R. and Philp, I. (2001) Carers in Europe, in I. Philp (ed.) *Family Care of Older People in Europe*. Amsterdam: IOS Press.

Borup, J.H. (1983) Relocation mortality research: assessment, reply, and the need to refocus on the issues, *The Gerontologist*, 23(3): 235–42.

Bosaquet, N. and Franks, P. (1998) *Stroke Care: Delivering the Burden of Disease*. London: Stroke Association.

Boss, P. (1988) *Family Stress Management*. Newbury Park, CA: Sage Publications.

Bowers, B.J. (1987) Inter-generational caregiving: adult caregivers and their ageing parents, *Advances in Nursing Science*, 9(2): 20–31.

Bowers, B.J. (1988) Family perceptions of care in a nursing home, *The Gerontologist*, 30(2): 361–7.

Bowling, A. (1995) *Measuring Disease: A Review of Disease-Specific Quality of Life Measurement Scales*. Buckingham: Open University Press.

Braithwaite, V. (2000) Contextual or generic stress outcomes: making choices through caregiving appraisals, *The Gerontologist*, 40(6): 706–17.

Brandon, D. and Jack, R. (1997) Struggling for services, in I.J. Norman and S.J. Redfern (eds) *Mental Health Care for Elderly People*. Edinburgh: Churchill Livingstone.

Brechin, A. (1998) What makes for good care?, in A. Brechin, J. Walmsley, J. Katz and S. Peace (eds) *Care Matters: Concepts, Practice and Research in Health and Social Care*. London: Sage Publications.

Brereton, L. (1997) Preparation for family caregiving: stroke as a paradigm case, *Journal of Clinical Nursing*, 6: 425–34.

Brereton, L. and Nolan, M.R. (2000) You do know he's had a stroke don't you? Preparation for family caregiving – the neglected dimension, *Journal of Clinical Nursing*, 9: 498–506.

Brereton, L. and Nolan, M.R. (2002) 'Seeking': a key activity for new family carers of stroke survivors, *Journal of Clinical Nursing*, 11: 22–31.

Briggs, K. and Askham, J. (1999) *The Needs of People with Dementia and Those Who Care for Them: A Review of the Literature*. London: Alzheimer's Society.

Brodaty, H., Pond, D., Kemp, N.M. *et al.* (2002) The GPCOG: a new screening test for dementia designed for general practice, *Journal of American Geriatrics Society*, 50(3): 530–4.

Brody, E.M., Dempsey, N.P. and Pruchno, R.A. (1990) Mental health of sons and daughters of the institutionalized aged, *The Gerontologist*, 30(2): 212–19.

Brooke, P. and Bullock, R. (1999) Validation of a 6 item cognitive impairment test with a view to primary care usage, *International Journal of Geriatric Psychiatry*, 14: 936–40.

Brown, L.J., Potter, J.F. and Foster, B.G. (1990) Caregiver burden should be evaluated during geriatric assessment, *Journal of the American Geriatrics Society*, 38(4): 455–60.

Brown, M.A. and Stetz, K. (1999) The labour of caregiving: a theoretical model of caregiving during potentially fatal illness, *Qualitative Health Research*, 9(2): 182–97.

Brubaker, E. and Brubaker, T.H. (1993) *Caregiving for adult children with mental retardation: concerns of elderly parents*. Newbury Park, CA: Sage Publications.

Brummel-Smith, K. (1994) Management of poststroke patient, *Hospital Practice (Office Edition)*, 30(2): 43–6, 49–52, 111–13.

Bunn, F. (1996a) The role of the primary healthcare team, in C. Wolfe, T. Rudd and R. Beech (eds) *Stroke Services and Research*. London: Stroke Association.

Bunn, F. (1996b) The needs of families and carers of stroke patients, in C. Wolfe, T. Rudd and R. Beech (eds) *Stroke Services and Research*. London: Stroke Association.

Burr, W.R., Klein, S.R. and associates (1994) *Re-examining Family Stress: New Theory and Research*. Thousand Oaks, CA: Sage Publications.

Bury, M. (1982) Chronic illness as biographical disruption, *Sociology of Health and Illness*, 4: 167–82.

Cameron, I., Curran, S., Newton, P., Petty, D. and Wattis, J. (2000) Use of Donepezil for the treatment of mild-moderate Alzheimer's disease: an audit of the assessment and treatment of patients in routine clinical practice, *International Journal of Geriatric Psychiatry*, 15: 887–91.

*Cancer Bulletin* (2002) *http://hebw.uwcm.ac.uk/cancers/chapter4.html* (accessed 22 July 2002).

Cardol, M., deJong, B.A., Van de Bos, G.A.M. *et al.* (2002) Beyond disability: perceived participation of people with chronic disability condition, *Clinical Rehabilitation*, 16: 27–35.

Cartwright, J.C., Archbold, P.G., Stewart, B.J. and Limandri, B. (1994) Enrichment processes in family caregiving to frail elders, *Advances in Nursing Sciences*, 17(1): 31–43.

Chappell, A. (1994) A question of friendship: community care and the relationships of people with learning difficulties, *Disability and Society*, 9(4): 419–33.

Chappell, N. (1996) The sociological meaning of caregiving and social support: issues for older people, the family and community, in V. Minchiello, V. Chappel, H. Kendig and A. Walker (eds) *Sociology of Aging: Interactional Perspectives*. Victoria, BC: International Sociological Association.

Charlesworth, G.M. (2001) Reviewing psychosocial interventions for family carers of people with dementia, *Aging and Mental Health*, 5(2): 104–6.

Charmaz, K. (2000) Grounded theory: objectivist and constructivist methods, in N.K. Denzin and Y.S. Lincoln (eds) *Handbook of Qualitative Research*, 2nd edition. Thousand Oaks CA: Sage Publications.

Chaston, D. and Shpylka, A. (1999) *Younger Person with Dementia*. Unpublished. Doncaster and South Humber Healthcare NHS Trust.

Chenitz, W.C. (1983) Entry into a nursing home as status passage: a theory to guide nursing practice, *Geriatric Nursing*, 4(2): 92–7.

Chesson, R., Macleod, M. and Massie, S. (1996) Outcome measures used in therapy departments in Scotland, *Physiotherapy*, 82(12): 673–9.

Clafferty, R. (1999) Alzheimer's disease – telling patients their diagnosis, *Progress in Neurology and Psychiatry*, 3(2): 12–13.

Clarke, C.L. (1999a) Partnerships in dementia care: taking it forward, in T. Adams and C.L. Clarke (eds) *Dementia Care: Developing Partnerships in Practice*. London: Balliere Tindall.

Clarke, C.L. (1999b) Dementia care partnerships: knowledge, ownership and exchange, in T. Adams and C.L. Clarke (eds) *Dementia Care: Developing Partnerships in Practice*. London: Balliere Tindall.

Clarke, C.L. (1999c) Professional practice with people with dementia and their family carers: help or hindrance, in T. Adams and C.L. Clarke (eds) *Dementia Care: Developing Partnerships in Practice*. London: Balliere Tindall.

Clarke, P.A. and Gladman, J.R.F. (1995) A survey of pre-discharge occupational therapy home assessment units for stroke patients, *Clinical Rehabilitation*, 9: 339–42.

Clarke, R.M. and Finucane, P. (1995) Care-receivers' and care-givers' experience and perceptions of respite care: implications for service provision, *Australian Journal on Ageing*, 13(4): 183–7.

Close, H.T. (1995) From home to nursing home: a ritual of transition, *American Journal of Family Therapy*, 23(1): 83–8.

Clyburn, L.D., Stones, M.J., Hadjistquropoulos, T. and Tuckko, H. (2000) Predicting caregiver burden and depression in Alzheimer's disease, *Journal of Gerontology, Social Sciences*, 5SB(1): S2–S13.

Coffman, R. (1981) Relocation and survival of institutionalized aged: a re-examination of the evidence, *The Gerontologist*, 21(5): 483–500.

Collins, C.E., Given, B.A. and Given, C.W. (1994) Interventions with family caregivers of persons with Alzheimer's disease, *Nursing Clinics of North America*, 29(1): 195–207.

Cooke, D.D., McNally, L., Mulligan, K.T., Harrison, M.J.G. and Newman, S.P. (2001) Psychosocial interventions for caregivers of people with dementia: a systematic review, *Aging and Mental Health*, 5(2): 120–35.

Corbin, J.M. and Strauss, A. (1988) *Unending Work and Care: Managing Chronic Illness at Home*. San Francisco, CA: Jossey-Bass.

Corr, S. and Bayer, A. (1992) Poor functional status of stroke patients after hospital discharge: scope for intervention?, *British Journal of Occupational Therapy*, 55: 383–5.

Cox, E.O. and Dooley, A.C. (1996) Care-receivers' perception of their role in the care process, *Journal of Gerontological Social Work*, 26(1/2): 133–52.

Coyle, J. (1999) Exploring the meaning of 'dissatisfaction' with healthcare: the importance of 'personal identity threat', *Sociology of Health and Illness*, 21(1): 95–124.

Coyle, J. and Williams, B. (2001) Valuing people as individuals: development of an instrument through a survey of person-centredness in secondary care, *Journal of Advanced Nursing*, 36(3): 450–9.

Croag, S.H., Sudilousky, A., Burleson, J.A. and Baune, R.M. (2001) Vulnerability of husband and wife caregivers of Alzheimer's disease patients to caregiving stressors, *Alzheimer's Disease and Related Disorders*, 15(4): 201–10.

Cummings, J.L., Donohue, J.A. and Brooks, R.L. (2000) The relationship between Donepezil and behavioural disturbance in patients with Alzheimer's disease, *American Journal of Geriatric Psychiatry*, 8(2): 134–40.

Czaja, S.J., Eisdorfer, C. and Schulz, R. (2000) Future directions in caregiving: implications of intervention research, in R. Schulz (ed.) *Handbook on Dementia Caregiving: Evidence-based Interventions for Family Caregivers*. New York, NY: Springer.

Darbyshire, P. (1987) Ask the family, *Nursing Times*, 83(37): 23–5.

Davies, B. (1995) The reform of community and long term care of elderly persons: an international perspective, in T. Scharf and G.C. Wenger (eds) *International Perspectives on Community Care for Older People*. Aldershot: Avebury.

Davies, L.L. (1992) Building a source of caring for caregivers, *Family and Community Health*, 15(2): 1–9.

Davies, S. (2001) Wanting what's best for them. Relatives' experiences of nursing home entry: a constructivist inquiry. PhD Thesis, University of Sheffield.

Davies, S., Nolan, M.R., Brown, J. and Wilson, F. (1999) *Dignity on the Ward: Promoting Excellence in the Acute Hospital Care of Older People*. London: Help the Aged/Order of St John's Trust.

Day, H. and Jankey, S.G. (1996) Lessons from the literatures: towards a holistic model of quality for life, in R. Renwick, I. Brown and M. Nagler (eds) *Quality of Life in Health Promotion and Rehabilitation: Conceptual Approaches, Issues and Applications*. Thousand Oaks, CA: Sage Publications.

Delaney, M. (1994) *Accommodating People with a Disability*. Sydney: The Disability Council of NSW.

De Lepeleire, J.A., Heyrman, J., Baro, F., Buntinx, F. and Lasuy, C. (1994) How do general practitioners diagnose dementia?, *Family Practice*, 11: 148–52.

Dellasega, C. (1991) Caregiving stress among community caregivers for the elderly: does institutionalization make a difference?, *Journal of Community Health Nursing*, 8(4): 197–205.

Dellasega, C. and Mastrian, K. (1995) The process and consequences of institutionalising an elder, *Western Journal of Nursing Research*, 17(2): 123–40.

Dellasega, C. and Nolan, M.R. (1997) Admission to care: facilitating role transition amongst family carers, *Journal of Clinical Nursing*, 6: 443–51.

DHSH (Department of Human Services and Health) (1994) *Your Guide to Residents' Rights in Nursing Homes*, 2nd ed. Canberra: DHSH.

Dickinson, D. (1996) Can elderly residents with memory problems be prepared for relocation?, *Journal of Clinical Nursing*, 5: 99–104.

Dilworth-Anderson, P. (2001) Family issues and the care of persons with Alzheimer's disease, *Aging and Mental Health*, 5(Supplement 1): S49–S51.

DoH (Department of Health) (1995) *Carers (Recognition and Services) Act*. London: HMSO.

DoH SSI (Social Services Inspectorate) (1996) *Carers (Recognition and Services) Act, Policy Guidelines*. London: HMSO.

DoH (1999) *The Carers National Strategy*. London: HMSO.

DoH (2000) *Carers and Disabled Children Act 2000*. London: HMSO.

DoH (2001a) *Making It Happen: A Guide to Delivering Mental Health Promotion*. London: HMSO.

DoH (2001b) *National Service Framework for Older People*. London: HMSO.

DoH (2001c) *Valuing People: A New Strategy for Learning Disability for the 21st Century*, Cm 5086. London: HMSO.

DoH (2001d) *The Expert Patient: A New Approach to Chronic Disease Management for the 21st Century*. London: The Stationery Office.

DoH (2001e) *Towards Person-Centred Approaches: Planning with People. Guidance for Implementation Groups*. London: The Stationery Office.

Doolittle, N.D. (1988) Stroke recovery: review of the literature and suggestions for future research, *Journal of Neuroscience Nursing*, 20: 169–73.

Doolittle, N.D. (1991) Clinical ethnography of lacunar stroke: implications for acute care, *Journal of Neuroscience Nursing*, 23: 235–40.

Doolittle, N.D. (1992) The experience of recovery following lacunar stroke, *Rehabilitation Nursing*, 17: 122–6.

Doolittle, N.D. (1994) A clinical ethnography of stroke recovery, in P. Benner (ed.) *Interpretive Phenomenology Embodiment, Caring and Ethics in Health and Illness*. Thousand Oaks, CA: Sage Publications.

Downs, M. (2000) Dementia in a socio-cultural context: an idea whose time has come, *Ageing and Society*, 20(3): 369–75.

Downs, M. (2002) How can we improve GPs' response to dementia?, *Journal of Dementia Care*, May/June: 18–19.

Drickamer, M.A. and Lachs, M.S. (1992) Should patients with Alzheimer's disease be told their diagnosis?, *New England Journal of Medicine*, 326(14): 947–51.

Ducharme, F., Levesque, L., Gendren, M. and Legault, A. (2001) Development process and qualitative evaluation of a program to promote the mental health of family caregivers, *Clinical Nursing Research*, 10(2): 182–201.

Duncan, M.T. and Morgan, D.L. (1994) Sharing the caring: family caregivers' views of their relationships with nursing home staff, *Gerontologist*, 34(2): 235–44.

Easterbrook, L. (1999) *When We Are Very Old: Reflections on Treatment, Care and Support of Older People*. London: King's Fund.

Eccles, M., Clarke, J., Livingstone, M., Freemantle, N. and Mason, J. (1998) North of England evidence-based guidelines development project: guideline for the primary care management of dementia, *British Medical Journal*, 317: 802–8.

Efraimsson, E., Höglund, I. and Sandman, P. (2001) 'The everlasting trial of strength and patience': transition in home care nursing as narrated by patients and family members, *Journal of Clinical Nursing*, 10(6): 813–19.

Ehrenfeld, M., Bergman, R. and Alpert, R. (1997) Family and staff involvement in tending dementia patients in nursing homes, *Journal of Clinical Nursing*, 6: 505–6.

Eldar, R. (2000) A conceptual proposal for the study of the quality of rehabilitation care, *Disability and Rehabilitation*, 22(4): 163–9.

Emmanuel, E.J. and Cass, F. (1993) Ethical and legal aspects of caring for patients with cancer, *Cancer Medicine*, 3rd edition, Vol.2: 2466–80. Pennsylvania, USA: Lea and Febiger.

Engelhardt, J.L., Lutzer, V.D. and Brubaker, T.H. (1987) Parents of adults with developmental disabilities: age and reasons for reluctance to use another caregiver, *Lifestyles*, 8: 47–54.

Enterlante, T.M. and Kern, J.M. (1995) Wives' reported role changes following a husband's stroke: a pilot study, *Rehabilitation Nursing*, 20: 155–60.

Eraut, M. (1994) *Developing Professional Knowledge and Competence*. London: Falmer Press.

Ericson, I., Hellström, I., Lundh, U. and Nolan, M.R. (2001) What constitutes good care for people with dementia? *British Journal of Nursing*, 10(11): 710–14.

Essex, E., Seltzer, M. and Krauss, M. (1997) Residential transitions of adults with mental retardation: predictors of waiting list use and placement, *American Journal on Mental Retardation*, 101: 613–29.

Etmanski, A. (2000) *A Good Life for You and Your Relative with a Disability*. Burnaby, British Columbia: Orwell Cove and Planned Lifetime Advocacy Network.

Evans, R.L., Griffith, J., Haselkorn, J.K. *et al.* (1992a) Poststroke family function: an evaluation of the family's role in rehabilitation, *Rehabilitation Nursing*, 17: 127–31; discussion 131–2.

Evans, R.L., Hendricks, R.D., Haselkorn, J.K., Bishop, D.S. and Baldwin, D. (1992b) The family's role in stroke rehabilitation: a review of the literature, *American Journal of Physical Medicine and Rehabilitation*, 71: 135–9.

Evans, R.L., Connis, D.S., Bishop, D.S., Hendricks, R.D. and Haselkorn, J.K. (1994) Stroke: a family dilemma, *Disability and Rehabilitation*, 16(3): 110–18.

Farquhar, M. (1995) Elderly people's definitions of quality of life, *Social Science and Medicine*, 41(10): 1439–46.

Farvis, M. (2001) Communication between clients, carers and staff in a dementia care facility, *American Journal of Nursing*, 9(4): 1–3.

Farzan, D.T. (1991) Reintegration for stroke survivors: home and community considerations, *Nursing Clinics of North America* 26: 1037–48.

Fawdry, M.K. (2001) An exploration of nursing and family caring for older adults, *Journal of Holistic Nursing*, 19(5): 285–96.

Fearnley, K., McLennan, J. and Weaks, D. (1997) *The Right to Know? Sharing the Diagnosis of Dementia*. Edinburgh: Alzheimer's Scotland – Action on Dementia.

Felce, D., Grant, G., Todd, S. *et al.* (1998) *Towards a Full Life: Researching Policy Innovation for People with Learning Disabilities*. Oxford: Butterworth Heinemann.

Ferguson, C. and Keady, J. (2001) The mental health needs of older people and their carers: exploring tensions and new directions, in M.R. Nolan, S. Davies and G. Grant (eds) *Working with Older People and their Families: Key Issues in Policy and Practice*. Buckingham: Open University Press.

Folkman, S. (1997) Positive psychological states and coping with severe stress, *Social Science and Medicine*, 45: 1207–21.

Fortinsky, R.H. (2001) Health care triads and dementia care: integrative framework and future directions, *Aging and Mental Health*, 5(Supplement 1): S35–S48.

Fossey, J. and Baker, M. (1995) Different needs demand different services, *Journal of Dementia Care*, 3(6): 22–3.

Freedman, R.I. and Freedman, D.N. (1994) Planning for now and the future: Social, legal and financial concerns, in M.M. Seltzer, M.W. Krauss and M.P. Janicki (eds) *Life Course Perspectives on Adulthood and Old Age*. Washington: American Association on Mental Retardation.

Freedman, R., Krauss, M. and Seltzer, M. (1997) Aging parents' residential plans for adult children with mental retardation, *Mental Retardation*, 35: 114–23.

Fruin, D. (1998) *A Matter of Chance for Carers? Inspection of Local Authority Support for Carers*. Wetherby: Social Services Inspectorate/Department of Health.

Fuller, K. and Lillquist, D. (1995) Geropsychiatric public sector nursing: placement challenges, *Journal of Psychosocial Nursing and Mental Health Services*, 33(8): 20–2.

Gattuso, S. and Bevan, C. (2000) 'Mother, daughter, patient, nurse':

women's emotion work in aged care, *Journal of Advanced Nursing*, 31(4): 892–9.

Gergen, K.J. (1994) *Realities and Relationships: Soundings in Social Construction*. Cambridge, MA: Harvard University Press.

Gilleard, C.J., Belford, E., Gilleard, E., Whittick, J.E. and Gledhill, K. (1984) Emotional distress amongst the supporters of the elderly mentally infirm, *British Journal of Psychiatry*, 145: 172–7.

Gilmour, J.A. (2002) Dis/integrated care: family caregivers and in-hospital respite care, *Journal of Advanced Nursing*, 39(6): 546–53.

Given, C.W., Given, B.A., Stomnel, M. and Azzouz, F. (1999) The imact of new demands for assistance on caregiver depression: Tests using an inception cohort, *The Gerontologist*, 39(1): 76–84.

Gladstone, J.W. (1995) The marital perceptions of elderly persons living or having a spouse living in long-term care institution in Canada, *The Gerontologist*, 35(1): 52–60.

Glaser, B.G. and Strauss, A.L. (1967) *The Discovery of Grounded Theory: Strategies for Qualitative Research*. Chicago, IL: Aldine.

Glaser, B.G. and Strauss, A.L. (1968) *Time for dying*. Chicago, IL: Aldine.

Glosser, G., Wexler, D. and Balmelli, M. (1985) Physicians and families' perspectives on the medical management of dementia, *Journal of American Geriatrics Societies*, 33(9): 383–91.

Gold, D. (1994) 'We don't call it a "Circle" ': the ethos of a support group, *Disability and Society*, 9(4): 435–52.

Goldberg, D.P. and Hillier, V.F. (1979) A scaled version of the General Health Questionnaire, *Psychological Medicine*, 9: 139–45.

Gouldner, A.W. (1960) The 'norm of reciprocity': a preliminary statement, *American Sociological Review*, 25: 161–78.

Grant, G. (1989) Letting go: decision making among family carers of people with mental handicap, *Australia and New Zealand Journal of Developmental Disabilities*, 15: 189–200.

Grant, G. (1993) Support networks and transitions over two years among adults with mental handicap, *Mental Handicap Research*, 6: 36–55.

Grant, G. (2001) Older people with learning disabilities: health, community inclusion and family caregiving, in M.R. Nolan, S. Davies and G. Grant (eds) *Working with Older People and their Families. Key Issues in Policy and Practice*. Buckingham: Open University Press.

Grant, G. and Nolan, M.R. (1993) Informal carers: sources and concomitants of satisfaction, *Health and Social Care*, 1(3): 147–59.

Grant, G. and Whittell, B. (1999) *Family Care of People with Learning Disabilities: Support for Family Coping*. Final report to the Wales Office of Research and Development for Health and Social Care. Bangor: Centre for Social Policy Research and Development, University of Wales, Bangor.

Grant, G. and Whittell, B. (2000) Differentiated coping strategies in families with children or adults with intellectual disabilities: the influence of gender, family composition and the life span, *Journal of Applied Research in Intellectual Disabilities*, 13: 256–75.

Grant, G. and Whittell, B. (2001) Do families and care managers have similar views of family coping?, *Journal of Learning Disabilities*, 5(2): 111–20.

Grant, G., McGrath, M. and Ramcharan, P. (1994) How family and informal supporters appraise service quality, *International Journal of Disability, Development and Education*, 41(2): 127–41.

Grant, G., McGrath, M. and Ramcharan, P. (1995) Community inclusion of older adults with learning disabilities: care in place, *International Journal of Networks and Community*, 2(1): 29–44.

Grant, G., Ramcharan, P., McGrath, M., Nolan, M.R. and Keady, J. (1998) Rewards and gratifications among family caregivers: towards a refined model of caring and coping, *Journal of Intellectual Disability Research*, 42(1): 58–71.

Grau, L., Teresi, J. and Chandler, B. (1993) Demoralization among sons, daughters, spouses, and other relatives of nursing home residents, *Research on Ageing*, 15(3): 324–45.

Greene, V. and Monahan, D. (1982) The impact of visitation on patient well-being in nursing homes, *The Gerontologist*, 22(4): 418–23.

Groger, L. (1994a) Decision as process: a conceptual model of black elders' nursing home placement, *Journal of Ageing Studies*, 8(1): 77–94.

Groger, L. (1994b) Limit of support and reaction to illness: an exploration of black elders' pathways to long-term care settings, *Journal of Cross Cultural Gerontology*, 9(4): 369–87.

Guberman, N., Nicholds, E., Nolan, M.R., Rembicki, D., Lundh, U. and Keefe, J. (in press) Impacts on practitioners of testing carer assessment tools: experiences from Britain, Canada and Sweden, with insights from Australia, *Journal of Health and Social Care in the Community*.

Gubrium, J.F. (1992) Qualitative research comes of age in gerontology [editorial], *The Gerontologist*, 32(5): 581–2.

Gubrium, J.F. (1995) Taking stock, *Qualitative Health Research*, 5(3): 267–9.

Gulliford, M., Morgan, M., Hughes, D. *et al.* (2001) *Access to Health Care*: Report of a Scoping Exercise for the National Coordinating Centre for NHS Service Delivery and Organisation R&D (NCCSDO). London: NCCSDO.

Gunstone, S. (1999) Expert practice: the interventions used by a Community Mental Health Nurse with carers of dementia sufferers, *Journal of Psychiatric and Mental Health Nursing*, 6: 21–7.

Haas, B.K. (1999) Clarification and integration of similar quality of life concepts, *Image*, 31(3): 215–20.

Häggström, T., Axelsson, K. and Norberg, A. (1994) The experience of living with stroke sequelae illuminated by means of stories and metaphors, *Qualitative Health Research*, 4: 321–37.

Hamel, G. (1995) Guilt: a hidden problem in caregiving, *Provider*, 21(11): 59–60.

Harel, Z. (1981) Quality of care, congruence and well-being among institutionalized elderly, *The Gerontologist*, 21(5): 523–31.

Harlan-Simmons, J., Holtz, P., Todd, J. and Mooney, M. (2001) Building social relationships through values roles: three adults and the community membership project, *Mental Retardation*, 39(3): 171–80.

Hart, E. (2001) System induced setbacks in stroke recovery, *Sociology of Health and Illness* 23(1): 101–23.

Harvath, T.A., Archbold, P.G., Stewart, B.J. *et al.* (1994) Establishing partnerships with family caregivers: local and cosmopolitan knowledge, *Journal of Gerontological Nursing*, 20(2): 29–35.

Hasselkus, B. (1988) Meaning in family caregiving: perspectives on caregiver/professional relationships, *The Gerontologist*, 28(5): 686–91.

Hasselkus, B.R., Dickie, V.A. and Gregory, C. (1996) Geriatric occupational therapy: the uncertain ideology of long-term care, *American Journal of Occupational Therapy*, 51(2): 132–9.

Hawkins, B. (1999) Rights, place of residence and retirement: lessons from case studies on aging, in S. Herr and G. Weber (eds) *Aging, Rights and Quality of Life*. Baltimore: MD Brookes.

Hawley, D.R. and DeHann, L. (1996) Toward a definition of family resilience: integrating life-span and family perspectives, *Family Process*, 35: 283–98.

Hayden, M.F. and Heller, T. (1997) Support, problem-solving/coping ability, and personal burden of younger and older caregivers of adults with mental retardation, *Mental Retardation*, 35: 264–372.

Heaton, J., Arksey, H. and Sloper, P. (1999) Carers' experience of hospital discharge and continuing care in the community, *Health and Social Care in the Community*, 7(2): 91–9.

Heinz, W.R. and Kruger, H. (2001) Life course: innovations and challenges for social research, *Current Sociology*, 49(2): 29–45.

Helff, C.M. and Glidden, L.M. (1998) More positive or less negative? Trends in research on adjustment of families having children with developmental disabilities, *Mental Retardation*, 36(6): 457–64.

Heller, T. and Factor, A. (1991) Permanency planning for adults with mental retardation living with family caregivers, *American Journal on Mental Retardation*, 96: 163–76.

Henwood, M. (1998) *Ignored and Invisible? Carers' Experience of the NHS*. Report of a UK research survey commissioned by Carers National Association, London.

Hertzberg, A. and Ekman, S.-L. (1996) How the relatives of elderly patients in institutional care perceive the staff, *Scandinavian Journal of Caring Science*, 10: 205–10.

Hertzberg, A., Ekman, S.-L. and Axelsson, K. (2001) Staff activities and behaviour are the source of many feelings: relatives' interactions and relationships with staff in nursing homes, *Journal of Clinical Nursing*, 10: 380–8.

High, D.M. and Rowles, G.D. (1995) Nursing home residents, families, and decision making: toward an understanding of progressive surrogacy, *Journal on Ageing Studies*, 9(2): 101–17.

Hirschfield, M.J. (1981) Families living and coping with the cognitively impaired, in L.A. Copp (ed.) *Care of the Ageing: Recent Advances in Nursing*. Edinburgh: Churchill Livingstone.

Hirschfield, M.J. (1983) Home care versus institutionalization: family caregiving and senile brain disease, *International Journal of Nursing Studies*, 20(1): 23–32.

Hirst, M. (2001) Trends in informal care in Great Britain during the 1990's, *Health and Social Care in the Community*, 9(6): 348–57.

Ho, D. (2000) Role of community mental health nurse for people with dementia, *British Journal of Nursing*, 9(15): 986–91.

Hochstenbach, J. (2000) Rehabilitation is more than functional recovery, *Disability and Rehabilitation*, 22(4): 201–4.

Hokenstadt, M.C. and Johansson, L. (1990) Caregiving for the elderly in Sweden: program challenges and policy initiatives, in D. Biegel and A. Blum (eds) *Ageing and Caregiving: Theory, Research and Policy*. Newbury Park, CA: Sage Publications.

Hooyman, N. (1983) Social support networks in services to the elderly, in J. Whittaker and J. Garbarino (eds) *Social Support Networks: Informal Helping in Human Services*. New York, NY: Aldine.

Horowitz, A. and Shindehan, L.W. (1983) Reciprocity and affection: past influences on current caregiving, *Journal of Gerontological Social Work*, 5(3): 5–20.

Howe, A. (1990) Nursing home care policy: from laissez faire to restructuring, in H. Kenig and J. McCallum (eds) *Grey Policy*. Sydney: Allen and Unwin.

Huberman, A. and Miles, M. (1994) Data management and analysis methods, in N. Denzin and Y. Lincoln (eds) *Handbook of Qualitative Methods*. Newbury Park CA: Sage Publications.

Hutchinson, S.A. (1986) Grounded theory: the method, in P.L. Munhall and C.J. Oiler (eds) *Nursing Research: A Qualitative Perspective*. Norwalk, CT: Appleton-Century-Crofts.

Hutchinson, S.A., Leger-Krall, S. and Wilson, H.S. (1997) Early probably Alzheimer's disease and awareness context theory, *Social Science and Medicine*, 45(9): 1399–409.

Iliffe, S. (1994) Why GPs have a bad reputation, *Journal of Dementia Care*, Nov/Dec: 24–5.

Iliffe, S., Wilcock, J., Austen, T. *et al.* (2002) Dementia diagnosis and management in primary care, *Dementia: The International Journal of Social Research and Practice*, 1(1): 11–23.

Jameson, C. (1998) Promoting long-term relationships between individuals with mental retardation and people in their community, *Mental Retardation*, 36(2): 116–27.

Janicki, M.P. (1996) *Help for caring – for older people caring for adults with developmental disability*. Albany, NY: New York State Developmental Disabilities Planning Council.

Jani-le Bris, H. (1993) *Family Care of Dependent Older People in the European Community*. Luxembourg: EU Publishers.

Jansson, W., Almberg, B., Grafström, M. and Winblad, B. (1998) The circle model: support for relatives of people with dementia, *International Journal of Geriatric Psychiatry*, 13: 674–81.

Jeon, Y.H. and Madjar, I. (1998) Caring for a family member with chronic mental illness, *Qualitative Health Research*, 8(5): 694–706.

Jette, A.M., Tennstedt, S. and Crawford, S. (1995) How does formal and informal community care affect nursing home use?, *Journals of Gerontology, Series B: Psychological Sciences and Social Sciences*, 50b(1): S4–S12.

Johansson, L. (1993) Swedes test new strategies, *Ageing International*, 2: 42–5.

Johansson, L. (2001) Recent developments in caregiver support in Sweden. Paper given at the 17th World Congress of the International Association of Gerontology, Vancouver, 3 July 2001.

Johnson, J. (1998) The emergence of care as policy, in A. Brechin, J. Walmsley, J. Katz and S. Peace (eds) *Care Matters: Concepts, Practice and Research in Health and Social Care*. London: Sage Publications.

Johnson, M.A. (1990) Nursing home placement: the daughter's perspective, *Journal of Gerontological Nursing*, 16(11): 6–11.

Jongbloed, L., Stanton, S. and Fousek, B. (1993) Family adaptation to altered roles following a stroke, *Canadian Journal of Occupational Therapy*, 60: 70–7.

Kadzin, A.E. (1999) The meanings and measurement of clinical significance, *Journal of Consulting and Clinical Psychology*, 67: 332–9.

Kahana, E. and Young, R. (1990) Clarifying the caregiving paradigm: challenges for the future, in D.E. Biegel and A. Blum (eds) *Ageing and Caregiving: Theory, Research and Policy*. Newbury Park, CA: Sage Publications.

Kahana, E., Biegel, D.E. and Wykle, M.L. (1994) (eds) *Family Caregiving across the Lifespan*. Thousand Oaks, CA: Sage Publications.

Kammer, C.H. (1994) Stress and coping of family members responsible for nursing home placement, *Research in Nursing and Health*, 17(2): 89–98.

Kaplan, I. and Ade-Ridder, L. (1991) Impact on the marriage when one spouse moves to a nursing home, *Journal of Women and Ageing*, 3: 81–101.

Kaufmann, A.V., Adams, J.P. and Campbell, V.A. (1991) Permanency planning for older parents who care for adult children with mental retardation, *Mental Retardation*, 29: 293–300.

Keady, J. (1999) The dynamics of dementia: a modified grounded theory study. PhD Thesis, University of Wales, Bangor.

Keady, J. and Nolan, M.R. (1994a) Working with dementia sufferers and their carers in the community: exploring the nursing role. Paper presented to International Nursing Conference, University of Ulster, Coleraine, N. Ireland, 30 August.

Keady, J. and Nolan, M.R. (1994b) Younger onset dementia: developing a longitudinal model as the basis for a research agenda and as a guide to interventions with sufferers and carers, *Journal of Advanced Nursing,* 19: 659–69.

Keady, J. and Nolan, M.R. (1995) A stitch in time. Facilitating proactive interventions with dementia caregivers: the role of community practitioners, *Journal of Psychiatric and Mental Health,* 2: 33–40.

Keady, J., Nolan, M.R. and Gilliard, J. (1995) Listen to the voices of experience, *Journal of Dementia Care,* 3(3): 15–7.

Kearney, G., Krishman, V. and Londhe, R. (1993) Characteristics of elderly people with a mental handicap living in a mental handicap hospital: a descriptive study, *British Journal of Developmental Disabilities,* 39: 31–50.

Keefe, J. and Fancey, P. (2000) The care continues: responsibility for elderly relatives before and after admission to a long-term care facility, *Family Relations,* 49(3): 235–44.

Kellett, O. (1996) Caring in nursing homes: the family perspective, *Geriaction,* 14(4): 18–23.

Kellett, U. (1997) *Creating Meaning, Responsibility and Choice: The Lived Experience of Family Carers in Nursing Homes.* Unpublished PhD Thesis. Melbourne: La Trobe University.

Kernich, C.A. and Robb, G. (1988) Development of a stroke family support and education program, *Journal of Neuroscience Nursing,* 20: 193–7.

King, R.B., Shade-Zeldow, Y., Carlson, C.E., Knafl, K. and Roth, E.J. (1995) Early adaptation to stroke: patient and primary support person, *Rehabilitation Nursing Research,* 4: 82–9.

King, S., Collins, C., Given, B. and Vredevoogd, J. (1991) Institutionalization of an elderly family member: reactions of spouse and non-spouse caregivers, *Archives of Psychiatric Nursing,* 5(6): 323–30.

Kirk, S. and Glendinning, G. (2002) Supporting 'expert' parents: professional support and family caring for a child with complex healthcare needs in the community, *International Journal of Nursing Studies,* 39: 625–35.

Kitwood, T. (1997) *Dementia Reconsidered: The Person Comes First.* Buckingham: Open University Press.

Kitwood, T. and Bredin, M. (1992) Towards a theory of dementia care: personhood and well-being, *Ageing and Society,* 12: 269–87.

Kivnick, H.Q. and Murray, S.U. (1997) Vital involvement: an overlooked source of identity in frail elders, *Journal of Aging and Identity,* 2(3): 205–25.

Kobayashi, S., Masaki, H. and Noguchi, M. (1993) Developmental process: family caregivers of demented Japanese, *Journal of Gerontological Nursing,* 19(10): 7–12.

Koch, T. (1993) Establishing rigour in qualitative research: the decision trail, *Journal of Advanced Nursing,* 19: 976–86.

Koch, T. (1996) Implementation of a hermeneutic inquiry in nursing: philosophy, rigour and representation, *Journal of Advanced Nursing,* 24: 174–84.

Kosloski, K. and Montgomery, R.J.V. (1995) Impact of respite use on nursing home placement, *The Gerontologist*, 35(1): 67–74.

Krause, A.M., Grant, L.D. and Long, B.C. (1999) Sources of stress reported by daughters of nursing home residents, *Journal of Aging Studies*, 13(3): 349–64.

Krauss, M. and Erickson, M. (1988) Informal support networks among aging persons with mental retardation: a pilot study, *Mental Retardation*, 26: 197–201.

Krauss, M., Seltzer, M. and Goodman, S. (1992) Social support networks of adults with mental retardation who live at home, *American Journal on Mental Retardation*, 96: 432–41.

Krauss, M., Seltzer, M., Gordon, R. and Friedman, D. (1996) Binding ties: the roles of adult siblings of persons with mental retardation, *Mental Retardation*, 34: 83–93.

Kuhn, D.R. (1998) Caring for relatives with early stage Alzheimer's disease: an exploratory study, *American Journal of Alzheimer's Disease*, 13(4): 189–96.

Kultgen, P., Harlan-Simmons, J. and Todd, J. (2000) Community membership, in M. Janicki and E. Ansello (eds) *Community Supports for Aging Adults with Lifelong Disabilities*. Baltimore, MD: Brookes.

Laitinen, D. (1992) Participation of informal caregivers in the hospital care of elderly patients and their evaluations of the care given: pilot study in three different hospitals, *Journal of Advanced Nursing*, 17: 1233–7.

Lavoie, J.P., White, D. and Zuniga, R. (2001) When caregiving means reciprocity: the multiple forms of reciprocity in providing care for a frail relative. Paper presented at 17th World Congress of the International Association of Gerontology, Vancouver, 3 July.

Lawrence, R.A., Tennstedt, S.L. and Assmann, S.F. (1998) Quality of the caregiver – care–recipient relationship: does it affect negative consequence of caregiving for family caregivers? *Psychology and Ageing*, 13(1): 150–8.

Lazarus, R.S. (1993) Coping theory and research: past, present and future, *Psychosomatic Medicine*, 55: 234–47.

Lazarus, R.S. and Folkman, S. (1984) *Stress, Appraisal and Coping*. New York, NY: Springer.

Lee, H.S., Brennan, P.F. and Daly, B.J. (2001) Relationships between empathy to appraisal, depression, life satisfactions and physical health of informal caregivers, *Research in Nursing and Health*, 24: 44–56.

Lemov, P. (1994) Nursing homes and common sense, *Governing*, 7(10): 44–9.

Levesque, L., Cossette, J. and Laurin, L. (1995) A multidimensional examination of the psychological and social well-being of caregivers of a demented relative, *Research on Aging*, 17(3): 322–60.

Levine, D. (1995) Your ageing parents: choosing a nursing home, *American Health: Fitness of Body and Mind*, 14(5): 82–5.

Lewinter, M. (2001) Reciprocity in caregiving relationships between elderly and family and elderly and home help in Denmark. Paper given at 17th World Congress of the International Association of Gerontology, Vancouver, 3 July.

Lewinter, M. and Mikkelsen, S. (1995a) Patients' experience of rehabilitation after stroke, *Disability and Rehabilitation*, 17(1): 3–9.

Lewinter, M. and Mikkelsen, S. (1995b) Therapists and the rehabilitation process after a stroke, *Disability and Rehabilitation*, 17(5): 211–16.

Lewis, M.B., Curtis, M.P. and Lundy, K.S. (1995) 'He calls me his angel of mercy': the experience of caring for elderly parents in the home, *Holistic Nursing Practice*, 9(4): 54–65.

Lewycka, M. (1998) *Finding and Paying for Residential and Nursing Home Care*, 2nd edition. London: Age Concern.

Liaschenko, J. (1997) Knowing the patient, in S.E. Thorne and V.E. Hays (eds) *Nursing Praxis: Knowledge and Action*. Thousand Oaks, CA: Sage Publications.

Liaschenko, J. and Fisher, A. (1999) Theorising the knowledge that nurses use in the conduct of their work, *Scholarly Inquiry for Nursing Practice: An International Journal*, 13(1): 29–41.

Lightbody, P. and Gilhooly, M. (1997) The continuing quest for predictions of breakdown of family care of elderly people with dementia, in M. Marshall (ed.) *State of the Art in Dementia Care*. London: Centre for Policy on Ageing.

Litvin, S. (2000) Appraisal of dependence versus independence among care-receiving elderly women, in R.L. Ruberstein, M. Moss and M.H. Kleban (eds) *The Many Dimensions of Aging*. New York, NY: Springer.

Litwak, E. (1985) *Helping the Elderly*. New York, NY: The Guilford Press.

Livingston, G., Watkins, V., Manela, M., Rosser, R. and Katona, C. (1998) Quality of life in older people, *Aging and Mental Health*, 2(1): 20–3.

Llewellyn, G., Gething, L., Cant, R. and Kendig, H. (2002) *Older Parent-carers of Adults with Intellectual Disability and Service Pathways*. Final report. Sydney: University of Sydney.

Llewellyn, G., Thompson, K. and Whybrow, S. (in press) Mothers as activists, in S. Esdaile and J. Olsen (eds) *Mothering Occupations: Challenge, Agency and Participation*. Philadelphia, PA: F.A. Davis Publishers.

Lothian, K. and McKee, K. (2000) *Informal Care in the United Kingdom: Who Cares?* COPE Country Report. Sheffield: University of Sheffield, Sheffield Institute for Studies on Ageing.

Low, J.T.S., Payne, S. and Roderick, P. (1999) The impact of stroke on informal carers: a literature review, *Social Science and Medicine*, 49(6): 711–25.

Lundh, U. (1999) Coping strategies among family carers in Sweden, *British Journal of Nursing*, 8(11): 735–40.

Lundh, U. (2001) Impact on professional carers of structured interviews with families, *British Journal of Nursing*, 10(10): 677–81.

Lundh, U. and Nolan, M.R. (2001) Närståendes vård av äldre anhörigas och professionellas perspektiv. Report to the Swedish National Board of Health and Welfare. *http://www.sos.se/plus/dokinfo.asp?valPubl_id=2001-124-6*

Lundh, U., Sandberg, J. and Nolan, M.R. (2000) 'I don't have any other choice': spouses' experiences of placing a partner in accommodation for older people in Sweden, *Journal of Advanced Nursing*, 32(5): 1178–86.

Lyons, K.S., Zarit, S.H., Sayer, A.G. and Whitlach, C.J. (2002) Caregiving as a dyadic process: perspectives from caregiver and care receiver, *Journal of Gerontology (Psychological Sciences)*, 57B(3): 195–204.

McAuley, W.J., Travis, S.S. and Safewright, M.P. (1997) Personal accounts of the nursing home search and selection process, *Qualitative Health Research*, 7(2): 236–54.

Maccabee, J. (1994) The effect of transfer from a palliative care unit to nursing homes – are patients' and relatives' needs met?, *Palliative Medicine*, 8(3): 211–14.

McCallion, P. and Tobin, S.S. (1995) Social workers' perceptions of older parents caring at home for sons and daughters with developmental disabilities. *Mental Retardation*, 33: 153–62.

McDerment, L., Ackroyd, J., Teale, R. and Sutton, J. (1997) *As Others See Us: A Study of Relationships in Homes for Older People*. London: Relatives' Association.

MacDonald, L.D., Higgs, P.F.D., MacDonald, J.S., Godfrey, E.L. and Ward, M.C. (1996) Carers' reflection on nursing home and NHS long stay care for elderly patients, *Health and Social Care in the Community*, 4(5): 264–70.

McFall, S. and Miller, B.H. (1992) Caregiver burden and nursing home admission of frail elderly persons, *Journal of Gerontology*, 47(2): S73–S79.

McGrath, M. and Grant, G. (1993) The life-cycle and support networks of families with a mentally handicapped member, *Disability, Handicap and Society*, 8(1): 25–41.

McHaffie, H.E. (1992) Coping: an essential element of nursing, *Journal of Advanced Nursing*, 17: 933–40.

McIntosh, I.B., Swanson, V., Power, K., Rae, G. and Catherine, A.L. (1999) General practitioners' and nurses' perceived roles, attitudes and stressors in the management of dementia. *Health Bulletin*, Vol.57, No.1, The Scottish Office.

McKee, K. (1999) This is your life: research paradigm in dementia care, in T. Adams and C.L. Clarke (eds) *Dementia Care: Developing Partnerships in Practice*. London: Balliere Tindall.

McLaughlin, E. and Ritchie, J. (1994) Legacies of caring: the experiences and circumstances of ex-carers, *Health and Social Care in the Community*, 2(4): 241–53.

McLean, J., Roper-Hall, A., Mayer, P. and Main, A. (1991) Service needs of stroke survivors and their informal carers: a pilot study, *Journal of Advanced Nursing*, 16: 559–64.

Magrill, D., Handley, P., Gleeson, S. and Charles, D. (1997) *Crisis Approaching: The Situation Facing Sheffield's Elderly Carers of People with Learning Disabilities*. Sheffield: Sharing Caring Project.

Mahon, M. and Mactavish, J. (2000) A sense of belonging, in M. Janicki and E. Ansello (eds) *Community Supports for Aging Adults with Lifelong Disabilities*. Baltimore, MD: Brookes.

Marcusson, J., Blennow, K., Skoog, I. and Wallin, A. (1995) *Demenssjukdomar* [Trans. *Dementia Diseases*]. Liber: Falköping.

Martin, G.W. and Younger, D. (2001) Person-centred care for people with dementia: a quality audit, *Journal of Psychiatric and Mental Health Nursing*, 8: 443–8.

Martini, T.S., Grusec, J.E. and Bernardine, S.C. (2001) Effects of interpersonal control, perspective taking and attributions on older mothers and adult daughters' satisfaction with their helping relationships, *Journal of Family Psychology*, 15(4): 688–705.

Maslow, K. and Whitehouse, P. (1997) Defining and measuring outcomes in Alzheimer's disease research: conference findings, *Alzheimer's Disease and Related Disorders*, 11(6): 186–95.

Matthiesen, V. (1989) Guilt and grief: when daughters place mothers in nursing homes, *Journal of Gerontological Nursing*, 15(7): 11–15.

May, D. (ed.) (2000) *Transition and Change in the Lives of People with Intellectual Disabilities*. London: Jessica Kingsley.

Mead, N. and Bower, P. (2000) Patient-centredness: a conceptual framework and review of the literature, *Social Science and Medicine*, 51: 1087–110.

Mendes del Leon, C., Glass, T., Beckett, L. *et al.* (1999) Social networks and transition across eight intervals of yearly data in the New Haven EPESE, *Journal of Gerontology*, 54(3): 162–72.

Mikhail, M.L. (1992) Psychological responses to relocation to a nursing home, *Journal of Gerontological Nursing*, 18(3): 35–9.

Miller, A. and Gwynne, G. (1972) *A Life Apart*. London: Tavistock.

Mills, M. (2000) Providing space for time: the impact of temporality on life course research, *Time and Society*, 9(1): 91–127.

Milne, B., Pitt, I. and Sabin, N. (1993) Evaluation of a carer support scheme for elderly people: the importance of 'coping', *British Journal of Social Work*, 23: 157–68.

Minichiello, V. (1987) Visitors to nursing homes: few or many?, *Australian Journal on Ageing*, 6(3): 31–5.

Mintz, S. and Marosy, J.P. (2000) Family caregivers and home care: a declaration of interdependence, *Caring Magazine*, June: 24–6.

Montgomery, R. (1982) Impact of institutional care policies on family integration, *The Gerontologist*, 22(1): 54–8.

Montgomery, R.J.V. and Kosloski, K.D. (1994) A longitudinal analysis of nursing home placement for dependent elders cared for by spouses vs adult children, *Journal of Gerontology*, 49(2): S62–S74.

Montgomery, R.J.V. and Kosloski, K.D. (2000) Family caregiving: change, continuity and diversity, in M.P. Lawton and R.L. Rubestein (eds) *Interventions in Dementia Care: Towards Improving Quality of Life.* New York, NY: Springer.

Montgomery, R.J.V. and Williams, K.N. (2001) Implications of differential impacts of caregiving for future research on Alzheimer care, *Aging and Mental Health,* 5(Supplement 1): S23–S34.

Moore, K. (1994) Stroke: the long road back, *Rehabilitation Nursing,* 57: 50–5.

Morgan, D., Reed, J. and Palmer, A. (1997) Moving from hospital into a care home: the nurse's role in supporting older people, *Journal of Clinical Nursing,* 6: 463–71.

Moriarty, J. (1999) Use of community and long-term care by people with dementia in the UK: a review of some issues in service provision and carer and user preferences, *Aging and Mental Health,* 3(4): 311–19.

Moriarty, J. and Levin, E. (1998) Respite care in homes and hospitals, in A. Jack (ed.) *Residential vs Community Care: The Role of Institutions in Welfare Provision.* Basingstoke: Macmillan.

Moriarty, J. and Webb, S. (2000) *Part of their Lives: Community Care for Older People with Dementia.* Bristol: The Policy Press.

Morse, J.M. (1994) 'Emerging from the data': the cognitive processes of analysis in qualitative inquiry, in J.M. Morse (ed.) *Critical Issues in Qualitative Research Methods.* London: Sage Publications.

Morse, J.M. and Field, P.G. (1994) *Nursing Research: The Application of Qualitative Approaches.* London: Chapman and Hall.

Morton, I. (2000) Just what *is* person-centred dementia care?, *Journal of Dementia Care,* 8(3): 28–9.

Motenko, A.K. (1989) The frustrations, gratifications and well-being of dementia caregivers, *Gerontologist,* 29(2): 166–72.

Mui, A.C. (1995) Caring for frail elderly parents: a comparison of adult sons and daughters, *The Gerontological Society of America,* 35(1): 86–93.

Murphy, B., Schofield, H. and Herrman, H. (1995) Information for family carers: does it help?, *Australian Journal of Public Health,* 19(2): 192–7.

Myers, F., Ager, A., Kerr, P. and Myles, S. (1998) Outside looking in: studies of the community integration of people with learning disabilities, *Disability and Society,* 13(3): 389–414.

Naleppa, M.J. (1996) Families and the institutionalized elderly: a review, *Journal of Gerontological Social Work,* 27(1/2): 87–111.

Narayan, S., Lewis, M., Tornatone, J., Hepburn, K. and Corcoran-Perry, S. (2001) Subjective responses to caregiving for a spouse with dementia, *Journal of Gerontological Nursing,* March: 19–28.

NAW (National Assembly for Wales) (2001) *Fulfilling the Promises: Proposals for a Framework for Services for People with Learning Disabilities.* Cardiff: Learning Disability Advisory Group.

National Board of Health and Welfare (2001) *Närståendes vård av äldre, anhörigas och professionellas perspectiv* [Trans. *Family care for older persons from the perspective of family carers and professionals*], Anhörig 300. Stockholm: Socialstyrelsen.

Nay, R. (1993) Benevolent oppression: lived experience of nursing home life. PhD Thesis, UNSW, Sydney.

Nay, R. (1995) Nursing home residents' perceptions of relocation, *Journal of Clinical Nursing*, 4(5): 319–25.

Nay, R. (1996) Nursing home entry: meaning making by relatives, *Australian Journal on Ageing*, 16(1): 24–9.

Nay, R. (1997) Relatives' experience of nursing home life: characterized by tension, *Australian Journal on Ageing*, 16(1): 24–9.

Nelson, H.W. (2000) Injustice and conflict in nursing homes: towards advocacy and exchange, *Journal of Aging Studies*, 14(1): 39–61.

Neufeld, A. and Harrison, M.J. (1995) Reciprocity and social support in caregiving relationships: variations and consequences, *Qualitative Health Research*, 5(3): 348–65.

Newbronner, E. and Hare, P. (2002) *Services to Support Carers of People with Mental Health Problems*. Consultation report for the National Coordinating Centre for NHS Services Delivery and Organization R&D. London: NCCSDO.

Nicholas, E. (2003) An outcomes focus in carer assessment and review: value and challenge, *British Journal of Social Work*, 33: 31–47.

Nolan, M.R. (1991) Timeshare beds: a pluralistic evaluation of rota bed systems in continuing care hospitals. PhD Thesis, University of Wales, Bangor.

Nolan, M.R. (1993) Carer/dependant relationships and the prevention of elder abuse, in P. Decalmer and F. Glendenning (eds) *The Abuse and Neglect of Elderly People: A Handbook*. London: Sage Publications.

Nolan, M.R. (1997) Health and social care: what the future holds for nursing. Keynote address at Third Royal College of Nursing Older Person European Conference and Exhibition, Harrogate, 5th November.

Nolan, M.R. (1998) Outcomes and effectiveness: beyond a professional perspective, *Clinical Effectiveness in Nursing*, 2(2): 57–68.

Nolan, M.R. (2001) Successful ageing: keeping the 'person' in person-centred care, *British Journal of Nursing*, 10(7): 450–4.

Nolan, M.R. and Dellasega, C. (1999) 'It's not the same as him being at home': creating caring partnerships following nursing home placement, *Journal of Clinical Nursing*, 8: 723–30.

Nolan, M.R. and Grant, G. (1989) Addressing the needs of family carers: a neglected area of nursing practice, *Journal of Advanced Nursing*, 14: 950–61.

Nolan, M.R. and Grant, G. (1992a) *Regular Respite: An Evaluation of a Hospital Rota Bed Scheme for Elderly People*. Age Concern Institute of Gerontology Research Papers, Series No. 6. London: Ace Books.

Nolan, M.R. and Grant, G. (1992b) Helping new carers of the frail elderly patient: the challenge for nursing in acute care settings, *Journal of Clinical Nursing*, 1: 303–7.

Nolan, M.R. and Keady, J. (1996) Training for long-term care: the road to better quality, *Reviews in Clinical Gerontology*, 6, 333–42.

Nolan, M.R. and Keady, J. (2001) Working with carers, in C. Cantley (ed.) *A Handbook of Dementia Care*. Buckingham: Open University Press.

Nolan, M.R. and Lundh, U. (1999) Satisfactions and coping strategies of family carers, *British Journal of Community Nursing*, 4(9): 470–5.

Nolan, M.R. and Philp, I. (1999) COPE: towards a comprehensive assessment of caregiver need, *British Journal of Nursing*, 8(20): 1364–72.

Nolan, M.R., Grant, G. and Ellis, N.C. (1990) Stress is in the eye of the beholder: reconceptualizing the measurement of carer burden, *Journal of Advanced Nursing*, 15: 544–55.

Nolan, M.R., Grant, G., Caldock, K. and Keady, J. (1994) *A Framework for Assessing the Needs of Family Carers: A Multi-disciplinary Guide*. Stoke-on-Trent: BASE Publications.

Nolan, M.R., Keady, J. and Grant, G. (1995) CAMI: a basis for assessment and support with family carers, *British Journal of Adult/Elderly Care Nursing*, 1(3): 822–6.

Nolan, M.R., Grant, G. and Keady, J. (1996a) *Understanding Family Care: A Multidimensional Model of Caring and Coping*. Buckingham: Open University Press.

Nolan, M.R., Walker, G., Nolan, J. *et al.* (1996b) Entry to care: positive choice or fait accompli? Developing a more proactive response to the needs of older people and their carers, *Journal of Advanced Nursing*, 24: 265–74.

Nolan, M.R., Booth, A. and Nolan, J. (1997) *New Directions in Rehabilitation: Exploring the Nursing Contribution*. Research Reports Series No. 6, English National Board for Nursing, Midwifery and Health Visiting, London.

Nolan, M.R., Grant, G. and Keady, J. (1998) *Assessing Carers' Needs: A Practitioner's Guide*. Brighton: Pavilion Publications.

Nolan, M.R., Davies, S. and Grant, G. (eds) (2001) *Working with Older People and their Families: Key Issues in Policy and Practice*. Buckingham: Open University Press.

Nolan, M.R., Ryan, T., Enderby, P. and Reid, D. (2002a) Towards a more inclusive vision of dementia care practice and research, *Dementia: The International Journal of Social Research and Practice*, 1(2): 193–211.

Nolan, M.R., Davies, S., Brown, J., Keady, J. and Nolan, J. (2002b) *Longitudinal Study of the Effectiveness of Educational Preparation to Meet the Needs of Older People and Carers: The AGEIN (Advancing Gerontological Education in Nursing) Project*. London: English National Board for Nursing, Midwifery and Health Visiting.

Norman, I.J. (1999) Person-centred dementia care, in S.J. Redfern and F.M. Ross (eds) *Nursing Older People*, 3rd edition. Edinburgh: Churchill Livingstone.

Nunley, B.L., Hall, L.A. and Rowles, G.D. (2000) Effects of the quality of dyadic relationships on the psychological well-being of elderly care recipients, *Journal of Gerontological Nursing*, December: 23–31.

Nussbaum, J.F. (1993) The communicative impact of institutionalization for the elderly: the admissions process. Special Issue: Discourse, Institutions, and the Elderly, *Journal of Ageing Studies*, 7(3): 237–46.

Nydevik, I. and Eller, B. (1995) Stroke patients in long-term care. The relatives' conception of functional capacity and appropriate care, *Scandinavian Journal of Caring Science*, 8(3), 155–61.

Nygaard, H.A. (1991) Who cares for the caregiver? Factors exerting influence on nursing home admissions of demented elderly, *Scandinavian Journal of Caring Sciences*, 5(3): 157–62.

O'Boyle, C.A. (1997) Measuring the quality of later life, *Philosophical Transactions of the Royal Society of London, Series B: Biological Sciences*, 352(136): 1871–9.

O'Connor, D. (1988) Do GPs miss dementia in their elderly patients?, *British Medical Journal*, 297: 1107–10.

O'Connor, D., Fertig, A., Grande, M.J. *et al.* (1993) Dementia in general practice: the practical consequences of a more positive approach to diagnosis, *British Journal of General Practice*, 43: 185–8.

O'Connor, S. (2000) Mode of care delivery in stroke rehabilitation nursing: a development of Kirkvold's unified perspective of the role of the nurse, *Clinical Effectiveness in Nursing*, 4: 180–8.

O'Donovan, S. (1999) The service needs of younger people with dementia, *Signpost to Older People and Mental Health Matters*, 4(3): 3–6.

Oldman, C., Quilgars, D. and Carlisle, J. (1998) *Living In a Home: The Experience of Living and Working in Residential Care in the 1990s*. Kidlington, Oxfordshire: Anchor Trust.

O'Neill-Conger, C. and Marshall, E.S. (1998) Recreating life: toward a theory of relationship development in acute home care, *Qualitative Health Research*, 8(4): 528–46.

Opie, A. (1994) The instability of the caring body: gender and caregivers of confused older people, *Qualitative Health Research*, 4(1): 31–50.

Orr, R.R., Cameron, S.J. and Day, D.M. (1991) Coping with stress in children who have mental retardation: an evaluation of the double ABCX model, *American Journal on Mental Retardation*, 95: 444–50.

Ory, M.G. (2000) Dementia caregiving at the end of the 20th century, in M.P. Lawton and R.L. Rubenstein (eds) *Interventions in Dementia Care: Towards Improving Quality of Life*. New York, NY: Springer.

Ory, M.G., Hoffman, R.R., Yee, J.L., Tennstedt, S. and Schulz, R. (1999) Prudence and impact of caregiving: a detailed comparison between dementia and non-dementia caregivers, *The Gerontologist*, 39(2): 177–85.

Osis, M. (2001) Partnering with families. Paper presented at 17th World Congress of the International Association of Gerontology, Vancouver, 3 July.

Palus, C.J. (1993) Transformative experiences of adulthood: a new look at the seasons of life, in J. Demeck, K. Bursik and R. Dibiase (eds) *Parental Development*. Hillsdale, NJ: Erlbaum.

Parker, C.J., Gladman, J.R.F. and Drummond, A.E.R. (1997) The role of leisure in stroke rehabilitation, *Disability and Rehabilitation*, 19(1): 1–5.

Paterson, B. (2001) Myth of empowerment in chronic illness, *Journal of Advanced Nursing*, 34(5): 574–81.

Pearlin, L.I. and Schooler, C. (1978) The structure of coping, *Journal of Health and Social Behaviour*, 19: 1–21.

Pearlin, L.I., Mullan, J.T., Semple, S.J. and Skaff, M.M. (1990) Caregiving and the stress process: an overview of concepts and their measures, *The Gerontologist*, 30(5): 583–94.

Pearlin, L.I., Harrington, C., Powell-Lawton, M., Montgomery, R.J.V. and Zarit, S.H. (2001) An overview of the social and behavioural consequences of Alzheimer's disease, *Aging and Mental Health*, 5 (Supplement 1): S3–S6.

Pender, N.J. (1996) *Health Promotion in Nursing Practice*, 3rd edition. Stanford, Connecticut: Appleton Lang.

Peters, D.J. (1995) Human experience in disablement: the impetus of the ICIDH, *Disability and Rehabilitation*, 17(214): 135–44.

Phillips, L.R. and Rempusheski, V.F. (1986) Caring for the frail elderly at home: towards a theoretical explanation of the dynamics of poor quality family care, *Advances in Nursing Science*, 8(4): 62–84.

Philp, I. (ed.) (2001) *Family Care of Older People in Europe*. Amsterdam: IOS Press.

Pickard, S. (1999) Coordinated care for older people with dementia, *Journal of Inter-professional Care*, 13(4): 345–54.

Pickard, S., Shaw, S. and Glendenning, G. (2000) Health care professionals' support for older carers, *Ageing and Society*, 20(6): 725–44.

Piercey, K.W. and Woolley, D.N. (1999) Negotiating worker–client relationships: a necessary step to providing quality home care, *Home Health Care Services Quarterly*, 18(1): 9–24.

Pillemer, K. (1996) Family caregiving: what would a martian say?, *The Gerontologist*, 36(2): 269–71.

Pillemer, K., Hegerman, C., Albright, B. and Henderson, C. (1998) Building bridges between families and nursing home staff: the Partners in Caregiving programme, *Gerontologist*, 38(4): 499–503.

Pilnick, A., Dingwall, R., Spencer, E. and Finn, E. (2000) *Genetic Counselling: A Review of the Literature*, Discussion Paper 00/01. Sheffield: Trent Institute for Health Services Research.

Pitkeathley, J. (1995) Carers' perspectives, *Nursing Times*, 91(42): 30–1.

Post, S.G. (2001) Comments on research in the social sciences pertaining to Alzheimer's disease: a more humble approach, *Aging and Mental Health*, 5(Supplement 1): S17–S19.

Pound, P., Bury, M., Gompertz, P. and Ebrahim, S. (1995) Stroke patients' view on their admission to hospital, *British Medical Journal*, 311: 18–22.

Prosser, H. and Moss, S. (1996) Informal care networks of older adults with learning disability, *Journal of Applied Research in Intellectual Disabilities*, 9(1): 17–30.

Pruchno, R.A. (2000) Caregiving research: looking backward, looking forward, in R.L. Ruberstein, M. Moss and M.H. Kleban (eds) *The Many Dimensions of Aging*. New York, NY: Springer.

Pryor, J. (2000) Creating a rehabilitative milieu, *Rehabilitation Nursing* 25(4): 141–4.

Pusey, H. and Richards, D. (2001) A systematic review of the effectiveness of psychosocial interventions for carers of people with dementia, *Aging and Mental Health*, 5(2): 107–19.

Qualls, S.H. (2000) Therapy with ageing families: rationale, opportunities and challenges, *Journal of Aging and Mental Health*, 4(3): 191–9.

Quayhagen, M.P. and Quayhagen, M. (1996) Discovering life quality in coping with dementia, *Western Journal of Nursing Research*, 18(2): 120–35.

Quine, L. and Pahl, J. (1991) Stress and coping in mothers caring for a child with severe learning difficulties: a test of Lazarus' transactional model of coping, *Journal of Community and Applied Social Psychology*, 1: 57–70.

Qureshi, H., Bamford, C., Nicholas, E., Patmore, C. and Harris, J.C. (2000) *Outcomes in Social Care Practice: Developing an Outcome Focus in Care Management and Use Surveys*. York: Social Policy Research Unit, University of York.

Rantz, M.J., Zwygart-Stauffacher, M., Popejoy, L., Grando, V.T., Mehr, D.R., Hicks, L.L. *et al*. (1999) Nursing home care quality: a multidimensional theoretical model integrating the views of consumers and providers, *Journal of Nursing Care Quality*, 14(1): 16–37.

Rapp, S.R., Shumaker, S., Schmidt, S., Naughton, M. and Anderson, R. (1998) Social resourcefulness: its relationship to social support and well-being among caregivers of dementia victims, *Aging and Mental Health*, 2(1): 40–8.

Raynes, N., Temple, B., Glenister, C. and Coulthard, L. (2001) *Quality at Home for Older People: Involving Service Users in Defining Home Care Specifications*. Bristol: The Policy Press.

Read, J. (2000) *Disability, the Family and Society. Listening to Mothers*. Buckingham: Open University Press.

Redfern, S. (1990) Care after a stroke, *Nursing: The Journal of Clinical Practice Education and Management*, 4: 7–11.

Reed, J. and Clarke, C.L. (1999) Nursing older people: considering need and care, *Nursing Inquiry*, 6: 208–15.

Reinders, J. (2002) The good life for citizens with learning disability, *Journal of Learning Disability Research*, 46(1): 1.

Reinhardy, J.R., Kane, R.A., Huch, S., Coll, K.T. and Shen, C.T. (1999) Beyond burden: two ways of looking at caregiver burden, *Research on Aging*, 21(1): 106–27.

Richardson, A. and Ritchie, J. (1989) *Letting Go: Dilemmas for Parents Whose Son or Daughter Has a Mental Handicap*. Milton Keynes: Open University Press.

Riddick, C.C., Cohen Mansfield, J., Fleshner, E. and Kraft, G. (1992) Caregiver adaptations to having a relative with dementia admitted to a nursing home, *Journal of Gerontological Social Work*, 19(1): 51–76.

Riessman, C.K. (1993) *Narrative Analysis*. Thousand Oaks, CA: Sage Publications.

Riorden, J.M. and Bennett, A.V. (1998) An evaluation of an augmented domiciliary service to older people with dementia and their carers, *Ageing and Mental Health*, 2(2): 137–43.

Robinson, C. (2000) Transition and change in the lives of families with a young disabled child: the early years, in T. May (ed.) *Transition and Change in the Lives of People with Intellectual Disabilities*. London: Jessica Kingsley.

Robinson, C. and Williams, V. (1999) *In their Own Right*. Bristol: Norah Fry Research Institute, Bristol University.

Robinson, C.A. and Thorne, S. (1984) Strengthening family interference, *Journal of Advanced Nursing*, 9: 597–602.

Rodgers, H. (2000) The scope of rehabilitation in severely disabled stroke patients, *Disability and Rehabilitation*, 22(4): 199–200.

Rodwell, M. (1998) *Social Work Constructivist Research*. New York, NY: Garland.

Roe, B., Wheltern, M., Young, H. and Dimond, M. (2001) Elders' perceptions of formal and informal care: aspects of getting and receiving help for their activities of daily living, *Journal of Clinical Nursing*, 10(3): 398–504.

Rolland, J.S. (1988) A conceptual model of chronic and life threatening illness and its impact on families, in C.S. Chilman, E.W. Nunnally and F.M. Cox (eds) *Chronic Illness and Disabilities*. Beverly Hills, CA: Sage Publications.

Rolland, J.S. (1994) *Families, Illness and Disability: An Integrative Treatment Model*. New York, NY: Basic Books.

Rose, L. (1998) Benefits and limitations of professional and family interactions: the family perspective, *Archives of Psychiatric Nursing*, XII(3): 140–7.

Rosenthal, S.G., Pituch, M.J., Greninger, L.O. and Metress, E.S. (1993) Perceived needs of wives of stroke patients, *Rehabilitation Nursing*, 18: 148–53, 167, 207–8.

Ross, H.M., Rosenthal, C.J. and Dawson, P. (1997) Spousal caregiving in the residential setting – visiting, *Journal of Clinical Nursing*, 6: 473–83.

Routledge, M. and Sanderson, H. (2002) *Towards Person Centred Approaches: Planning with People. Guidance for Implementation Groups*. London: Department of Health.

Rowland, D. (1991) *Ageing in Australia*. Melbourne: Longman Cheshire.

Rubin, A. and Shuttlesworth, G.E. (1983) Engaging families as support resources in nursing home care: ambiguity in the subdivision of tasks, *The Gerontologist*, 23(6): 632–6.

Russell, C.K., Phillips, L.R., Cromwell, S.L. and Gregory, D.M. (1999) Elder caregiver care negotiations as chances of dependency, *Scholarly Inquiry for Nursing Practice; An International Journal*, 13(4): 283–98.

Ruston, A., Clayton, J. and Calnan, M. (1998) Patients' action during their cardiac event: qualitative study exploring differences and modifiable factors, *British Medical Journal*, 316: 1060–5. Cited in NCCSDO (National Co-ordinating Centre for NHS Services Delivery and Organization R&D) (2001) *Access to Health Care*. London: Department of Public Health Sciences.

Rutter, M. (1996) Transitions and turning points in developmental psychopathology: as applied to the age span between childhood and mid-adulthood, *International Journal of Behavioural Development*, 19(3): 603–26.

Ryan, A. and Scullion, H.F. (2000) Family and staff perceptions of the role of families in nursing homes, *Journal of Advanced Nursing*, 32(3): 626–34.

Safford, F. (1989) 'If you don't like the care, why don't you take your mother home?' Obstacles to family/staff partnerships in the institutional care of the aged, *Journal of Gerontological Social Work*, 13(3/4): 1–7.

Sällström, C. (1994) Spouses' experiences of living with a partner with Alzheimer's disease. Unpublished PhD thesis, Department of Advanced Nursing, Geriatric Medicine and Psychiatry, University of Umeå, Sweden.

Sandberg, J. (2001) Placing a spouse in a care home for older people: (Re)-constructing roles and relationships. Published PhD thesis, Department of Neuroscience and Locomotion, Division of Geriatrics, Linköping University.

Sandberg, J., Lundh, U. and Nolan, M.R. (2001) Placing a spouse in a care-home: the importance of keeping, *Journal of Clinical Nursing*, 10(3): 406–11.

Sandberg, J., Nolan, M.R. and Lundh, U. (2002a) Moving into a care home: the role of adult children in the placement process, *International Journal of Nursing Studies*, 39(3): 353–62.

Sandberg, J., Nolan, M.R. and Lundh, U. (2002b) The role of community staff in care home placement in Sweden, *Journal of Clinical Nursing*, 11: 1–10.

Sandberg, J., Nolan, M.R. and Lundh, U. (2002c) 'Entering a new world': empathic awareness as the key to positive family/staff relationships in care homes, *International Journal of Nursing Studies*, 39(5): 507–15.

Santacruz, K.S. and Swagerty, D. (2001) Early diagnosis of dementia, *American Family Physician*, 63: 703–13.

Schmall, V.L. (1995) Family caregiving education and training: enhancing self-efficacy, *Journal of Case Management*, 4(4): 156–62.

Schneewind, E.H. (1990) The reaction of the family to the institutionalization of an elderly member: factors influencing adjustment and suggestions for easing the transition to a new life phase, *Journal of Gerontological Social Work*, 15(1/2): 121–36.

Schofield, H., Bloch, S., Herman, H. *et al.* (1998) *Family Caregivers. Disability, Illness and Ageing.* Melbourne: Allen and Unwin Victorian Health Promotion Foundation.

Schultz, C., Smyrnios, K., Grbich, C. and Schultz, N. (1993) Caring for family caregivers in Australia: a model of psychoeducational support, *Ageing and Society,* 13: 1–25.

Schulz, R. (2001) Some critical issues in caregiver intervention research, *Aging and Mental Health,* 5(Supplement 1): S112–S115.

Schulz, R. and Williamson, G.M. (1997) The measurement of caregiver outcomes in AD research, *Alzheimer's Disease and Related Disorders,* 11(Supplement 6): 1–6.

Schulz, R., O'Brien, A., Czaja, S. *et al.* (2002) Dementia caregiver intervention research: in search of clinical significance, *The Gerontologist,* 42(5): 589–602.

Schumacher, K.L., Stewart, B.J., Archbold, P.G., Dodd, M.J. and Dibble, S.L. (1998) Family caregiving skill: development of the concept, *Image: Journal of Nursing Scholarship,* 30(1): 63–70.

Schumacher, K.L., Stewart, B.J., Archbold, P.G., Dodd, M.J. and Dibble, S.L. (2000) Family caregiving skill: development of a concept, *Research in Nursing and Health,* 23: 191–203.

Scorgie, K. and Sobsey, D. (2000) Transformational outcomes associated with parenting children who have disabilities, *Mental Retardation,* 38(3): 195–206.

Seale, C. (1996) Living alone towards the end of life, *Ageing and Society,* 16(1): 75–91.

Secrest, J. (2000) Transformation of the relationship: the experience of primary support persons of stroke survivors, *Rehabilitation Nursing,* 25(5): 93–9.

Seltzer, G.B., Begun, A., Seltzer, M.M. and Krauss, M.W. (1991) Adults with mental retardation and their aging mothers: impacts of siblings, *Family Relations,* 310–17.

Seltzer, M. and Krauss, M. (1994) Aging parents with co-resident adult children: the impact of lifelong caring, in M. Seltzer, M. Krauss and M. Janicki (eds) *Life Course Perspectives on Adulthood and Old Age.* Washington, DC: American Association of Mental Retardation.

Shakespeare, T. (2000) The social relations of care, in G. Lewis, S. Gewirtz and J. Clarke (eds) *Rethinking Social Policy.* Thousand Oaks, CA: Sage Publications.

Shuttlesworth, G.E., Rubin, A. and Duffy, M. (1982) Families versus institutions: incongruent role expectations in the nursing home, *The Gerontologist,* 22(2): 200–8.

Shyu, Y.C. (2002) A conceptual framework for understanding the process of family caregiving to frail elders in Taiwan, *Research in Nursing and Health,* 25: 111–21.

Silva, E.B. and Smart, C. (2000) *The New Family?* London: Sage Publications.

Simpson, M. (2000) Programming adulthood: intellectual disability and adult services, in D. May (ed.) *Transition and Change in the Lives of People with Intellectual Disabilities*. London: Jessica Kingsley.

Skeie, G. (1989) Contact between elderly people with mental retardation living in institutions and their families, *Australia and New Zealand Journal of Developmental Disabilities*, 15: 201–6.

Smagt-Duijnstree, M., Harners, J.P.H. and Abu-Sead, H.H. (2000) Relatives of stroke patients: their experiences and needs in hospital, *Scandinavian Journal of Nursing Sciences*, 14: 44–51.

Smale, G., Tilson, G., Biehal, N. and Mars, P. (1993) *Empowerment, Assessment, Care Management and the Skilled Worker*. National Institute for Social Work Practice and Development Exchange. London: HMSO.

Smallegan, M. (1981) Decision making for nursing home admission: a preliminary study, *Journal of Gerontological Nursing*, 7(5): 280–5.

Smith, G.C. (1997) Ageing families of adults with mental retardation: patterns and correlates of service use, need and knowledge, *American Journal on Mental Retardation*, 102: 13–26.

Smith, G.C. and Tobin, S.S. (1993) Practice with older parents of developmentally disabled adults, *Clinical Gerontologist*, 14: 59–77.

Smith, G.C., Fullmer, E.M. and Tobin, S.S. (1994) Living outside the system: an exploration of older families who do not use day programs, in M.M. Seltzer, M.W. Krauss and M.P. Janicki (eds) *Life Course Perspectives on Adulthood and Old Age*. Washington, DC: American Association on Mental Retardation.

Smith, G.C., Tobin, S.S. and Fullmer, E.M. (1995) Elderly mothers caring at home for offspring with mental retardation: a model of permanency planning, *American Journal on Mental Retardation*, 99(5): 487–99.

Snyder, J.R. (2000) Impact of caregiver–receiver relationship quality on burden and satisfaction, *Journal of Women and Aging*, 12(1/2): 147–67.

Socialdepartementet (1999) *Nationell handlingsplan för äldrepolitiken: Mål, inriktning och förslag till åtgärder* (*prop. 1997/1998: 113*). Stockholm: Norsteds. [Trans. The Ministry of Health and Social Affairs (1999) *National plan of action for the care of older people: Aim, direction and recommendation for actions.*]

Socialstyrelsen (1998) *Ädel utvädering 96:5. Nya förutsättningar, hättre incitament – högre effekitivitet efter Ädel?* Stockholm: Socialstyrelsen. [Trans. The National Board of Health and Welfare (1998) *Evaluation of the Ädel reform 96:5. New conditions, better incentives – higher efficiency after Ädel?*]

Socialstyrelsen (1999) *Socialstyrelsens meddelandeblad nr 2/99. 'ANHÖRIG 300' – 300 miljner för utveckling av stöd till anhöriga*. Stockholm: Socialstyrelsen. [Trans. The National Board of Health and Welfare (1999) *Memorandum number 2/99. "RELATIVE 300" – 300 million for development of support for relatives.*]

Socialstyrelsen (2001) *Närståendes vård av aldre, anhörigas och professionellas perspectiv*, Anhörig 300. Stockholm: Socialstyrelsen. [Trans. National Board of Health and Welfare (2001) *Family care for older persons from the perspective of family carers and professionals*.]

Socialstyrelsen (2001) *Statistik – Socialtjänst 2001:3, Äldre – vård och omsorg år 2000*. Stockholm: Socialstyrelsen. [Trans. The National Board of Health and Welfare (2001) *Statistics – Social Services 2001: 3, Older people – care and service in 2000*.]

Sörenson, S., Pinquart, M. and Duberstein, P. (2002) How effective are interventions with caregivers? An updated meta-analysis, *The Gerontologist*, 43(3): 356–72.

SOU (1997) *Brister I omsorg – en fråga om bemötande av Äldre Delbetänkande av Utredningen om bemötande av äldre*. Stockholm: Socialdepartementet. [Trans: Swedish Government Official Reports (1997: 51) *Deficiencies in care – a matter of encountering older people. Interim report, part of the official report of encountering older people.*]

Sperlinger, D. and Furst, M. (1994) The services experiences of people with presenile dementia: a study of carers in one London borough, *International Journal of Geriatric Psychiatry*, 9: 47–50.

Stainton, T. and Besser, H. (1998) The positive impact of children with an intellectual disability on the family, *Journal of Intellectual and Developmental Disability*, 23: 57–70.

Stanley, D. and Reed, J. (1999) *Opening Up Care: Achieving Principled Practice in Health and Social Care Institutions*. London: Arnold.

Steinmetz, S.K. (1988) *Duty Bound: Elder Abuse and Family Care*. Newbury Park, SA: Sage Publications.

Stephens, M.A.P., Kinney, J.M. and Ogrocki, P.K. (1991) Stressors and well-being among caregivers to older adults with dementia: the in-home versus nursing home experience, *The Gerontologist*, 31(2): 217–23.

Stevens, J. (1995) A career with older people: do nurses care for it?, PhD Thesis, UNSW, Sydney.

Stewart, B.J., Archbold, P.G., Harvath, T.A. and Nkongho, N.O. (1993) Role acquisition in family caregivers of older people who have been discharged from hospital, in S.G. Funk, E.H. Tornquist, M.T. Champagne and R.A. Weise (eds) *Key Aspects of Caring for the Chronically Ill: Hospital and Home*. New York, NY: Springer.

Summers, J.A., Behr, S.K. and Turnbull, A.P. (1989) Positive adaptation and coping strengths of families who have children with disabilities, in G.H.S. Singer and L.K. Irvin (eds) *Support for Caregiving Families: Enabling Positive Adapation to Disability*. Baltimore, MD: Brookes.

Szabo, V. and Strang, V.R. (1999) Experiencing control in caregiving, *Image*, 31(1): 71–6.

Tamm, M. (1999) Relatives as a help or hindrance: a grounded theory study seen from the perspective of the occupational therapist, *Scandinavian Journal of Occupational Therapy*, 6: 36–45.

Tebb, S. and Jivanjee, P. (2000) Caregiver isolation: an ecological model, *Journal of Gerontological Social Work*, 34(2): 51–71.

Thomas, C. (1999) *Female Forms. Experiencing and Understanding Disability.* Buckingham: Open University Press.

Thompson, W. (1990) *Ageing is a Family Affair: A Guide to Quality Visiting, Long Term Care Facilities and You*, 3rd edition. Toronto: NC Press.

Thompson, C. and Briggs, M. (2000) *Support for Carers of People with Alzheimer's Type Dementia.* Oxford: *Cochrane Review*, Issue 4.

Thorne, S.E. (1993) *Negotiating Health Care: The Social Context of Chronic Illness.* Newbury Park, CA: Sage Publications.

Thorne, S.E., Nyhlin, K.T. and Paterson, D.L. (2000) Attitudes towards patient expertise in chronic illness, *International Journal of Nursing Studies*, 37: 303–11.

Thorslund, M. (1991) The increasing number of very old people will change the Swedish model of the welfare state, *Social Science and Medicine*, 32: 455–64.

Thorslund, M. (1998) De allra äldstas situation. I Socialvetenskapliga Forskningsrådet (ed.) *Äldreeomsorgens vardag.* Stockholm: Social-högskolan. [Trans. The situation of the oldest old. In: Swedish Council for Social Research (ed) *Ordinary days in eldercare.*]

Thorslund, M. and Parker, M. (1994) Care of the elderly in the changing Swedish welfare state, in D. Challis, B. Davies and K. Traske (eds) *Community Care: New Agendas and Challenges from the UK and Overseas.* Aldershot: Arena.

Tickle, E.H. and Hull, K.V. (1995) Family members' roles in long-term care, *MEDSURG Nursing*, 4(4): 300–4.

Tilse, C. (1994) Long term marriage and long term care: 'We thought we'd be together till we died', *Australian Journal on Ageing*, 13(4): 172–4.

Tindall, L. and Manthorpe, J. (1997) Early onset dementia: a case of ill-timing?, *Journal of Mental Health*, 6(3): 237–49.

Todd, S. and Shearn, J. (1996a) Identities at risk: the relationships parents and their co-resident adult offspring have with each other and their social worlds, *European Journal of Mental Disability*, 3: 47–60.

Todd, S. and Shearn, J. (1996b) Struggles with time: the careers of parents with adult sons and daughters with learning disabilities, *Disability and Society*, 11(3): 379–401.

Todd, S., Shearn, J., Beyer, S. and Felce, D. (1993) Careers in caring: the changing situation of parents caring for offspring with learning difficulties, *Irish Journal of Psychology*, 14: 130–53.

Townsend, P. (1962) *The Last Refuge.* London: Routledge and Kegan Paul.

Traustadottir, R. and Johnson, K. (2000) *Women with intellectual disabilities. Finding their place in the world.* Philadelphia, PA: Jessica Kingsley.

Tresolini, C.P. and the Pew-Fetzer Task Force (1994) *Health Professions Education and Relationships-Centred Care: A Report of the Pew-Fetzer Task Force on Advancing Psychosocial Education.* San Francisco, CA: Pew Health Professions Commission.

Turnbull, A.P. and Turnbull, H.R. (1993) Participatory research in cognitive coping: from concepts to research planning, in A.P. Turnbull, J.M. Patterson, S.K. Behr, D.L. Murphy, J.G. Marquis and M.J. Blue-Banning (eds) *Cognitive Coping, Families and Disability*. Baltimore, MD: Brookes.

Twigg, J. and Atkin, K. (1994) *Carers Perceived: Policy and Practice in Informal Care*. Buckingham: Open University Press.

Tyson, S.F. (1995) Stroke rehabilitation: what is the point?, *Physiotherapy*, 81(8): 430–2.

Uehara, E.S. (1995) Reciprocity reconsidered: Gouldner's 'moral norm of reciprocity' and social support, *Journal of Social and Personal Relationships*, 12(4): 483–502.

Vårdalstylesen (1999) *Vårda Och Vårdas. Ett Program För Stöd Till Forskning Om Äldrre Cch Deras Närstående Vårdare*. Stockholm: Vårdalstifttelsens Rapportserie, 4. [Trans. The Vardal Foundation for Health Care Sciences and Allergy Research (1999) *Care and being cared for. A programme of support for research about older people and their carers*. Stockholm: Vardal Foundation]

Victor, C.R. (1997) *Community Care and Older People*. Cheltenham: Stanley Thorne.

Vinton, L. and Mazza, N. (1994) Aggressive behavior directed at nursing home personnel by residents' family members, *The Gerontologist*, 34(4): 528–33.

Walker, A. (1995) Integrating the family in the mixed economy of care, in I. Allen and E. Perkins (eds) *The Future of Family Care for Older People*. London: HMSO.

Walker, A. and Walker, C. (1998a) *Uncertain Future: People with Learning Difficulties and their Ageing Family Carers*. Brighton: Pavilion Publishing and Joseph Rowntree Foundation.

Walker, A. and Walker, C. (1998b) Age or disability? Age based disparities in service provision for older people with intellectual disabilities in Great Britain, *Journal of Intellectual and Developmental Disability*, 23(1): 25–40.

Walmsley, J. (1996) Doing what Mum wants me to do: looking at family relationships from the point of view of adults with learning disabilities, *Journal of Applied Research in Intellectual Disabilities*, 9(4): 324–41.

Ward-Griffin, C. (2001) Negotiating care of frail elders: relationships between community nurses and family carers, *Canadian Journal of Nursing Research*, 33(2): 63–81.

Ward-Griffin, C. and McKeever, P. (2000) Relationships between nurses and family caregivers: partners in care, *Advances in Nursing Science*, 22(3): 89–103.

Warfield, M.E. (2001) Employment, parenting and well-being among mothers of children with disabilities, *Mental Retardation*, 39(4): 297–309.

Warner, C. and Wexler, S. (1998) *Eight Hours a Day and Taken for Granted?* London: The Princess Royal Trust for Carers.

Weightman, G. (1999) *A Real Break: A Guidebook for Good Practice in the*

*Provision of Short-term Breaks as a Support for Care in the Community.* London: Department of Health.

Wellwood, I., Dennis, M. and Warlow, C. (1995) Patients' and carers' satisfaction with acute stroke management, *Age and Ageing*, 20: 519–24.

Welsh Office (1983) *All Wales Strategy for the Development of Services for Mentally Handicapped People.* Cardiff: Welsh Office.

Whitehouse, P. and Maslow, K. (1997) Defining and measuring outcomes in Alzheimer's disease research: introduction and overview, *Alzheimer's Disease and Related Disorders*, 11(Supplement 6): 1–6.

White-Means, S. and Chollet, D. (1996) Opportunity wages and the workforce adjustments: understanding the cost of in-home elder care, *Journal of Gerontology: Social Sciences*, 51B(2): S82–S90.

Whitlach, C.J. (2001) Including the person with dementia in family care-giving research, *Aging and Mental Health*, 5(Supplement 1): S20–S22.

Whitlach, C.J., Schur, D., Noelker, L.L., Ejaz, F.K. and Loorman, W.J. (2001) The stress process in family caregiving in institutional settings, *The Gerontologist*, 41(4): 462–73.

Wilkinson, P. (1996) Longer term care, in C. Wolfe, T. Rudd and R. Beech (eds) *Stroke Services and Research.* London: Stroke Association.

Williams, J. (1994) The rehabilitation process for older people and their carers, *Nursing Times*, 90(29): 33–4.

Willoughby, J. and Keating, N. (1991) Being in control: the process of caring for a relative with Alzheimer's disease, *Qualitative Health Research*, 1(1): 27–50.

Wilson, H.S. (1989a) Family caregivers: the experience of Alzheimer's disease, *Applied Nursing Research*, 2(1): 40–5.

Wilson, H.S. (1989b) Family caregiving for a relative with Alzheimer's dementia: coping with negative choices, *Nursing Research*, 38(2): 94–8.

Wilson, P.M. (2002) The expert patient: issues and implications for community nurses, *British Journal of Community Nursing*, 7(10): 514–19.

Wolfe, C. (1996) The burden of stroke, in C. Wolfe, T. Rudd and R. Beech (eds) *Stroke Services and Research.* London: Stroke Association.

Wolfe, L.E., Woods, J.P. and Reid, J. (1995) Do general practitioners and old age psychiatrists differ in their attitudes to dementia?, *International Journal of Geriatric Psychiatry*, 10: 63–9.

Wood, J. and Skiles, L. (1992) Planning for the transfer of care. Who cares for the developmentally disabled adult when the family can no longer care? *Generations*, Winter: 61–2.

Woods, B. *et al.* (1999) *Partners in Care. A Training Guide for Staff and Relatives and Friends of People with Dementia Living in Long-term Care.* Produced as part of a project funded by the European Commission, 'The interface between family caregivers and institutional care for people with Alzheimer's disease and related disorders: developing relevant training resources', coordinated by Professor B. Woods, University of Wales, Bangor.

Woods, R.T. (2001) Discovering the person with Alzheimer's disease: cognitive, emotional and behavioural aspects, *Aging and Mental Health*, 5(Supplement 1): S7–S16.

Wright, F. (1998) *Continuing to Care. The Effect on Spouses and Children of an Older Person's Admission to a Care Home*. York: York Publishing Services Ltd.

Wuest, J. (2000a) Repatterning care: women's proactive management of family caregiving demands, *Health Care for Women International*, 21: 393–411.

Wuest, J. (2000b) Negotiating with helping systems: an example of grounded theory evolving through emergent fit, *Qualitative Health Research*, 10(1): 51–70.

Wuest, J. and Stern, P.N. (2001) Connected and disconnected support: the impact on the caregiving process in Alzheimer's Disease, *Health Care for Women International*, 22: 115–30.

Wuest, J., Ericson, P.K. and Stern, P.N. (1994) Becoming strangers: the changing family caregiving relationship in Alzheimer's disease, *Journal of Advanced Nursing*, 20: 437–43.

Wyller, T.B. (2000) Rehabilitation after severe stroke: an enthusiastic approval and a cautionary tale, *Disability and Rehabilitation*, 22(4): 193–5.

Young, H. (1990) The transition of relocation to a nursing home, *Holistic Nursing Practice*, 4(3): 74–83.

Young, J.B. and Gladman, J.R.F. (1995) Future directions in stroke rehabilitation, *Reviews in Clinical Gerontology*, 5: 329–37.

Zarit, S.H. and Leitsch, S.A. (2001) Developing and evaluating community based intervention programes for Alzheimer's patients and their caregivers, *Aging and Mental Health*, 5(Supplement 1): S84–S98.

Zarit, S.H. and Whitlatch, C.J. (1993) Effects of placement in nursing homes on family caregivers: short and long term consequences, *Irish Journal of Psychology*, 14(1): 25–37.

Zarit, S.H., Reever, K.E. and Bach-Peterson, J. (1980) Relatives of the impaired elderly: correlates of feelings of burden, *The Gerontologist*, 20(6): 649–55.

Zarit, S.H., Todd, P.A. and Zarit, J.M. (1986) Subjective burden of husbands and wives as caregivers: a longitudinal study, *The Gerontologist*, 26(3): 260–6.

Zarit, S.H., Gaugler, J.E. and Jarrott, S.E. (1999) Useful services for families: research findings and directions, *International Journal of Geriatric Psychiatry*, 14: 165–77.

Zerubavel, E. (1981) *Hidden Rhythms: Schedules and Calendars in Social Life*, Berkeley, CA: University of California Press.

Zetlin, A. (1986) Mentally retarded adults and their siblings, *American Journal of Mental Deficiency*, 91: 217–25.

Zgola, J.M. (1999) *Care That Works: A Relationship Approach to Persons with Dementia*. Baltimore, MD: Johns Hopkins University Press.

# Index

Page numbers in *italics* refer to tables.

# UNDERSTANDING FAMILY CARE
## A MULTIDIMENSIONAL MODEL OF CARING AND COPING

### Mike Nolan, Gordon Grant and John Keady

- How are the burdens and difficulties of caregiving balanced by the satisfactions experienced?
- How do the demands of caregiving change over time and what are the policy and practice implications of such changes?
- How is a balance achieved between the needs of the caregiver and the cared-for person?

The importance of family (informal) care both in making a reality of community care policies and in helping to sustain the quality of life of people who require support to remain within their homes is beyond doubt. However, whilst considerable research and practice literature has developed in this area over the last ten years there remains much to learn about caring at both conceptual and practice levels. There is in particular a need to develop more dynamic models which account for the changing nature of care over time and integrates the perspectives of carer, cared-for person and the formal service network.

Based on several years research conducted by the authors, *Understanding Family Care* integrates a number of theories and perspectives in order to provide a more holistic understanding of the needs of carers. Emphasis is placed on providing a balanced picture which recognizes both the burdens and satisfactions of caring, in addition to the coping effects that carers employ. A new longitudinal model of caring is described and the various stages and processes are explored. Although the focus is primarily on the carer the perspectives of the cared-for person are not ignored and a model is presented which aids the integration of disparate viewpoints. In addition to theoretical and methodological debates, implications for policy and practice are fully explored.

*Understanding Family Care* is recommended reading for practitioners and managers in the health and social services, as well as students of social science, nursing, gerontology and social work.

### Contents
*Acknowledgements – Introduction: Family caregiving – The need for a multidimensional approach – Caring in context – Towards a more holistic conceptualization of caring – Stress and coping: implications for family caregiving – Satisfactions of caring: the neglected dimension – Family caregiving: a temporal perspective – Integrating perspectives – Reaching the end or a new beginning? – Appendices – References – Index.*

208pp    0 335 19574 1 (Hardback)    0 335 19573 3 (Paperback)

# WORKING WITH OLDER PEOPLE AND THEIR FAMILIES
## KEY ISSUES IN POLICY AND PRACTICE

**Mike Nolan, Sue Davies and Gordon Grant (eds)**

Addressing the needs of older people and their carers is an essential element of both policy and practice in the fields of health and social care. Recent developments promote a partnership and empowerment model, in which the notion of 'person-centred' care figures prominently. However, what 'person-centred' care means and how it can be achieved is far from clear.

*Working with Older People and their Families* combines extensive reviews of specialist literatures with new empirical data in an attempt at a synthesis of themes about making a reality of 'person-centred' care. Uniquely, it seeks to unite the perspectives of older people, family and professional carers in promoting a genuinely holistic approach to the challenges of an ageing society.

*Working with Older People and their Families* is recommended reading for students on health related courses such as nursing, medicine and the therapies. It is also of relevance to students of social work and social gerontology, researchers, managers and policy makers.

### Contents
*The changing face of health and social care – Quality of life, quality of care – Who's the expert: redefining lay and professional relationships – Acute and rehabilitative care for older people – Community care – The care needs of older people and family caregivers in continuing care settings – Palliative care and older people – The mental health needs of older people and their carers: exploring tensions and new directions – Older people with learning disabilities, health, community inclusion and family caregiving – Integrating perspectives – Appendix 1: Literature review: Methodology – Bibliography – Index.*

224pp     0 335 20560 7 (Paperback)     0 335 20561 5 (Hardback)

# openup
ideas and understanding
in social science

www.**openup**.co.uk

 **Browse, search and
order online**

 **Download detailed
title information and
sample chapters***

*for selected titles

www.**openup**.co.uk